Minimally Invasive Surgical Procedures for Pain

Minimally Invasive Surgical Procedures for Pain

EDITED BY

Dawood Sayed

Alaa Abd-Elsayed

Steven Falowski

Timothy Deer

OXFORD
UNIVERSITY PRESS

OXFORD
UNIVERSITY PRESS

Oxford University Press is a department of the University of Oxford. It furthers the University's objective of excellence in research, scholarship, and education by publishing worldwide. Oxford is a registered trade mark of Oxford University Press in the UK and certain other countries.

Published in the United States of America by Oxford University Press
198 Madison Avenue, New York, NY 10016, United States of America.

Library of Congress Cataloging-in-Publication Data
Names: Sayed, Dawood, editor. | Abd-Elsayed, Alaa, editor. |
Falowski, Steven M., editor. | Deer, Timothy R., editor.
Title: Minimally Invasive Surgical Procedures for Pain /
[edited by] Dawood Sayed, Alaa Abd-Elsayed, Steven Falowski, Timothy Deer.
Description: New York, NY : Oxford University Press, [2024] |
Includes bibliographical references and index.
Identifiers: LCCN 2022044657 (print) | LCCN 2022044658 (ebook) |
ISBN 9780197616734 (paperback) | ISBN 9780197616758 (epub) |
ISBN 9780197616765 (online)
Subjects: MESH: Spinal Diseases—surgery | Chronic Pain |
Minimally Invasive Surgical Procedures
Classification: LCC RD768 (print) | LCC RD768 (ebook) | NLM WE 727 |
DDC 617.5/6059—dc23/eng/20230118
LC record available at https://lccn.loc.gov/2022044657
LC ebook record available at https://lccn.loc.gov/2022044658

DOI: 10.1093/med/9780197616734.001.0001

Printed by Integrated Books International, United States of America

MIX
Paper
FSC FSC® C183721

I dedicate this book to my parents, Jan and Gulnar Sayed, my wife, Lindsey Sayed, and my three children, Zahra, Farah, and Sabrina. I am also eternally grateful to my patients for allowing me to take care of them in their greatest times of need. Above all else, I thank our Creator for giving me the health and capacity to work on this project.
—Dawood Sayed, MD

I dedicate this book to God, my parents, my wife, my daughter, Maro, and my son, George.
—Alaa Abd-Elsayed, MD, MPH

I dedicate this work to the continued education and further advancement of our space. As always, I offer a special dedication to my wife and children, who give unwavering strength and support.
—Steven Falowski, MD

This book is dedicated to God, from whom all blessings flow, my wife, Melissa, who has been on this journey with me for many years, and to my patients, who suffer as we try to find solutions.
—Tim Deer, MD

Contents

Preface

In the last decade, a significant paradigm shift has occurred in the way complex spinal disorders are treated. Historically, after patients failed conservative treatments—largely consisting of therapy, medications, and injections—they would be left with only highly invasive open surgical options. Now, with the development of minimally invasive surgical techniques, patients often have significantly more effective and safer treatment options available. Many of the minimally invasive approaches can be done percutaneously and under image guidance, instead of with open approaches under direct visualization. For those of us trained as interventional pain physicians, many of the minimally invasive surgical techniques have become an integral part of our treatment algorithms. However, although these approaches are less invasive and safer, they are not without risk and complications. Furthermore, significant gaps exist in training programs for interventionalists with regard to minimally invasive surgical approaches. To continue to improve innovation in the field of minimally invasive spine surgery, improved educational resources are vitally important, not only for interventionalists but also for physicians from traditional surgical backgrounds, such as neurosurgery and orthopedics. This text aims to convey an understanding of the basic concepts of spinal surgical approaches combined with an in-depth approach to the various techniques, with the overall goals of enhancing physician knowledge and leading to improved patient outcomes and safety.

Dawood Sayed, MD
Alaa Abd-Elsayed, MD, MPH
Steven Falowski, MD
Timothy Deer, MD

Contributors

Alaa Abd-Elsayed, MD, MPH
Anesthesiology and Pain Medicine
University of Wisconsin School of Medicine and Public Health
Madison, WI, USA

Nomen Azeem, MD
Department of Neurology
University of South Florida
Florida Spine and Pain Specialists
Tampa, FL, USA

Steven Bhutra, MD
Department of Anesthesiology
University of Virginia
Charlottesville, VA, USA

Patrick Buchanan, MD
Spanish Hills Interventional Pain Specialists

Timothy Deer, MD
The Spine and Nerve Center of The Virginias
Charleston, WV, USA

Jack Diep, MD
Lakeside Spine & Pain

Erica R. Eldon
Icahn School of Medicine at Mount Sinai
Department of Rehabilitation and Human Performance
New York, NY, USA

Alyson M. Engle, MD
The Spine and Nerve Center of The Virginias
Charleston, WV, USA

Alexander Escobar, MD
The University of Toledo
Department of Anesthesiology
Toledo, OH, USA

Steven M. Falowski, MD
Director of Functional Neurosurgery
Neurosurgical Associates of Lancaster
Lancaster, PA, USA

Vinicius Tieppo Francio, MD, MS
The University of Kansas Medical Center (KUMC)
Department of Anesthesiology and Pain Medicine
Department of Physical Medicine & Rehabilitation
Kansas City, KS, USA

Priyanka Ghosh, MD
Remedy Medical Group
San Francisco, CA, USA

Anthony Giuffrida, MD
Cantor Spine Center at the Paley Orthopedic & Spine Institute
Fort Lauderdale, FL, USA

Johnathan Goree, MD
Department of Anesthesiology
University of Arkansas for Medical Sciences
Little Rock, AR, USA

Mayank Gupta, MD
Kansas Pain Management
Overland Park, KS, USA

Jonathan M. Hagedorn, MD
Department of Anesthesiology and Perioperative Medicine
Division of Pain Medicine, Mayo Clinic
Rochester, MN, USA

Corey W. Hunter
Ainsworth Institute of Pain
Mount Sinai Hospital
Department of Rehabilitation and Human Performance
New York, NY, USA

Nasir Hussain, MD, MSc
Department of Anesthesiology
Wexner Medical Center
The Ohio State University
Columbus, OH, USA

Sameer Jain, MD
Pain Treatment Centers of America
Little Rock, AR, USA

Jessica Jameson MD, FASA
Axis Spine Center
Coeur D'Alene, ID

Navdeep Singh Jassal, MD
Spine & Pain Institute of Florida
Lakeland, FL, USA
Assistant Clinical Professor—University of South Florida, Department of Neurology
Assistant Clinical Professor—University of Central Florida, Department of Physical Medicine & Rehabilitation

Hermant Kalia, MD, MPH, FIPP, FACPM
Rochester Regional Health System
University of Rochester
Rochester, NY, USA

Brian Y. Kim, MD
Department of Anesthesiology and Pain Medicine
The University of Kansas Medical Center
Kansas City, KS, USA

David H. Kim, MD, MS
Department of Anesthesiology and Pain Medicine
The University of Kansas Medical Center
Kansas City, KS, USA

Lynn Kohan, MD
Professor of Anesthesiology and Pain Management
Department of Anesthesiology
University of Virginia
Charlottesville, VA, USA

Christopher M. Lam, MD
Department of Anesthesiology and Pain Medicine
The University of Kansas Medical Center
Kansas City, KS, USA

Sean Li, MD
Premiere Pain Centers
Shrewsbury, NJ, USA

Mark Malinowski, DO, FIPP
Adena Spine Center
Adena Health System
Chillicothe, OH, USA

Behnam Myers DO, MPH
Nova Southeastern University
Broward Health

Arti Ori, MD
North Shore Pain Management

Jeffrey D. Petersohn, MD
PainCare, PC
Englewood, CO and Linwood, NJ, USA

Bethany Potere, MD MSc
The Ohio State University
Wexner Medical Center, Department of Anesthesiology
Columbus, OH, USA

Andrew Sack, MD
University of Kansas Medical Center
Kansas City, KS, USA

Salman Sagarwala, MD
Department of Anesthesiology and Pain Medicine
The University of Kansas Medical Center
Kansas City, KS, USA

Dawood Sayed, MD
Professor of Anesthesiology and Pain Medicine
The University of Kansas Medical Center
Kansas City, KS, USA

Harry Sukumaran, MD
Wayne State University School of Medicine
Detroit, MI, USA

Umar M. Syed, MS-III
Kansas City University
Kansas City, MO, USA

Jacqueline Weisbein, DO
Napa Valley Orthopaedic Medical Group
Napa, CA, USA

Benjamin D. Westerhaus, MD
Cantor Spine Center at the Paley Orthopedic & Spine Institute
West Palm Beach, FL, USA

Steven Zhou, MD
Department of Anesthesiology
Wexner Medical Center
The Ohio State University
Columbus, OH, USA

PART 1

Minimally Invasive Spine Surgery for the Interventional Pain Physician

1

The Interventionalist's Perspective

Dawood Sayed

The practice of interventional pain medicine (IPM) has seen a dramatic evolution over the last 10 years. Historically, the majority of an IPM physician's practice was dealing with steroid injections and medications to manage the pain arising from spinal disorders, and a significant proportion of patients treated with only these palliative measures did not experience success, as defined by level of function and subjective pain scores. Referral of the patient suffering from chronic spinal disorders for surgical solutions can also be challenging, in that many patients are either not candidates for, or are not interested in pursuing, traditional open surgical treatments. The escalating risks of opioids and the current opioid epidemic have further compounded the challenges for patients with chronic spinal disorders. Fortunately, recent innovation in minimally invasive spine techniques has led to a paradigm shift in the way patients with spinal disease are treated. Although not comprehensive, the following major factors will continue to drive the paradigm shift toward more patient-centered and minimally invasive techniques:

1. The aging population: From 2000 to 2030, the percentage of the population over the age of 65 is projected to increase from 12% to over 20%. Because the incidence of spinal disorders is directly correlated with age, the demand for care for spinal disorders is expected to increase at the same rate.[1]
2. Advancements in minimally invasive techniques and safety.
3. Movement away from long-term medical management of spinal disorders with opioids.

With these factors in play, it will be of paramount importance for current and future generations of IPM physicians to continue to advance education and training in the evaluation for, and treatment using, minimally invasive surgical approaches. Equally as important as hands-on training in the techniques will be acquiring the acumen to diagnose and select patients for the interventions and applying the best available evidence in deciding not to pursue treatment if the risks outweigh the benefits in a particular scenario.

Similar to the shift in care of patients with cardiac disease that was ushered in by Dr. Gruentzig's first balloon angioplasty in the mid-1970s from more percutaneous approaches versus open cardiac revascularization, a similar shift is occurring in the care of those with spinal disorders.[2] As minimally invasive approaches continue to evolve, many of the approaches are developed to fit the profile of the image-guided approaches currently performed by physicians in IPM. Of note, recent surgical procedures, such as percutaneous interlaminar decompression (PILD) and indirect lumbar decompression with spinous process spacers for spinal stenosis, have been developed in an entirely percutaneous and image-guided approach.[3,4] Additionally, evolution in surgical techniques for the percutaneous approaches to permanent implantation of spinal cord stimulators has led to the majority of these surgical procedures being performed by anesthesiologists (63%) rather than neurosurgeons (22%).[5] Increasing experience and comfort with the surgical procedures contribute to surgical procedures in development.

The shift of minimally invasive surgical spinal procedures into the realm of IPM has to be done with patient safety and interests in mind above all else. The paradigm shift needs to be grounded in scientific evidence and patient safety and not to be based on political "turf battles." Future studies and product validations need to incorporate IPM physicians if the end user of a potential technology is going to be the IPM physician rather than classically trained spine surgeon, or a combination of both. Additionally, collaboration between interventionalists and surgeons is vitally important in improvement of surgical approaches, safety, and management of complications when they arise. The specialty of IPM must also critically evaluate each individual surgical procedure and decide if fits into the evolving scope of practice. A proposed guideline for determining if a procedure should be performed in IPM includes the questions:

1. Can the surgical procedure be performed in a largely percutaneous approach?
2. Is the technical skill required to perform the procedure similar to that required for current procedures?
3. Does the available evidence indicate the procedure has an overall low incidence of complications?
4. Can most potential complications be managed by an IPM physician, and is there a process in place for referral of more rare and serious complications?
5. Does the surgical procedure allow for more invasive approaches if a therapeutic response is not achieved ("no bridges burned")?

The future of minimally invasive surgical procedures holds much promise for patients suffering from spinal disorders. Techniques like intraoperative surgical navigation and spinal robotics are advancements that will draw increased interest and research in hopes of improving minimally invasive surgical options. Training of the future generation of physicians may also evolve over time from the current paradigm of primary specialties, such as anesthesiology, neurosurgery, orthopedics, and physical medicine with fellowship training, to a unique specialty in minimally invasive spinal medicine.

References

1. O'Lynnger TM, Zuckerman SL, Morone PJ, Dewan MC, Vasquez-Castellanos RA, Cheng JS. Trends for spine surgery for the elderly: implications for access to healthcare in North America. *Neurosurgery.* 2015;77(suppl 4):S136–S141. doi:10.1227/NEU.0000000000000945.
2. Mueller RL, Sanborn TA. The history of interventional cardiology: cardiac catheterization, angioplasty, and related interventions. *Am Heart J.* 1995;129(1):146–172. doi:10.1016/0002-8703(95)90055-1. PMID: 7817908.
3. Staats PS, Chafin TB, Golovac S, Kim CK, Li S, Richardson WB, Vallejo R, Wahezi SE, Washabaugh EP 3rd, Benyamin RM; MiDAS ENCORE Investigators. Long-term safety and efficacy of minimally invasive lumbar decompression procedure for the treatment of lumbar spinal stenosis with neurogenic claudication: 2-year results of MiDAS ENCORE. *Reg Anesth Pain Med.* 2018;43(7):789–794. doi:10.1097/AAP.0000000000000868. PMID: 30199512; PMCID: PMC6319572.
4. Nunley PD, Patel VV, Orndorff DG, Lavelle WF, Block JE, Geisler FH. Superion Interspinous Spacer treatment of moderate spinal stenosis: 4-year results. *World Neurosurg.* 2017;104:279–283. doi:10.1016/j.wneu.2017.04.163. PMID: 28479526.
5. Hussaini SMQ, Murphy KR, Han JL, et al. Specialty-based variations in spinal cord stimulation success rates for treatment of chronic pain. *Neuromodulation.* 2017;20(4):340–347. doi:10.1111/ner.12582.

2

A Surgeon's Perspective

Steven M. Falowski

The treatment of chronic pain can be very challenging and may not always have a clear algorithm. It is important that the spine surgeon be able to treat patients throughout their disease process. The days of having a hammer and everything looking like a nail are gone. In addition, a radiographically and technically successful surgery does not always translate into the patient results that one desires. It is known that at least 30% to 40% of spine surgery patients will develop postlaminectomy syndrome/failed back syndrome (FBS).[1,2] It has therefore become apparent that surgeons will be faced with the challenges of dealing with chronic pain patients along the treatment continuum.

Proper follow-up care is necessary to ensure maintenance and success of an implemented therapy. It is important that the treating spine surgeon be able to offer therapies to patients when pain persists after surgery, or perhaps when pain is present without a surgical pathology. This is a very important point as we begin to realize that surgery is only one piece of the algorithm in treating patients. Not all patients are surgical candidates or may benefit from spinal surgery. In addition, not all pathologies on imaging correlate with the patient's pain pattern and warrant surgery. Offering your patient options not only fosters the doctor–patient relationship, but also serves as an important treatment modality in patient care.

In order to ensure optimal care, surgeons and interventional pain physicians need to embrace minimally invasive therapies, new technologies, and approaches that have overlap between the specialties. The landscape is changing, and lines are becoming blurred on where division of services starts. Our space is evolving and is undergoing changes similar to those that were witnessed in cardiology and in vascular neurosurgery, in that procedures can be performed by multiple specialties; therefore, interspecialty relationships will need to be formed. The evolving interventions described throughout this text overlap between surgeons and interventional pain physicians. All physicians treating patients with spine pain must embrace these technologies and support interspecialty relationships and overlapping skill sets.

Surgeons need to set up a proper referral network. Referral depends on whether the surgeon decides to perform the therapy or is instead willing to work with someone else who performs the therapy. Surgeons who are not interested in minimally invasive and/or percutaneous procedures need to establish a network with physicians who undertake these procedures, whether they are other spine surgeons or interventional pain physicians. Not offering proper therapy is just as bad for patient care as performing unwarranted surgery. Several models exist for integrating care among specialties and for delivering appropriate care to patients. A spine surgeon can quickly become known for offering advanced therapies, or at least for indicating the appropriate pathway to obtain them.

A spine surgeon in the community will receive many referrals for an evaluation for candidacy for spinal surgery, and the majority of patients will not be candidates for spinal surgery. Serendipitously, these patients may also be the same patients who would benefit from interventional pain therapies, minimally invasive spinal procedures, or neuromodulation. In response to this pattern, spine surgeons can therefore diversify their offerings, develop a niche practice, and create a patient-centric referral network, all while delivering more cases to their practice.

Earlier intervention in appropriate patients leads to success in neuromodulation. These patients receive care among many specialties, and identification of candidates for neuromodulation throughout their course of treatment is of the utmost importance. Education, awareness, and relationships are paramount in delivering these therapies. Surgeons, specifically, have the ability to identify candidates early in the process and to offer options that will alleviate patients' pain and prevent potential long-term sequelae.

As their field is evolving, interventional pain physicians are adopting a new surgical skill set, including minimally invasive spinal decompressive procedures, vertebral augmentation, spinal implants (such as interspinous spacers) and fusions, sacroiliac fixation, and neuromodulation procedures. In response, surgeons have three primary concerns:

1. *Surgeons are losing patients.* The majority of the interventional pain procedures just listed are meant for patients who are not candidates for open surgical procedures, such as patients at advanced age, who have multiple comorbidities, and who are deemed unable to undergo open spinal approaches. On the other end of the spectrum are patients who are displaying mild symptoms, or who have mild to moderate imaging findings, but are considered early in the treatment algorithm. In both scenarios, there is little overlap with patients who are candidates for open spinal surgery. An initial surgical referral rectifies this.
2. *Interventional pain physicians may not be able to deal with complications.* The safety profile of these procedures reveals that they have extremely low rates of adverse events. In addition, any adverse outcomes are usually treated conservatively. Many of the procedures do not involve neural structures, and large published studies have demonstrated that the majority are extremely safe.
3. *Surgeons will need to perform revision surgery when the interventional pain procedure does not work.* Data show that many of these procedures have high success rates and, in some cases, success rates far better than those for open spinal surgery. In addition, the

revision and reoperation rates for minimally invasive procedures are much lower than those for open surgery. The majority of these procedures, such as interspinous spacer placement, do not alter anatomy and do not incur bone removal, therefore allowing surgeons access to unaltered spinal structures.

Thus, despite their concerns, spine surgeons should begin to embrace interventional pain therapies and the overlap within specialties. This is not about being competitive, but about being collaborative. The patients are the center of the algorithm, and they need access to these therapies. Surgeons need to understand the changing landscape and how to adapt together. Ultimately, patients can be offered minimally invasive percutaneous procedures with extremely safe profiles and high chances of success. This warrants collaboration among all who care about patients' welfare.

References

1. Kumar K, Taylor RS, Jacques L, et al. PROCESS Study SCS vs CMM for FBSS. *Pain* 2007;132(1-2):179–188.
2. Kumar K, et al. Spinal cord stimulation in treatment of chronic benign pain: challenges in treatment planning and present status, a 22-year experience. *Neurosurgery*. 2006;58(3):481–496.

3

Surgical Instruments

Salman Sagarwala, Brian Y. Kim, and David H. Kim

Preoperative Phase: Operating Room Setup, Equipment Check, Team Check

Settings can be highly variable, ranging from the most advanced, in-hospital, fully equipped operating rooms, to ambulatory surgery center operating rooms, to outpatient clinic procedure rooms. Key issues to identify are anesthesiology support, anesthetic type, availability of neurosurgery or orthopedic spine surgery backup, and setting transfer arrangements or care capabilities for emergency events. Disposition and recovery phase capabilities and lengths of stay of the facility should be known.

The cursory equipment check involves visually confirming that there is a ventilator, patient monitors (such as a pulse oximeter, blood pressure cuff, and electrocardiogram leads), emergency airway equipment, and emergency medications and equipment. Although this equipment is typically the responsibility of the anesthesiologist, the equipment check serves to ensure both the appropriateness of the procedure in the given setting and the intraoperative communication between the proceduralist and the anesthesia team (Figure 3.1). For example, a prone spine procedure requiring moderate to heavy sedation incurs elevated airway management risks. Another example is the problem that arises when a procedure undertaken in an outpatient procedure suite where no ventilator or appropriate equipment and medications are present, yet intolerable amounts of intraoperative patient movement require conversion to general anesthesia.

The operating room table should be inspected and adjusted appropriately depending on the type. Three main types of tables are utilized in minimally invasive spine procedures: the standard surgical table, a table with a Jackson frame, and a table with a Wilson frame (Figure 3.2). Depending on the anticipated positioning of the patient, preoperative table adjustments should be made. These include arm board attachment, positioning of pads, supply of additional padding or pillows, and use of head positioning equipment,

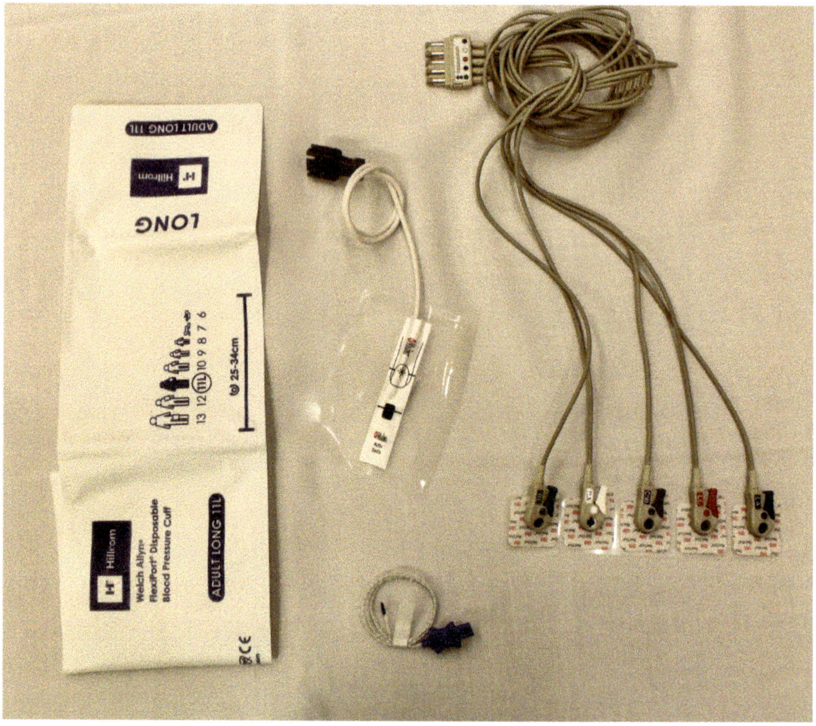

FIGURE 3.1. Standard blood pressure cuff, pulse oximeter, electrocardiography cables and leads, and temperature probe.

such as head cradles, Gardner-Wells tongs and counterweights, and Mayfield head holder. Particular attention should be paid to preventing peripheral nerve injuries by ensuring appropriate pad placement or padding at chest and hips, appropriate positioning of arm boards to not overextend the upper extremities, and appropriate padding and support of the lower extremities. Additionally, restraint devices, such as a safety belt and arm straps, should be attached and ready for use. Sequential compression devices should be positioned, and sleeves should be available for attachment. Blankets or forced-air blanket warmers are also useful depending on the length of the procedure and anticipated heat loss.

Basic operating equipment should be adjusted in the preparation phase. A crucial aspect of preparation is testing and adjustment of overhead surgical lighting and headlights, given the potential to have nonfunctioning lighting or the inability to reach or adjust the light once fully gowned and draped with a patient under anesthesia. Cautery type, whether Bovie, bipolar, or Harmonic, typically should be adjusted to appropriate settings and a fresh grounding pad should be available. Suction should also be confirmed, as well as blood-scavenging capabilities if desired. The availability of the correct draping materials and preferred antiseptic preparation is also important, given the wide varieties of materials. Staples, such as draping towels, antimicrobial iodine-impregnated skin drapes, half sheets, C-arm drapes, alcohol, chlorhexidine solution, and iodine solution, are examples of such necessities.

(a)

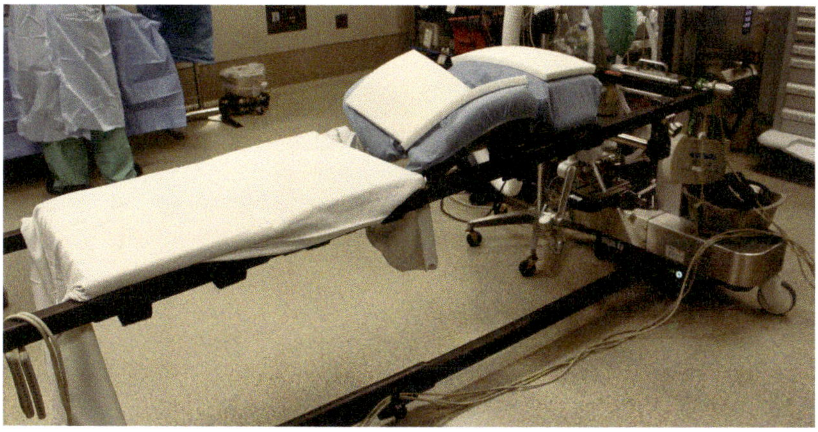

(b)

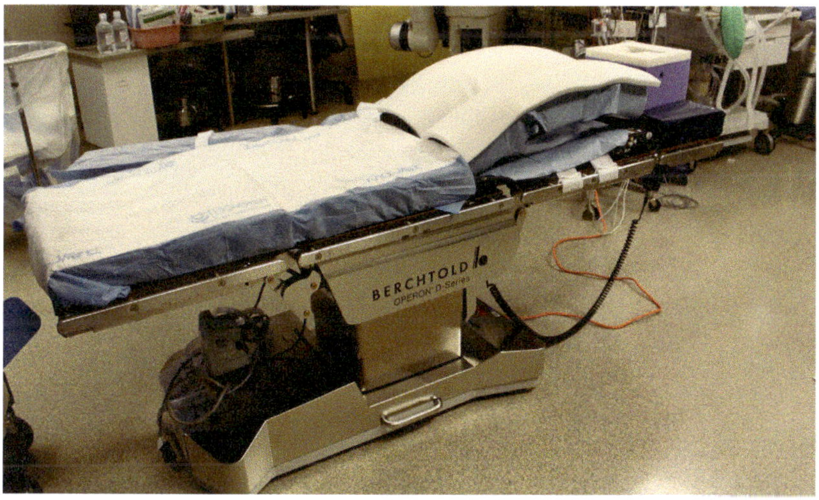

FIGURE 3.2. A, Operating table with the Jackson frame. B, Table with Wilson frame.

Intraoperative imaging is a particularly important domain. Minimally invasive interventional spine procedures typically rely on an advanced form of imaging rather than direct visualization. Modalities include fluoroscopy, computed tomography (CT), magnetic resonance imaging (MRI), intraoperative surgical navigation systems, video endoscopy, and surgical microscopy (Figure 3.3). With regard to fluoroscopy, ensuring the availability of the C-arm itself as well as a radiology technician is a basic step that is often overlooked. Appropriate draping of the C-arm as well as availability of appropriate draping for lateral views is needed. A test maneuver from anterior-posterior to lateral views is suggested if there is any uncertainty before the patient enters the room. Intraoperative CT can be utilized, although it is uncommon for minimally invasive interventional spine procedures. MRI done preoperatively may be used for intraoperative surgical navigation. Video endoscopic equipment should be inspected, with confirmation that both the monitor and the

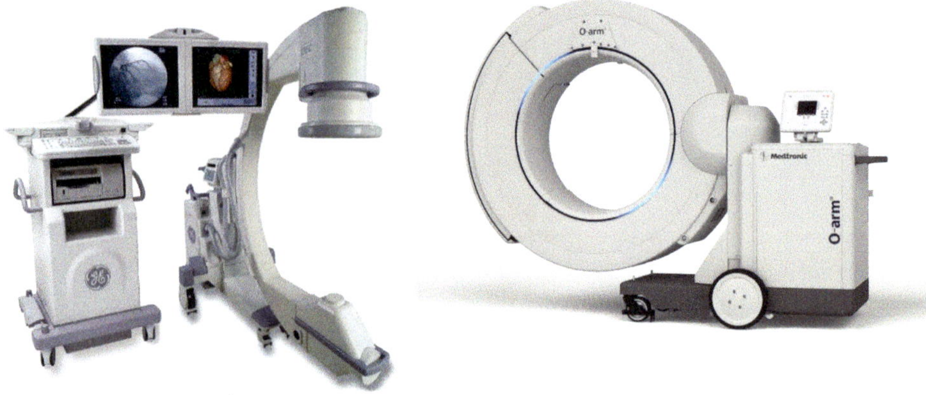

FIGURE 3.3. Left, C-arm fluoroscope. Right, O-arm fluoroscope.

endoscope are functioning and available. If surgical intraoperative microscopy will be used, the microscope should be confirmed to be able to focus appropriately, with functioning lighting, and should be draped before the patient enters the room. A key component of imaging is to directly review relevant imaging preoperatively and to have the imaging available for viewing intraoperatively. This may involve downloading the images, loading a disc or drive, or placing physical radiographs or CT/MRI physical images on an illuminator.

The operating team's presence and readiness are of the utmost importance before heading back to the operating room. Members of the team, including proceduralist, assistant if needed, industry representative, surgical scrub technician or nurse, circulating nurse, anesthesiologist, and nurse anesthetists, should be confirmed prior to bringing the patient to the operating room. While confirming presence and readiness of team members, secondary checks, such as ensuring agreement on the anesthetic plan, availability of correct surgical instruments or trays, and availability of implants or devices, can be performed with minimal interruption or delay of operating room flow.

Intraoperative Phase: Surgical Instruments

Surgical instruments and devices for the spine are innumerable. A comprehensive review of every possible surgical instrument for all spine interventions is beyond the scope of this publication, but key categories of instruments are reviewed here.

Surgical scalpels typically either have blade attachments to a reusable handle or a disposable retractable system. Typical blades include the 10 blade or 15 blade (Figure 3.4). Depending on user preference, the 10 blade is typically utilized for larger incisions or cutting in soft tissue while the 15 blade is typically utilized for shorter and precise incisions. For minimally invasive spine procedures, a pencil grip is typically recommended. This will allow for precise, short movements. A fingertip grip would be more useful for longer incisions given maximal blade contact with the skin. A palm grip would generally be very forceful and unnecessary for a typical minimally invasive spine procedure. Regardless of

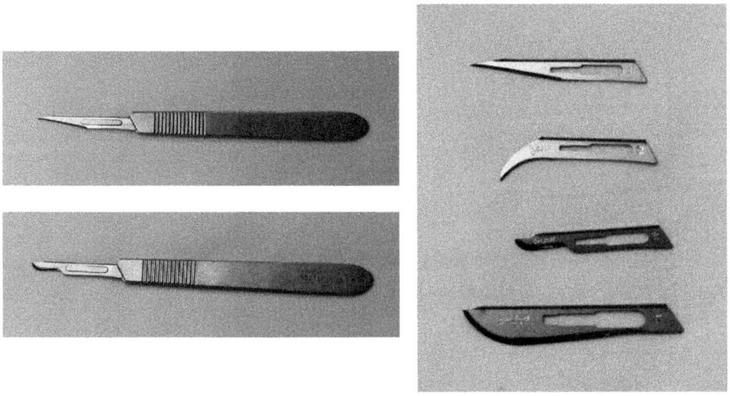

FIGURE 3.4. Top left, 11 blade on scalpel handle. Bottom left, 15 blade on scalpel handle. Right (top to bottom), Surgical blades 11, 12, 15, 21.

grip preferences, proceduralists should be aware of various scalpel manipulations, such as press cutting, stab incisions, slide cutting, sawing, and scraping. In addition, key concepts, such as planning and marking, skin stabilization, depth control, watching movements, direction, and blade angle, are important.

Scissors come in a wide variety of types and applications. It is important to realize that there are major categories of scissors, such as blunt or sharp tip, blunt or sharp blade, and straight or curved, which result in a numerous variety of scissor types. Particular examples that are useful include Metzenbaum scissors and Mayo scissors (Figure 3.5). Straight or curved Metzenbaum scissors are utilized typically for delicate tissue or blunt dissection. Another common dissecting scissor variant is the Toennis-Adson. In the setting of minimally invasive spine surgery, Mayo scissors would typically be utilized as the straight version for suture cutting. Variants of scissor grip include thumb–ring finger, thumb–middle finger, thumb–index finger, and backhand grip. The thumb–ring finger grip offers the most stability and control and is recommended. Precision of cut is greatest with cuts closer to the tip of the scissor blades rather than the fulcrum.

Forceps are a common surgical instrument category, and several useful varieties are commonly used in minimally invasive spine procedures. The forceps are designed as a grasping tool that is nonlocking and is usually held in the nondominant hand. The purpose of forceps use is highly variable, and typical applications include grasping tissue, retraction, stabilization of tissue or skin layers during suturing, packing with sponges, and extraction of free objects. Common variants utilized are Adson tissue forceps with or without teeth, DeBakey forceps, tissue forceps, and Gruenwald bayonet forceps (Figure 3.6). Given the minimal tissue trauma and incision size associated with minimally invasive spine surgery, Adson forceps are adequate for the level of tissue handling and suturing that one might encounter. If larger degrees of tissue handling are needed, DeBakey forceps are appropriate. In the Gruenwald bayonet forceps, the tips are set off-axis from the grip, which allows better visualization of the tips, which is useful when packing or removing packing. Proper technique for forceps use is to hold the instrument in the pencil position. When they are not in

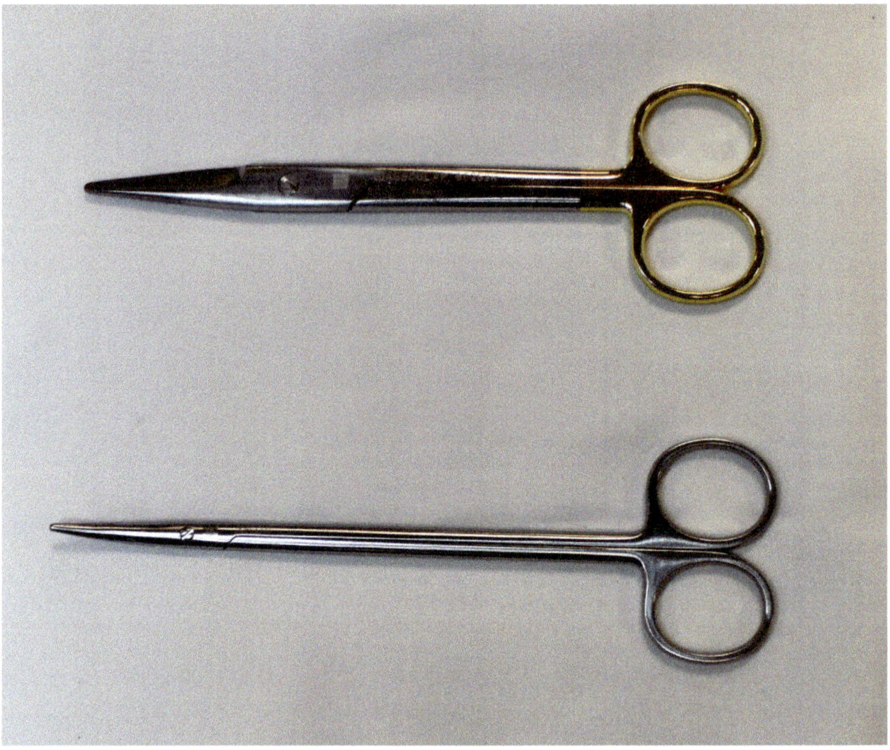

FIGURE 3.5. Top, Mayo scissors. Bottom, Metzenbaum scissors.

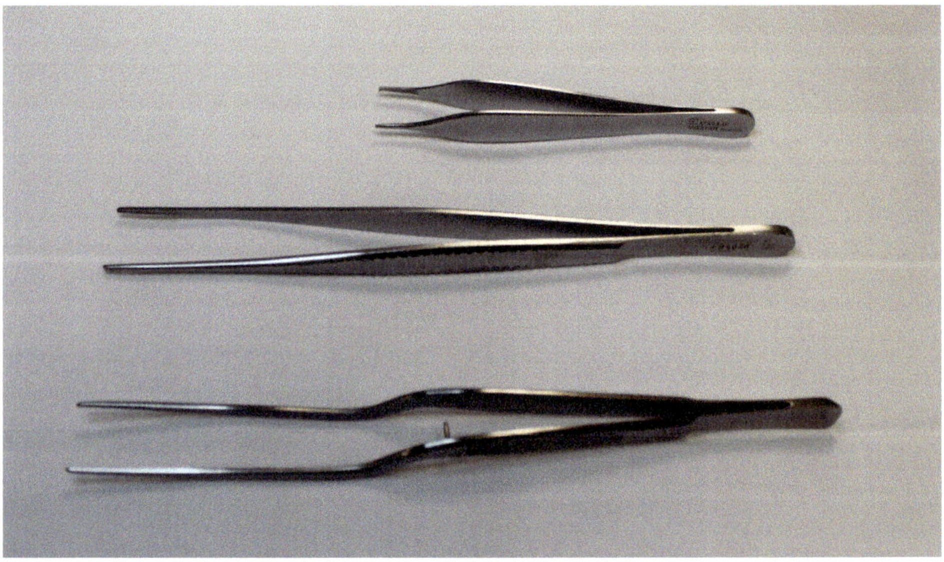

FIGURE 3.6. Top to bottom: Adson tissue forceps, DeBakey forceps, and Gruenwald bayonet forceps.

use, the forceps can be palmed with the fourth and fifth fingers, allowing for some use of the nondominant hand thumb, first digit, and second digit. The instrument can be transitioned between the fourth and fifth finger palming position and the pencil grip position with minimal interruption or use of the dominant hand.

Clamps are similar to forceps in concept but differ in terms of locking capability. The purpose of clamps is highly variable. Typical applications in minimally invasive spine procedures include hemostasis, blunt dissection, clamping of drape materials, retraction, ligature passage, and suture tagging. Three principal models are widely applicable to spine surgery: Crile straight or curved hemostat, Kelly straight or curved clamp, and Kocher clamp (Figure 3.7). The indications for each of these commonly used models are different. The hemostat is typically used for small arterial bleeding and can be used to clamp off sources of bleeding until passage of ligature and control of bleeding are achieved or cautery is applied either directly or via the hemostat. Additionally, the hemostat can be utilized as a fine blunt dissector. The Kelly clamp can typically be utilized as a blunt dissection tool,

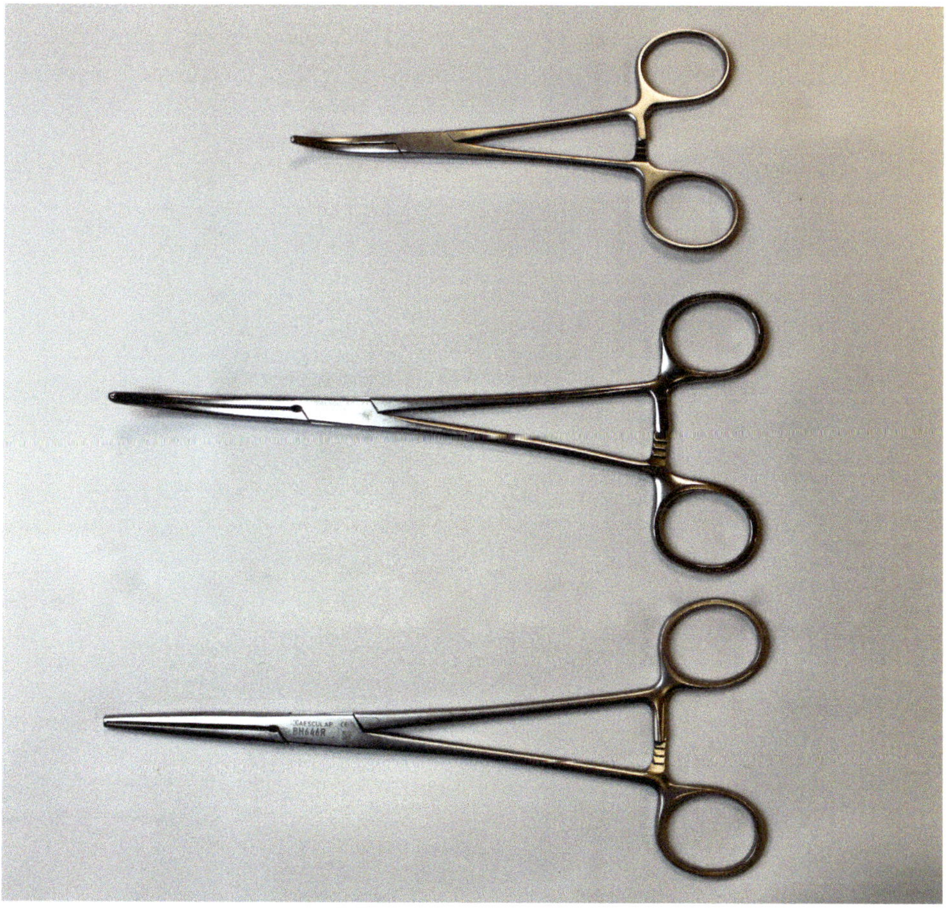

FIGURE 3.7. Top to bottom: Crile curved hemostat, Kelly curved clamp, and Kocher clamp.

which is particularly useful for opening up larger potential spaces within fascial planes for insertion of devices like intrathecal medical pumps or spinal cord stimulator implantable pulse generator. The Kocher clamp, although less frequently used in minimally invasive spine procedures, has an excellent grasping and locking capability and can be used to secure tissue that will be removed or that needs to be mobilized. Towel clamps are useful draping adjuncts and an alternative to skin staples. In addition, a hemostat can be used to remove skin staples prior to undraping. Like the grip for scissors, a thumb–ring finger grip is recommended for best accuracy and stability. With curved clamps, having the curvature point downward or upward is a balance between accuracy and minimal surrounding tissue damage versus wider effect but potential for greater surrounding tissue damage.

Needle holders are a close variant of clamps and are principally used to drive needles during suturing. Common variants include the Mayo Hegar needle holder and Olsen Hegar needle holder, which come in a variety of lengths and sizes (Figure 3.8). The principal difference between these two very common variants is that the Mayo Hegar needle holder has short, strong jaws utilized solely for needle driving, whereas the Olsen Hegar needle holder combines both needle holder and suture scissors. With combined tools, the suture placement and subsequent cut can be performed without changing instruments or having an assistant cut. However, this can lead to inadvertent cutting of the suture. Misuse or inefficient use of needle holders is a large component of intraoperative delay and poor wound closure.

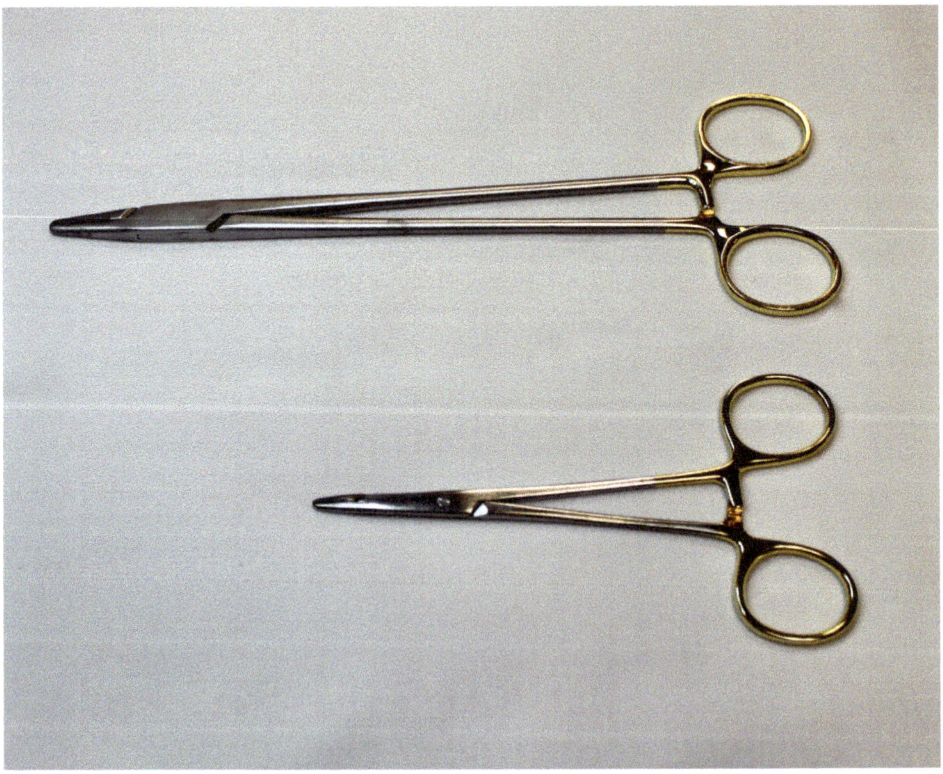

FIGURE 3.8. Two different sizes of Mayo Hegar needle holders.

Interrupted or nonproductive repetitive movements explain why the use of this particular instrument type can lead to large amounts of time wasted. Vital steps include correctly positioning the needle, grasping the needle holder efficiently, using an entry angle that is orthogonal to tissue, accomplishing needle release and regrasping without need for repositioning in the needle holder, and leaving the correct suture tail length through the wound for tying. Various problems, such as not positioning the needle at an optimal angle, inefficient or awkward grasp, poor tissue entry angle, needle release and regrasping, and too long or too short of a suture tail, can cause a myriad of problems. In addition, inaccurate needle driving through inappropriate layers can cause problems like dehiscence due to nonfascial needle bites or infection due to inadvertent skin puncture with suture tracking from the skin surface to deeper layers. Among grip types, several are acceptable depending on user preferences, such as the palmed grip, thenar grip, thumb–ring finger grip, and pencil grip. The palmed grip in particular is useful because it allows performing an unlimited arc of motion by manipulating the needle holder within the palm as well as delivering a significant amount of force. However, other grips are acceptable depending on the type of needle holder, clinical indications, and preferences.

Needle choices are myriad. Needles can be classified by point geometry, such as tapered point, blunt tapered point, reverse cutting, conventional cutting, taper cutting, blunt point, and spatulated. The most common variants are tapered and conventional cutting. The conventional cutting needle has the cutting edge facing the inside of the curved needle and can be utilized for tougher tissues, such as fascia or skin. Tapered needles are typically used for softer tissues or organs but can be used in muscle layers. Needle shape, such as 1/4, 3/8, 1/2, and 5/8 circle shapes, J shapes, compound curve, and straight, are all common variants. Curved needles are used most, whereas straight needles may be used for skin or subcuticular applications. Needle size is another variable as well. The needle point geometry, size, and type will depend on the application.

Suture choices are also highly variable. The principal suture choices include absorbable or nonabsorbable, braided or monofilament, natural or synthetic materials, and size. Nonabsorbable sutures will retain the majority of their tensile strength after 60 days. Common variants of sutures include a braided absorbable suture type, such as Vicryl, ranging in size from 0 to 2-0 for fascial or deep closures utilizing deep dermal sutures. Absorbable monofilaments like Monocryl in a size 3-0 or 4-0 can be utilized for subcuticular closures. Nonabsorbable monofilament, such as nylon 2-0, is useful for vertical mattress or horizontal mattress sutures. Nonabsorbable braided sutures, such as silk 2-0, or nonabsorbable monofilament, such as Ethilon 2-0. Overall, the choice of suture is largely driven by clinical application and user preference. However, braided sutures can increase the risk of infection, with in vitro modeling demonstrating increased bacterial adherence to Vicryl sutures, for example.[1] Additionally, in vitro modeling has demonstrated a significant drop in tensile strength of polyglactin, polyglycolic acid, and polyglycolidcaprone sutures with exposure to moisture or simulated saliva.[2] This supports a key concept of wound closure, which is to err on the side of thoroughness and strength rather than speed, in anticipation of possible suture breakage and dehiscence given tensile strength loss over time before tissues have a chance to completely heal. Certain suture types, such as nylon monofilament, can be kept in place in a vertical mattress or horizontal mattress configuration with less anticipated tensile strength loss or risk of infection. In addition, braided sutures may not be suitable in the presence of infection such as a washout or debridement.

Skin staplers can be used for superficial closure and have several advantages and disadvantages. Advantages for skin closure include technical ease and speed. A meta-analysis has demonstrated that between sutures and staples, an over 5-minute closure time difference exists between groups over a broad spectrum of nonorthopedic surgeries.[3] With regard to the technique of skin staple use, appropriately approximating tissue edges with the help of an assistant or applying the stapler itself so that the tissue is everted appropriately is important to prevent future wound contraction and eventual inversion or breakdown. However, this concept has been questioned and has been subjected to a randomized controlled trial in dermatologic surgery, which demonstrated no significant difference in scar assessment by patients or observers.[4] Everted or planar repair using a stapler may not be as important as previously assessed. However, inverted incision closure is not recommended for two reasons: it creates a linear skin depression that can trap microbes and that can be difficult to cleanse for wound care without disrupting the healing incision, and there is no assurance that underlying tissues do not have an undue amount of tension causing the inversion itself. The risk of infection, postoperative pain, and poor cosmetic appearance after staple closure are definite considerations against the use of skin staples. Both the previously mentioned nonorthopedic surgery meta-analysis and an orthopedic meta-analysis have noted higher rates of infection associated with staple closure.[3,5] Thinner, atrophic skin types in more elderly patients that are more likely to receive minimally invasive spine procedures may not be ideal for the use of staples.

Skin glue or adhesive can be utilized to maintain approximated suture edges. Skin glue is usually a cyanoacrylate compound, and it is theorized to also provide a microbial barrier postoperatively. The infection-preventive effect of skin glue has been supported by clinical evidence from cardiothoracic surgery and neurologic surgery. A meta-analysis from cardiothoracic surgery examined prevention of sternal wound infections with preoperative and postoperative glue application, and infections decreased from 10.8% to 2.7% and 4.3% to 2.1%, respectively.[6] A neurosurgical study of 90 children with primary ventriculoperitoneal shunt placement demonstrated a reduction of the wound dehiscence rate from 24% to 2% and the infection rate from 17% to 0% with the use of skin glue instead of nonabsorbable skin sutures for final layer closure.[7] Proper use of skin glue or adhesive is to ensure that incision edges are approximated well and then to cleanse the skin before application of skin glue. With regard to postoperative care, skin glue can cause dermatitis or itching that may be confounded with infectious or allergic complications. The skin glue does not need to be removed and will naturally peel off after 1 to 2 weeks.

Retractors are broadly subdivided into hand-held and self-retaining formats. The hand-held retractors include several well-known examples, such as the Army-Navy retractor, Richardson retractor, Volkman rake retractor, Cloward hand-held retractor, Caspar hand-held retractor, and Senn retractor (Figure 3.9). Self-retaining retractors applicable to spine surgery include the Weitlaner retractor, Harvey Jackson retractor, McCulloch

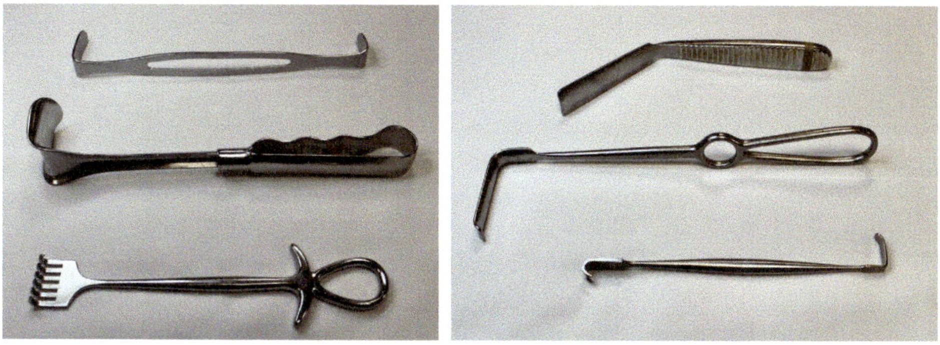

FIGURE 3.9. Left (top to bottom), Army-Navy, Richardson, and Volkman rake retractors. Right (top to bottom), Cloward hand-held, Caspar hand-held, and Senn retractors.

retractor, Caspar double hinge retractor, and Cloward double hinge retractor (Figure 3.10). A multitude of tubular retraction systems exist. Spinal endoscopy or access cannulas can be considered a subdivision of tubular retractors. The basic principle is to provide steady tissue retraction during a portion of surgery, typically for visualization. Ideally, the retraction approach should be self-retaining to avoid fatigue and to allow assistants to use their hands for other tasks. However, manual retraction may be indicated for brief tissue mobilization, such as aiding in implantation of a device or for care around vulnerable tissue. The principal hazards with any retraction system are ischemia and tissue damage. Key concepts, such as traction and countertraction and appropriate tissue tension for dissection, are invaluable. Of the hand-held retractors, typically an Army-Navy or Richardson retractor is used for moderately sized incisions or tissue mobilization. Fine manipulation or retraction may require a Senn retractor. The Cloward and Caspar hand-held retractors allow for deep layer retraction and have double-hinged self-retaining formats. The Weitlaner retractor is useful for superficial retraction. The Harvey Jackson retractor can be utilized for retraction

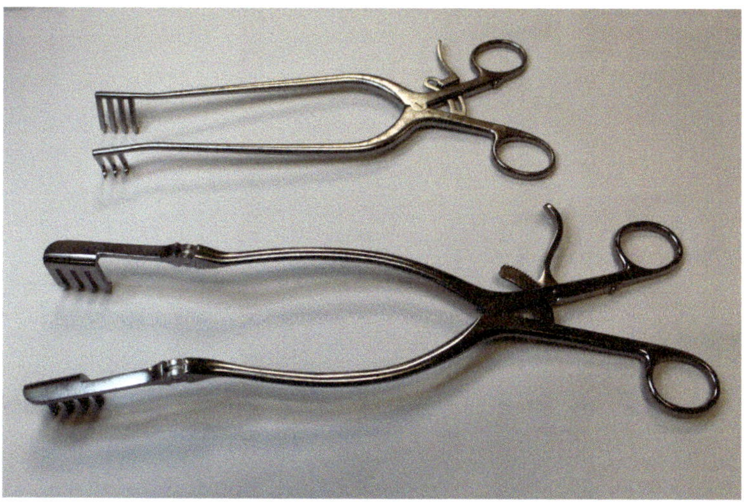

FIGURE 3.10. Top, Weitlaner retractor. Bottom, Harvey Jackson retractor.

of deeper layers. The McCulloch retractor is particularly useful for minimally invasive spine surgery given the deep nature of the blades and relatively modular design, allowing for a small incision site and deep retraction. Similarly, the Cloward and Caspar self-retaining retractors are useful in cervical spine surgery. Tubular retractors and spinal endoscopy cannulas both provide an access pathway to the spine but differ in relative size and visualization method. Tubular retractors will typically be larger than spinal endoscopy cannulas and utilize direct visualization, usually aided by microscopy. Endoscopic cannulas are typically smaller and utilize indirect visualization, via cameras or fluoroscopy.

Suction tips vary in size, angle, and control. Two common variants are the Yankauer suction tube and the Fergusson or Frazier suction tube. The Yankauer is a much larger suction tube and does not have a manual keyhole to control suction flow. It is useful for larger amounts of bleeding or fluid suction, typically during incision. The Fergusson and Frazier suction tubes are thin and angled, with a manual keyhole for suction interruption. A Poole suction tube has a straight design and is indicated for large amounts of fluid in an open field, which is unlikely to be applicable to minimally invasive spine procedures (Figure 3.11).

Electrosurgery is an invaluable tool. Electrosurgery began in 1926, when it was invented by William T. Bovie. The key concept of electrosurgery is to apply high-frequency alternating electrical current through tissue, causing tissue destruction, dehydration, coagulation, or vaporization. (On the other hand, electrocautery is electric current applied to a metal resistor, which generates heat, thus becoming essentially a heated tool applied to tissue.) The electrosurgical unit converts electrical energy from the main supply to a

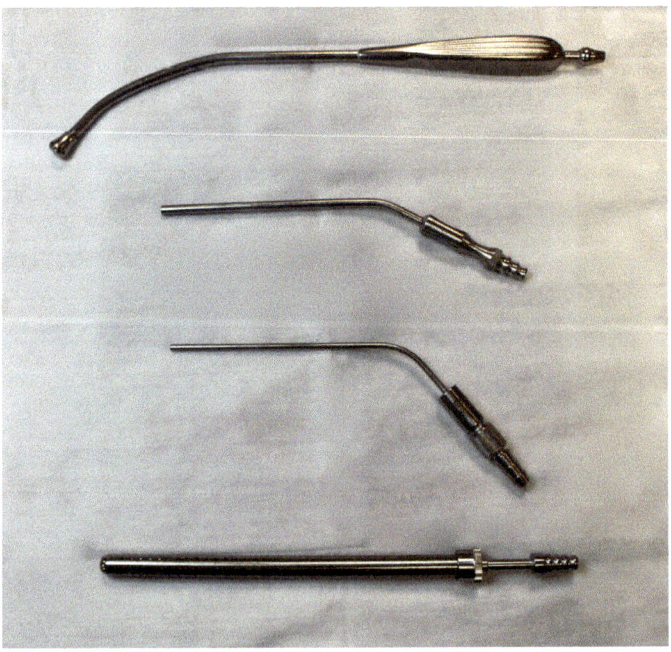

FIGURE 3.11. Top, Yankauer suction tube. Middle, two variations of Fergusson/Frazier suction tubes. Bottom, Poole suction tube.

high-frequency current, which is then applied into an active electrode. The energy density of this active electrode is what causes the desired electrosurgical effect. The circuit is completed by a neutral electrode. Monopolar and bipolar forceps are the two most common electrosurgery configurations (Figure 3.12). The monopolar electrosurgical unit utilizes a large dispersive electrode that is attached to the patient. The small active electrode that applies the concentrated current creates the clinical effect of electrosurgery, with the current passing through the patient into a large dispersive neutral electrode that is attached to the electrosurgical unit. It is important to note that it is the larger area and thus lower energy density of the neutral electrode that prevents any tissue damage at the site of the neutral electrode. Thus, using inappropriately sized grounding pads or not fully attaching grounding pads with maximal skin contact may result in burns at the pad site. Interfering factors at the grounding pad can include excessive hair, adipose tissue, bony prominences, fluid, incomplete adhesion, or scar. The electrosurgical unit with a monopolar device will not function without the circuit completed by the grounding pad appropriately attached to the patient and the electrosurgical unit. The grounding pad's placement may be affected by avoiding having the current path cross the heart or implanted devices. The monopolar has two main settings, cut and coagulate. The cut setting will vaporize and cut tissue. The coagulation setting will reduce the current-flow time or interrupt the waveform to produce

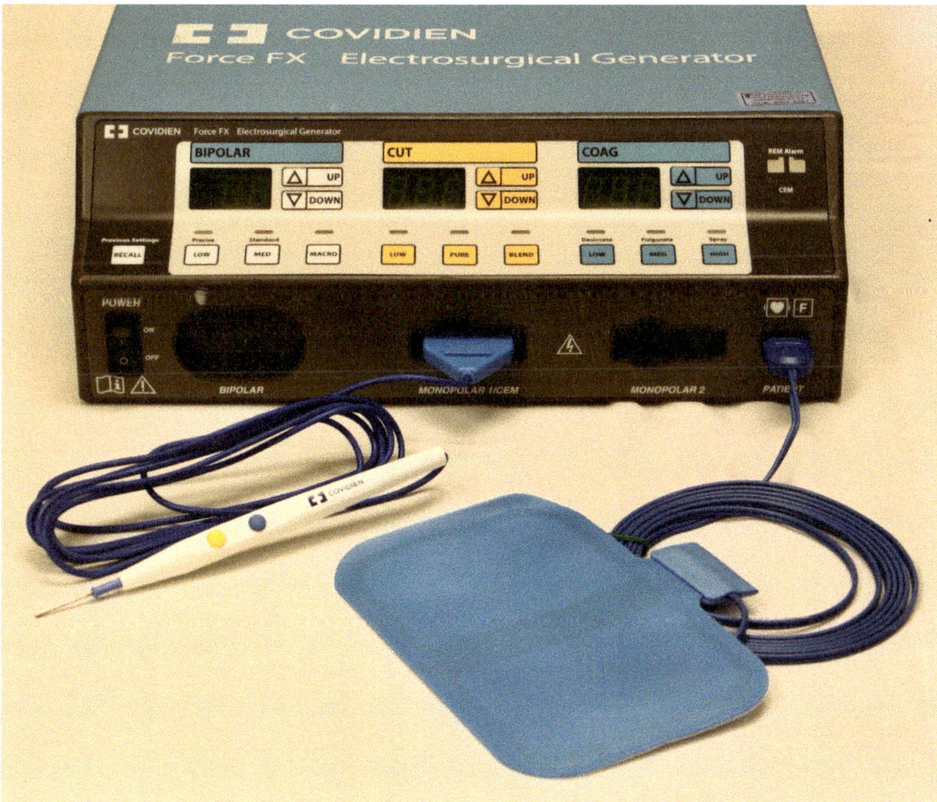

FIGURE 3.12. Electrosurgical generator with Bovie electrocautery pen and grounding pad.

less overall heat and thus coagulate. For a monopolar, typical default settings are 30-30 cut-coagulate. The bipolar electrode mounts both active and neutral electrodes on the hand-held forceps. Thus, the bipolar only targets tissue located between the two electrodes. The clinical implication of the bipolar unit is that it can work in a wet field, whereas with a monopolar unit, current would be dispersed by conducting fluid. The bipolar electrodes have three main types of operation: precise, standard, and macro. A grounding pad is not needed for bipolar electrosurgery because the active and neutral electrodes are contained in the forceps. In addition, if electromagnetic interference is a concern, the bipolar is an excellent alternative to monopolar electrosurgery.[8,9]

Orthopedic instruments for spine surgery and spinal instrumentation are numerous. Blunt instruments that are particularly of use in spine surgery are dissectors, such as the Penfield Nos. 1 to 5. These all have different heads and can be utilized for dissection and exploration. The Penfield No. 4 in particular is used widely in spine surgery. The Daubenspeck bone curette is a hand-held device with a sharp-edged scoop head that is an excellent instrument with which to atraumatically scrape and expose bone surfaces. The Cobb elevator is an instrument that can be used to remove periosteum and to detach ligaments and muscles from bone. The Langenbeck rib raspatory is another instrument that is particularly useful for removal of periosteum and for bone exposure. Osteotomes are utilized to chisel bone but are generally not applicable to minimally invasive spine surgery because they are utilized more commonly in facetectomy, laminectomy, or larger deformity repairs, such as posterior column osteotomy, pedicle subtraction, or vertebral column resection (Figure 3.13).

Rongeurs are varied, with common variants like the Caspar rongeur, Echlin bone rongeur, and Roettgen-Ruskin rongeur (Figure 3.14). The Caspar rongeur is specifically designed for intervertebral disks and has fenestrated and serrated grasping jaws attached to a long shaft and handle. A similar design is used for pituitary rongeurs. The Echlin bone rongeur and the Roettgen-Ruskin rongeur have angled heads and are attached to plierlike handles. A similar instrument is the Leksell bone rongeur, which has a light curvature. However, it is unlikely that a minimally invasive spine procedure would involve bone rongeurs, which require a wider exposure to allow use of the wide handle arms. The Kerrison bone punch, a very commonly used tool with a long neck, allows precise removal of bone fragments with a stamping or punch grasping action (Figure 3.14). Many of the

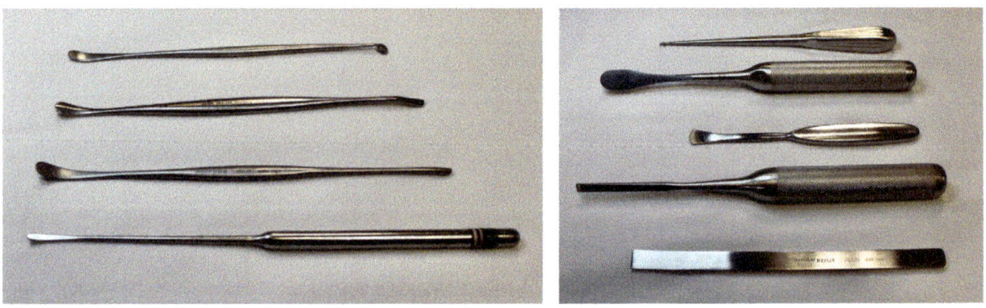

FIGURE 3.13. Left (top to bottom), Penfield #1–4 (top to bottom). Right (top to bottom), Daubenspeck bone curette, Cobb elevator, Langenbeck raspatory, Hibbs osteotome, and Lambotte osteotome.

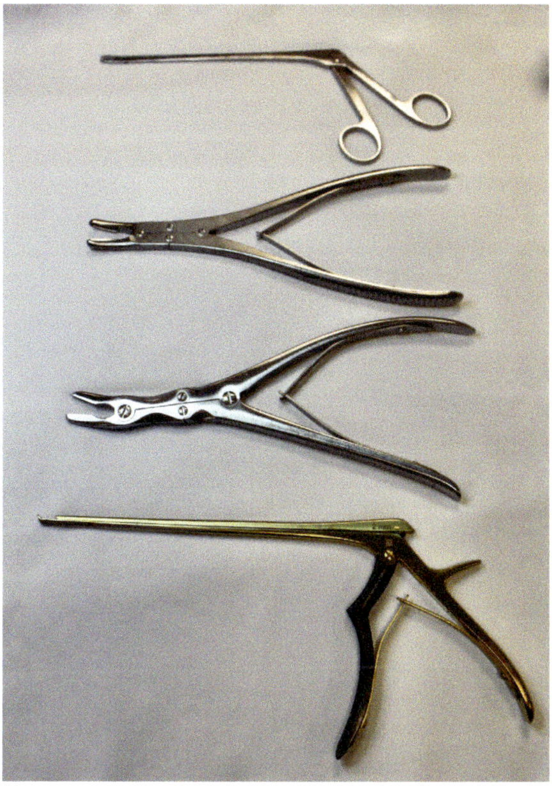

FIGURE 3.14. Top to bottom: Caspar rongeur, Roettgen-Ruskin rongeur, Echlin rongeur, and Kerrison bone punch.

long-neck rongeur variants are in common use in both fluoroscopically guided and endoscopic minimally invasive spine surgery. High-speed drills and shavers for endoscopic surgery are another set of tools converted from use in open spine surgery for use in minimally invasive spine procedures. These instruments have a large variety of endoscopic drill heads, head-angle adjustments, speeds, and manufacturers.

References

1. Masini BD, Stinner DJ, Waterman SM, Wenke JC. Bacterial adherence to suture materials. *J Surg Educ.* 2011;68(2):101–104. doi:10.1016/j.jsurg.2010.09.015.
2. Khiste SV, Ranganath V, Nichani AS. Evaluation of tensile strength of surgical synthetic absorbable suture materials: an in vitro study. *J Periodont Implant Sci.* 2013;43(3):130–135. doi:10.5051/jpis.2013.43.3.130.
3. Iavazzo C, Gkegkes ID, Vouloumanou EK, Mamais I, Peppas G, Falagas ME. Sutures versus staples for the management of surgical wounds: a meta-analysis of randomized controlled trials. *Am Surg.* 2011;77(9):1206–1221.
4. Kappel S, Kleinerman R, King TH, Sivamani R, Taylor S, Nguyen UT, Eisen DB. Does wound eversion improve cosmetic outcome? Results of a randomized, split-scar, comparative trial. *J Am Acad Dermatol.* 2015;72(4):668–673. doi:10.1016/j.jaad.2014.11.032.
5. Smith TO, Sexton D, Mann C, Donell S. Sutures versus staples for skin closure in orthopaedic surgery: meta-analysis. *BMJ.* 2010;340:c1199. doi:10.1136/bmj.c1199.

6. Chambers A, Scarci M. Is skin closure with cyanoacrylate glue effective for the prevention of sternal wound infections? *Interact Cardiovasc Thorac Surg.* 2010;10(5):793–796. doi:10.1510/icvts.2009.230425.
7. Eymann R, Kiefer M. Glue instead of stitches: a minor change of the operative technique with a serious impact on the shunt infection rate. *Acta Neurochir Suppl.* 2010;106:87–89. doi:10.1007/978-3-211-98811-4_14.
8. Cordero I. Electrosurgical units—how they work and how to use them safely. *Community Eye Health.* 2015;28(89):15–16.
9. Munro MG. Fundamentals of electrosurgery part I: principles of radiofrequency energy for surgery. In: Feldman L., Fuchshuber P., Jones D, eds. *The SAGES Manual on the Fundamental Use of Surgical Energy (FUSE).* New York, NY: Springer; 2012. https://doi.org/10.1007/978-1-4614-2074-3_2.

4

Perioperative Considerations

Brian Y. Kim

The Preoperative Evaluation

Preoperative Testing

As the average patient population grows older and exhibits increasing medical complexity, it is important to identify patients who require optimization before undergoing any surgical procedure. A thorough preoperative evaluation is paramount in ensuring patient safety and should begin with a complete but efficient history and physical examination. Although minimally invasive spinal procedures may be less invasive than traditional open surgeries, it is important to risk-stratify every patient to maximize patient safety and to avoid poor outcomes.

Tests, including basic labs (complete blood count, basic metabolic panel, urinalysis, blood gas analysis), electrocardiogram, echocardiography, chest x-ray, and pulmonary function tests, are often employed to help guide preventative measures. Multiple validated guidelines, including those of the National Institute for Health and Care Excellence (NICE),[2] American Heart Association (AHA),[3] and American Society of Anesthesiologists (ASA),[4,5] however, caution against the routine use of tests in healthy patients. In a 2013 systematic review including 101 randomized controlled and observational studies, Johansson et al failed to find significant correlation between preoperative testing and risk of morbidity, mortality, or adverse events in healthy individuals undergoing noncardiac surgery.[6]

Similarly, a 2012 practice advisory by the ASA was released with updated evidence on preanesthesia evaluation of patients undergoing surgery. The findings indicated that routine perioperative tests intended to discover a disease or disorder in an asymptomatic patient do not make an important contribution to the perioperative assessment. However, selective perioperative tests (tests ordered after consideration of specific patient information obtained in review of medical records, patient interview, and physical exam, as well as

TABLE 4.1. ASA Practice Advisory for Preanesthesia Evaluation: Abnormal Test Findings in Asymptomatic Patients[5]

Perioperative Test	Incidence of Abnormal Findings in Asymptomatic Patients	Incidence of Case Management Changes or Cancellations due to Findings
ECG	4.6%–44.9%	0.46%–2.6%
Echocardiography	25%	NA
Stress test	24%	2%
Chest x-ray	0.3%–60.1%	0.6%–20.3%
Spirometry	14.0%–51.7%	NA
Hemoglobin	0.5%–65.4%	2.4%–28.6%
Hematocrit	0.2%–38.9%	20.0%
CBC	2.9%–9.0%	2.9%
Coagulation tests	0.06%–21.2%	0.0%–4.0%
Sodium	1.9%	NA
Potassium	0.2%–16.0%	NA
Glucose	0.9%–40.4%	NA
Urinalysis (not UPT)	0.7%–42.0%	2.3%–75.0%
Urine Pregnancy Test	0.3%–1.3%	100%

invasiveness of planned procedure) may assist in decision-making for the perioperative process. The ASA review found that abnormal ECG findings in asymptomatic or nonselected patients ranged from 4.6% to 44.9% (category B2 evidence), while abnormal transthoracic echocardiography results were found in 25% of asymptomatic patients (category B2 evidence).[5] Abnormal chest radiography findings in asymptomatic or nonselected patients occurred in 0.3% to 60.1% and resulted in postponement, cancellations, or changes in management of 0.6% to 20.3% of cases found to be abnormal (category B2 evidence). Abnormal hemoglobin findings were reported in 0.5% to 65.4% of asymptomatic patients, resulting in case cancellation or management changes in 2.4% to 28.6% of cases with abnormal findings (category B2 evidence), while abnormal coagulation studies (bleeding time, prothrombin time, partial prothrombin time, or platelet count) were found in 0.06% to 21.2% of asymptomatic patients, resulting in 0.0% to 4.0% of patients having their management changed or cases cancelled (category B2 evidence).[5] A summary of rates of abnormal findings from perioperative tests in asymptomatic patients is shown in Table 4.1.

Thus, testing derived from pathological conditions in the patient's past medical history or physical examination may be warranted. The following sections explore specific medical conditions that warrant further evaluation and consultation to improve patient safety and outcomes.

Anesthetic Techniques

While many pain interventions can be performed under conscious sedation with nursing supervision, some procedures require the assistance of anesthesiology colleagues to optimize surgical conditions, patient positioning, and patient comfort. The two main anesthetic plans are general anesthesia and monitored anesthesia care (MAC) with local anesthetic infiltration. Most patients with significant cardiopulmonary disease benefit from the avoidance of the hemodynamic changes associated with the induction of general anesthesia and endotracheal intubation/extubation. MAC provides the same general standard of care and monitoring, including safe sedation and analgesia, but also provides rescue airway techniques by an anesthesia provider in case of oversedation.[7] MAC techniques have also been shown to aid in enhanced postoperative recovery times due to the use of relatively low doses of sedative medications compared to general anesthetics. Another benefit of the MAC technique is the possibility to maintain patient cooperation in basic neurologic examinations for higher risk procedures.

While MAC is generally a safe option, even for the elderly and patients with high disease burden, relative contraindications to MAC techniques do exist. These contraindications are often related to some of the most common complications associated with the technique, including airway obstruction, hypoxia, and cardiovascular collapse.[8] One study analyzing thyroidectomies under MAC listed specific contraindications, such as patient refusal, communication/language barrier, allergy to local anesthetics, morbid obesity, sleep apnea, and anticipated difficult airway.[9] Pain procedures requiring prone positioning, such as vertebroplasty and discography, however, have historically been found to be highly amenable to the technique.[10–12] Ultimately, patient selection based on unique individual patient factors and clinical judgment should be utilized in requesting an anesthetic plan that optimizes conditions for both the patient and proceduralist.

Medical Comorbidities

Cardiac Disease

Heart disease is the leading cause of mortality in the United States, affecting an estimated 121.5 million people or 48% of American adults.[13] Although heart disease is highly prevalent, studies have shown that routine cardiac consultation or testing leads to overutilization of healthcare resources without significant effect on outcomes, especially before low-risk surgical procedures.[14,15] In the setting of decompensated heart failure, acute coronary syndrome, or moderate to severe valvulopathy, however, patients may require consultation, testing, and further management before undergoing an elective procedure safely.

Validated risk assessment tools, such as the Revised Cardiac Risk Index (RCRI) created by the American College of Cardiology/American Heart Association (ACC/AHA) and the surgical risk calculator of the American College of Surgeons National Surgical Quality Improvement Program (ACS NSQIP), can provide a quick and effective assessment to guide appropriate risk stratification and triage of procedural candidates.[16] The RCRI was first published in 1977 after a multivariate discriminant analysis was performed at Massachusetts General Hospital (MGH) evaluating surgical outcomes of patients over the age of 40 receiving surgery at MGH.[17] The result of the analysis was the formulation of a scoring system that estimates the risk of major adverse cardiac events (MACE) based on six elements in the patient's past medical history (Table 4.2). Studies since have demonstrated that the RCRI score is able to discriminate low versus high MACE risk after noncardiac surgery, but the

TABLE 4.2. Revised Cardiac Risk Index for Preoperative Risk[17,23]

Variable	Points
History of ischemic heart disease	1
History of congestive heart disease	1
History of cerebrovascular disease	1
Use of insulin therapy for diabetes	1
Preoperative serum creatinine > 2.0 mg/dL	1
High-risk surgery*	1

Defined as intraperitoneal, intrathoracic, or suprainguinal vascular surgery.

system may have limited predictive value in MACE risk after vascular noncardiac surgery. Furthermore, the predictive value of the system is specific for MACE and not overall mortality.[18] Depending on the RCRI score, patients may have up to 15.0% risk for perioperative MACE (Table 4.3).[19]

Meanwhile, the ACS NSQIP calculator determines overall risk of any type of postoperative complications.[20] This scoring system was compiled from clinical data (1,414,006 patients) from the 393 ACS NSQIP hospitals that were subsequently used for regression model analysis to predict eight outcomes based on patient perioperative risk factors.[21] Outcomes predicted include risk of mortality, morbidity, pneumonia, cardiac complications, surgical site infections (SSIs), urinary tract infections, deep venous thrombus, and renal failure. The calculator consists of 22 questions based on the patient's medical history and planned surgical procedure. ACS NSQIP recommends cardiac consultation and/or testing if the patient's cardiac risk exceeds 1%. The ACS NSQIP calculator includes a subjective surgeon adjustment score to help capture complications not predicted by the calculator. Further analysis has found that universal and procedure-specific calculators have similar predictions. While internal evaluation of the calculator has shown it to have good accuracy, external validation studies have found it to be inconsistent. However, it remains useful as a general predictive tool to guide discussions with patients.[22]

Patient assessment of functional capacity can be classified using metabolic equivalents (METs). First proposed by researchers at Duke University, METs are a means for determining peak oxygen uptake and cardiovascular demand utilizing a self-administered

TABLE 4.3. Estimated Risk of Major Adverse Cardiac Events (MACE) Based on RCRI Score[19]

Total RCRI Score	Risk Estimate (%)	95% CI for risk estimate
0	3.9	2.8%–5.4%
1	6.0	4.9%–7.4%
2	10.1	8.1%–12.6%
≥3	15.0	11.1%–20.0%

TABLE 4.4. Correlation of Metabolic Equivalents (METs) and Activity[25]

METs	Activity
1	Resting
2	Level walking 2 mph
4	Level walking 4 mph
5	Chopping wood (4.9 METs)
6	Aerobic or ballet dancing
7	Fast swimming
10	Jogging 10 min mile (10.2 METs)
12	Rope skipping

brief questionnaire.[24] Subsequent studies have helped identify activities that approximate METs based on maximum exercise tolerated by patients (Table 4.4).[25] If a patient reports more than one element listed in the RCRI as present and the patient's functional capacity is diminished below 4 METs, the ACC/AHA recommend further investigation and testing, because the MACE risk exceeds 0.9%. Additionally, the ACC/AHA recommend that elective surgery be delayed at least 60 days after myocardial infarction, regardless of intervention.[23] Special clinical situations requiring anticoagulation for coronary stents and valve prosthetics must be considered and are discussed further in the hematology section of this chapter.

Cardiac Devices

Cardiac implantable electronic devices (CIED) are increasingly common and present unique considerations for the proceduralist and the anesthetic team. CIEDs include permanent pacemakers (PPM), implantable cardioverter-defibrillators (ICD), cardiac resynchronization therapy (CRT) devices, and implanted loop recorders. In many facilities, the standard management for these devices is to apply a magnet to the device, but this is not always reliable. In the patient with any CIED who is undergoing a surgical procedure requiring electrocautery, it is important to have a specific management plan to ensure maintenance of a nonmalignant rhythm and prevention of inappropriate shock.

In 2011, the Heart Rhythm Society, ASA, AHA, and Society of Thoracic Surgeons presented an expert consensus statement regarding perioperative CIED management.[26] The panel suggested several risk-mitigation strategies to effectively reduce the incidence of adverse events related to electromagnetic interference (EMI). First, the operative team should identify all sources of potential EMI, including monopolar cautery (the most common source in the OR), radiofrequency ablation, transcutaneous electrical nerve stimulation, spinal cord stimulators, and even intraoperative monitors. In cases of monopolar cautery use, surgery sites > 6 inches from the CIED pulse generator or below the level of the umbilicus are unlikely to cause electrical events. Grounding pads should be placed strategically to avoid passage of current through the cardiac device. It is important to note, however, that bipolar cautery does not cause EMI unless it is applied directly to a CIED generator or lead. Cautery use should be limited to bursts of 5 seconds or less to minimize EMI.

In cases where device interrogation and reprogramming are not performed preoperatively, rescue magnet placement can be utilized to suspend ICD shock therapy and place pacemaker activity into a default "asynchronous" or VOO mode. This mode allows for ventricular pacing at manufacturer-specific rates regardless of the patient's underlying rhythm, while sensing and inhibition functions of the pacemaker are temporarily halted. Prior to magnet placement, care should be taken to identify the maker and model of the device, because each company has a unique asynchronous mode setting that, if unaccounted for, could prove to be harmful or fatal to a patient. If there is any question at all, case delay with device interrogation is strongly encouraged. Although EMI can lead to serious complications, adverse electrical events can be avoided with simple preoperative planning.

Respiratory Disease

When assessing a patient's ability to tolerate a surgical procedure under anesthesia, assessment of the patient's baseline pulmonary function is considered just as important as cardiac function. In fact, several large cohort studies report equivalent rates of serious pulmonary and cardiac complications and suggest both systems contribute similarly to morbidity, mortality, and length of stay.[27–30] The most important respiratory complications contributing to morbidity include atelectasis, pneumonia, respiratory failure, and exacerbation of chronic lung disease.

In 2011, the American College of Physicians and Smetana et al performed a systematic review of preoperative pulmonary risk stratification to identify specific risk factors that contribute to perioperative respiratory morbidity.[31] A total of 27 studies with 10,960 pulmonary complications among 324,648 patients were included for analysis. Preoperative testing, such as chest radiography and spirometry, was examined, but little evidence to support their routine use was found, and no change in management as a result of these tests was observed. Patient risk factors, however, including age greater than 60, history of chronic obstructive pulmonary disease (COPD) or smoking, higher ASA class (> ASA class 2), functional dependence on activities of daily living, and history of congestive heart failure, were associated with significant increases in the odds ratio for postoperative complications. Counterintuitively, obesity, presence of restrictive lung disease, and asthma were not found to be significant risk factors for pulmonary complications. Another study by the National Surgical Quality Improvement Project of 2012 examined unanticipated hospital admissions among 53,667 ambulatory surgical cases.[32] After adjusting for confounders, the authors found that history of COPD was a major risk factor, with an odds ratio of 3.46 ($P < .0001$).

Smoking

Many pulmonary diseases, such as COPD and restrictive lung disease, are relatively fixed in severity and are considered immutable. Cigarette smoking, however, is unique in that it is a readily modifiable risk factor for postoperative pulmonary complications. Studies have consistently shown that appropriately timed cessation counseling and patient cooperation result in significant decreases in morbidity. In a meta-analysis of 25 cohort and randomized controlled studies, Wong et al concluded that smokers who quit more than 4 or 8 weeks before surgery had significantly lower risks of pulmonary complications than those who did not (RR 0.77, 95% CI 0.61 to 0.96; and RR 0.53, 95% CI 0.37 to 0.76, respectively).[33]

Cigarette smoking has also been implicated in delayed postoperative wound healing. Nicotine's vasoconstrictive effects decrease tissue oxygenation and reduce both the inflammatory and proliferative healing responses to tissue injury.[34] Wong et al examined wound-healing complications in patients who quit smoking 3 to 4 weeks before surgery versus complications in those who did not and found significantly lower risk of complications in the former group (RR 0.69; 95% CI 0.56 to 0.84). Another study examined 295 patients undergoing aesthetic or reconstructive surgery and found that smokers developed wound-healing complications (defined as wound dehiscence, infection, or atypical scar formation) in 48.2% of cases, while nonsmokers and patients who quit for 6 weeks experienced complications in only 21% and 30.8% of cases, respectively.[35] The authors concluded that elective surgeries should be performed on smokers only if a 6-week abstinence period has been undertaken.

Finally, many medical providers view the perioperative period as an optimal time to create the necessary momentum for smoking cessation. Several studies report increased rates of long-term smoking cessation in both major and minor ambulatory surgery patients.[36,37] Because smoking is implicated in development of chronic low back pain and worsened disability associated with chronic pain, perioperative care presents an opportunity to optimize patients for long-term success.[38]

Central Nervous System Disease

Before a patient undergoes any interventional procedures involving the central or peripheral nervous system, a basic neurologic examination should be performed. The exam should always begin with a pertinent history, including past symptoms of common neurologic pathologies, such as cerebrovascular accident, peripheral neuropathy, Parkinson's disease, and dementia. This not only informs the proceduralist of baseline neurologic function, but also alerts the provider to the patient's possible increased susceptibility to perioperative neurologic injury. Although some patients may provide specific histories, many will require neurologic examination to detect subtle sensory and motor deficits.

A baseline neurologic examination should be gathered and documented in the patient's medical record before any surgical intervention. The basic tenets of a neurologic exam should be similar for all patients regardless of pathology to maximize consistency. The most commonly tested muscle groups in evaluating important spinal nerve roots include shoulder abductors, elbow flexors, elbow extensors, wrist extensors, finger flexors, hand intrinsics, hip flexors, knee extensors, dorsiflexors, great toe extensors, and plantar flexors. The American Spinal Injury Association publishes a reference manual for myotome assessment (Table 4.5) and sensory nerve assessment.[39] The exam should be focused on neurologic structures based on the principal area of intervention. For example, in a patient undergoing cervical spine intervention, documentation of strength and sensation scores in the upper arms along axillary, radial, median, and ulnar nerve distributions is important for postoperative comparison.

TABLE 4.5. American Spinal Injury Association (ASIA) Myotome Assessment[39,40]

Spinal Nerve	Motor Function
C5	Elbow flexion
C6	Wrist extension
C7	Elbow extension
C8	Finger flexion
T1	Finger abduction
L2	Hip flexion
L3	Knee extension
L4	Ankle dorsiflexion
L5	Hallux extension
S1	Ankle plantar flexion

Neurologic injury is a rare but possible complication of any minimally invasive pain procedure. Examination for common pain procedures should primarily consist of baseline motor and sensory function. The most accepted method for motor strength evaluation is the Medical Research Council Manual Muscle Testing scale.[41] The method involves testing specific muscle groups from both upper and lower extremities and is graded on a 0 to 5 scale (Table 4.6). Sensation should be tested systematically in key dermatomal distributions. Although mechanical nerve injury by direct surgical trauma is possible, peripheral stretch injuries from poor patient positioning are much more common (optimal positioning for common procedures is discussed in the "Patient Positioning" section of this chapter). Regardless of their etiology, elucidation of new injuries is an important aspect of postsurgical management.

Implanted Neuromodulation Devices

Neuromodulation is broadly defined as targeted stimulation of specific areas to alter neural activity. The concept of neuromodulation has been theorized and practiced across several cultures for centuries, but its modern use began in 1967 with the first implantation of a

TABLE 4.6. Medical Research Council Manual Muscle Testing Scale[41]

Grade	Description
0	No muscle activation
1	Trace muscle activation, such as a twitch, without achieving full range of motion
2	Muscle activation with gravity eliminated, achieving full range of motion
3	Muscle activation against gravity, full range of motion
4	Muscle activation against some resistance, full range of motion
5	Muscle activation against examiner's full resistance, full range of motion

neuromodulatory device for intractable pain via dorsal column stimulation.[42] Since then, the field has evolved and grown significantly, with more recent application in medication-resistant pathologies. Like CIEDs, these generators are susceptible to EMI that may alter or damage their function. It is important for the pain proceduralist to have a basic understanding of common indications and anatomical placements of existing devices to avoid both direct and indirect interference.

Stimulation of specific intracranial targets has been FDA approved for refractory Parkinson's disease, essential tremor, dystonia, major depression, and epilepsy. Although the basic principles of electrode and generator implantation are similar to those for spinal cord stimulation, the location of generator placement and lead tunneling differ. Deep brain stimulation (DBS) and vagal nerve stimulation generators are generally placed in the left subclavian subcutaneous tissue. The leads are generally tunneled along the anterior chest wall and extend through the anterolateral neck adjacent to the vagus nerve or further cephalad through the postauricular scalp and into bilateral burr holes. Newer devices providing lower esophageal sphincter stimulation for refractory gastroesophageal reflux have fewer available data but are usually placed subcutaneously in the left upper or lower quadrants of the abdomen and are inserted directly into the lower esophageal sphincter muscle.[43]

DBS or peripheral generators and leads are susceptible to dysfunction and can cause patient harm.[44] Cases of severe central nervous system thermal injury and death secondary to EMI, even in the setting of preoperative generator shutdown, have been reported.[45,46] Avoidance of devastating outcomes with existing stimulators requires preoperative and intraoperative precautions similar to those for CIED management. Device shutdown before start of surgery, consultation of device representatives for programming, use of bipolar instead of monopolar cautery, and grounding pad placement away from existing devices are of high importance. It is also important to note that many devices can become reprogrammed or dysfunctional with external magnet placement and should be interrogated postoperatively to ensure their proper function before discharge.[44,47] Finally, a low threshold for perioperative device consultation and management should be maintained, especially if EMI is anticipated.

Gastrointestinal Disorders

One of the most concerning complications associated with deep sedation is pulmonary aspiration of gastric contents following emesis. This complication is associated with a high level of morbidity and mortality in certain populations. One study analyzing all National Service hospitals over a 1-year period in the United Kingdom reported that > 50% of airway-related deaths in anesthesia were as a result of aspiration.[48] In 2017, the ASA released perioperative practice guidelines with the intention of reducing the risk and severity of complications related to pulmonary aspiration.[49] Fasting parameters for the ingestion of specific materials were established to help minimize gastric volumes (Table 4.7).[49] Of note, these guidelines do not apply to patients with conditions that affect gastric emptying, such as pregnancy, morbid obesity, uncontrolled diabetes, or hiatal hernia, or to emergency surgeries. Pain proceduralists should be well versed in these basic fasting guidelines both to ensure patient safety and to minimize case cancellations or delays.

TABLE 4.7. ASA Recommended Preoperative Fasting Guidelines[49]

Ingested Material	Minimum Fasting Period (hours)
Clear liquids	2
Breast milk	4
Infant formula	6
Nonhuman milk	6
Light meal	6
Fried foods, fatty foods, meat	≥ 8

Hematologic Disease

Thrombocytopenia is defined as a platelet count below 150×10^9 cells/L, with a reported prevalence as high as 10.3% in some studies.[50,51] Although routine laboratory testing is not recommended, patients may present with symptoms of diminished clotting function (e.g., petechial rash, excessive bruising, bleeding from gums, blood in stool or urine) that may warrant further investigation. The risk of bleeding is not linear with platelet count, but the consensus in most clinical practice guidelines for the platelet count cutoff for major non-neuraxial surgeries remains 50×10^9 cells/L.[52,53] Given the noncompressible nature of bleeding events related to paraspinal trauma, however, most experts agree with a higher platelet count threshold prior to neuraxial procedures (e.g., spinal cord stimulator placement, epidural steroid injection). Multiple retrospective studies cite that in the absence of additional bleeding risk factors, neuraxial procedures may be safely performed with platelet counts above 70 to 80×10^9 cells/L.[54–56] In patients with a history of thrombocytopenia, it may be prudent to assess platelet count prior to surgical intervention.

Modern pain interventions largely have low risk of mortality and morbidity related to large-volume blood loss with transfusion requirements. Traumatic manipulation of tissue in the perivertebral space, however, does place patients at risk for catastrophic complications, namely acute epidural hematoma with resultant paralysis. A literature review performed by Domenicucci et al analyzing 959 cases of spinal epidural hematoma published between 1869 and 2012 listed coagulopathy as one of the primary risk factors for this patient population.[57] The authors further specified that 41.7% of coagulopathy was caused by iatrogenic factors like anticoagulant and antiplatelet therapy, while 21.8% was related to non-iatrogenic factors, such as inherited and/or metabolic coagulopathy, suggesting the need for a careful review of bleeding history and anticoagulant medications.

The addition of coagulopathy greatly increases the complexity of perioperative management, which may influence clinical outcomes and complications. Etiologies vary widely, each with differing treatment parameters. Thus, with patients who have known hematologic disease, it may be prudent to consult the patient's hematologist to discuss perioperative optimization prior to the planned intervention. In patients on anticoagulation medications, pain-specific procedural guidelines for medication-specific holding and restarting parameters are available. In guidelines published in 2015 and updated in 2018, the American

TABLE 4.8. American Society of Regional Anesthesia and Pain Medicine Procedural Risk Stratification[58]

High-Risk Procedures	Intermediate-Risk Procedures*	Low-Risk Procedures*
▪ Spinal cord stimulation trial and implant ▪ Dorsal root ganglion stimulation ▪ Intrathecal catheter and pump implant ▪ Vertebral augmentation ▪ Percutaneous decompression laminectomy ▪ Epiduroscopy and epidural decompression	▪ Interlaminar epidural steroid injections (C, T, L, S) ▪ Transforaminal epidural steroid injections (C, T, L, S) ▪ Intradiscal procedures (C, T, L) ▪ Sympathetic blocks ▪ Trigeminal and sphenopalatine ganglia blocks	▪ Peripheral nerve blocks ▪ Peripheral joints and musculoskeletal injections ▪ Trigger point injections (including piriformis) ▪ Sacroiliac joint injections ▪ Thoracic and lumbar facet MBB and RFA ▪ Peripheral nerve stimulation trial and implant† ▪ Pocket revision and IPG/ITP replacement

Abbreviations: C, cervical; T, thoracic; L, lumbar; S, sacral.
* Patients with risk factors for high risk of bleeding (old age, history of bleeding tendency, concurrent use of anticoagulants/antiplatelets, liver cirrhosis, advanced liver disease, and advanced renal disease) undergoing low- or intermediate-risk procedures should be treated as intermediate or high risk, respectively.
† Peripheral neuromodulation is low or intermediate risk, depending on the location of the targeted nerve in relation to critical vessels and invasiveness of the procedure.

Society of Regional Anesthesia and Pain Medicine collaborated with several international societies to establish the gold standard of preprocedural anticoagulation management in pain medicine.[58] The authors acknowledged the wide spectrum of risk in pain procedures, ranging from minimally invasive procedures with high-risk targets (e.g., percutaneous Spinal Cord Stimulation (SCS) lead placement, vertebral augmentation, deep visceral nerve blocks) to low-risk peripheral nerve blocks (Table 4.8). The delineation of low-, moderate-, and high-risk procedures is important in that it allows the pain proceduralist to identify scenarios in which the patient risk outweighs benefit.

Special Considerations

The BRIDGES study was a double-blind multicenter randomized controlled trial evaluating the rate of perioperative thromboembolic events in patients on chronic anticoagulant (warfarin) for atrial fibrillation who were bridged with low-molecular-weight heparin (LMWH) or placebo. The placebo group was found to be noninferior to the bridged group for rates of arterial thromboembolism. Further, there was no statistically significant difference among rates of all-cause mortality, myocardial infarct, deep vein thrombosis, or pulmonary embolism. However, patients who were on LMWH had a statistically significant increase in risk of major bleeding (1.3% versus 3.2% with Number Needed to Harm (NNH) = 50) and minor bleeding (12.0% versus 20.9%).[59] The applicability of the results of this study has been criticized because only 3% of patients in the study had a CHADS2 score of 5 or 6. Thus, certain patient populations have unique thromboembolic risk that requires special consideration that falls outside the spectrum of routine care.

For patients with high thromboembolic risk, the time during which anticoagulation is held should be minimized. The patient's anticoagulation prescribing physician should consulted to discuss the need for bridging with heparin or LMWH during the washout period of the oral anticoagulant. The high-risk patient population also includes those who have recently undergone cardiac catheterization with coronary stent placement. The ACC and AHA assert that elective procedures requiring disruption of dual antiplatelet therapy (DAPT) should be delayed for a minimum of 30 days for coronary bare metal stent placement and 6 months for coronary drug-eluting stent placement.[60]

Pancytopenia

Pancytopenia is a relatively common triad of findings characterized by a decrease in hemoglobin, platelet count, and leukocytes. Pancytopenia has a bimodal presentation, commonly presenting in childhood or in adults in their third and fourth decades, with a female predominance.[61] It is important to view the condition not as a disease entity, but as a manifestation of an underlying condition. The differential diagnosis can be broad and extensive, making evaluation of the condition challenging. This section provides a wide overview of common causes of acquired, adult-onset pancytopenia and aims to inform the pain interventionist when emergency hematologic consultation is needed before an elective procedure.

The etiology of pancytopenia in adults falls roughly into two categories: impaired production or increased destruction of blood cells. Common conditions leading to impaired blood cell production broadly include aplastic anemia, viral infection (e.g., cytomegalovirus, Epstein-Barr virus, parvovirus, human immunodeficiency virus [HIV]), malignancy (e.g., leukemia, lymphoma, multiple myeloma), myelofibrosis, myelodysplastic syndrome, granulomatous disorders, and nutritional deficiencies (e.g., vitamin B_{12}, folic acid, copper). Common causes of increased cell destruction include splenomegaly, paroxysmal nocturnal hemoglobinuria, complement-mediated blood cell destruction, sepsis, drugs (e.g., methotrexate, anticonvulsants, chemotherapeutics), and autoimmune disease, such as systemic lupus erythematosus (SLE).[62]

Prompt hematology and oncology consultation with cancellation of elective procedures are warranted in any patient with incidentally discovered pancytopenia. If laboratory studies do not elucidate etiology, bone marrow biopsy may be necessary. Medical emergencies that require immediate treatment include fever in the neutropenic patient, life-threatening anemia, and thrombocytopenia with signs or symptoms of bleeding present.[63]

Thromboelastography

The thromboelastogram (TEG) provides qualitative information about platelet function, the coagulation cascade, clot strength, and fibrinolysis in whole blood. Thromboelastography can be a powerful tool in assessing the etiology of coagulopathy as well as in guiding corrective resuscitative efforts before and after invasive procedures. Huang et al tested this hypothesis and found no neurologic complications in 24 parturients undergoing neuraxial anesthesia with platelet counts greater than 56×10^9 cells/L and a normal TEG.[64] Based on the 2015 anticoagulation guideline for interventional spine procedures, the American Society of Regional Anesthesia and Pain Medicine agrees that TEG with the addition of Adenosine Diphosphate (ADP) or arachidonic acid mapping assays should be considered when possible, specifically in cases of an inadequate washout period for P2Y12 antagonists like clopidogrel.[58] A few small studies have also shown a significant correlation between dabigatran plasma concentration and TEG *R*-values.[65,66] TEG may show promise in specific clinical scenarios, but further appropriately powered studies are necessary.

Although TEG can be an important objective tool in reducing unnecessary transfusion, it is important to note that most of its evidence is for the cardiac, liver, or trauma surgery patient population. Multiple studies analyzing its use in patients taking warfarin have found a lack of correlation between INR and TEG, indicating unreliability and insensitivity in detecting bleeding risk in patients receiving external anticoagulation.[67–69] Furthermore, aspirin and clopidogrel have been reported to have little effect on TEG values.[70] Ultimately, TEG should not replace clinical judgment or recommendations from current intervention-specific evidence-based guidelines, but it may be a supplemental tool in clinically complex circumstances that fall outside the parameters set by these guidelines.

Endocrine Disease: Diabetes

Diabetes is one of the most common metabolic disorders in the general population and has significant effects on all organ systems. Preoperative tests like the hemoglobin A_{1c} (HbA_{1c}) and fasting blood glucose can detect insulin resistance and alter management choices in patients with diabetes. NICE recommends that any patient with a history of diabetes should at least have a documented HbA_{1c} test result within 3 months of surgery to best represent recent glycemic control.[71] Furthermore, optimal glycemic control may also have anti-inflammatory benefit that can positively impact perioperative management of pain.

In the surgical patient, poor glycemic control has significant implications for morbidity, such as impaired wound healing and incidence of infection secondary to depressed immune function, collagen production, and tissue circulation. Studies across multiple surgical subspecialties have shown this relationship, suggesting the benefit of tighter control (FBG < 200 mg/dL and HbA_{1c} < 7%).[72] A 2017 meta-analysis included 6 retrospective studies analyzing patients with and without perioperative prosthetic joint infection and found an odds ratio of 3.27 ($P = .000$) and 2.37 ($P = .000$) when comparing increased HbA_{1c} and fasting blood glucose, respectively.[73] Zerr et al demonstrated a reduced rate of sternal SSI in euglycemic postoperative cardiac surgery patients (1.5%) compared to a hyperglycemic control group (2.4%).[74] McConnell et al demonstrated a significant decrease in the rates of SSI 48 hours postoperatively in colorectal surgical patients with a mean capillary glucose concentration of ≤ 200 mg/dL compared to those with concentrations > 200 mg/dL (14.3% versus 29.7%).[75] Perioperative glycemic control is likely an important modifiable factor in preventing wound complications after interventional surgery. Interestingly, a 2017 multicenter retrospective review of spinal cord stimulator implants by Hoelzer et al did not find patients with chronic tobacco use, diabetes, or obesity to have an increased overall infection rate compared to control patients without these comorbidities.[76] Taking these studies into account, glycemic control should be discussed with patients to help minimize periprocedural complications.

Infectious Disease

In 1982, the CDC modified the original 1964 National Academy of Sciences and National Research Council Cooperative Research study's surgical wound classification system, which is widely used today.[77] Many pain procedures fall into the category of a "clean" operative wound in which the incision is closed by primary closure and neither the respiratory tract, alimentary tract, genitourinary tract, nor oropharyngeal cavity is entered. However, certain patient populations have increased susceptibility to pathogenic bacteria, leading to increased risk of SSI and may require different antibiotic treatment strategies.

Chronic Antibiotic Use and Multidrug-Resistant Organisms

While antibiotics have significantly improved morbidity and mortality in modern healthcare, antibiotic stewardship has become an urgent worldwide public health concern. Despite this concern, certain patient populations, such as patients with cystic fibrosis or those on immunosuppressive therapy, may require chronic antibiotic therapy. If the patient is on chronic scheduled cefazolin, clindamycin, or vancomycin therapy (three of the most commonly used perioperative antibiotics for skin flora), it is imperative to use an agent from a different class, rather than to increase the dosage of the current antibiotic, for surgical prophylaxis. Moreover, patients in these populations may develop multidrug-resistant organism (MDRO) infections more often than the general population, given their chronic antibiotic exposure. MDRO-associated infections have increased mortality and hospital readmission rates compared to infections caused by other organisms.[78] MDRO infections are often difficult to treat and contribute significantly to perioperative morbidity and mortality. The most common MDROs include methicillin-resistant *Staphylococcus aureus* (MRSA), vancomycin-resistant enterococci (VRE), and extended-spectrum beta-lactamase gram-negative bacilli, such as *Klebsiella*, *Escherichia coli*, and *Pseudomonas*. According to the guidelines for perioperative antibiotic selection and administration from the Surgical Care Improvement Project (SCIP), in the case of beta-lactam allergy or MRSA history, clindamycin is considered a first-line prophylactic agent and vancomycin is the second-line agent, due to risk of "prolonged infusion times, potential bacterial resistance, and red man syndrome."[79] Although rough guidelines exist, infectious disease specialist consultation may be appropriate in the setting of significant MDRO history, patients on chronic antibiotics, or patients on prolonged antibiotics. The local hospital antibiogram should also be referenced when targeting susceptibility patterns to optimize coverage and to practice antibiotic stewardship.

Special Consideration

In 2007, the AHA published a set of perioperative guidelines for the prevention of infective endocarditis (IE) in specific high-risk individuals (e.g., patients with a history of prosthetic cardiac valve, unrepaired congenital heart disease, or the like).[80] Although a concerning history may warrant broader prophylaxis in certain high-risk procedures, general pain procedures are considered low risk. The guidelines state that the cost and risk of adverse reactions exceed the benefit of additional antibiotic coverage above the standard prophylactic regimen.

Intraoperative Considerations

Procedural Concerns

Bone Density

Osteopenia and osteoporosis are defined as reductions in bone mass due to the inability to form bone at the rate of bone resorption. The two conditions are quantitatively differentiated through bone densitometry testing or DEXA scan at the spine, hip, or forearm in which T-scores are assigned, with normal scores ranging from -1 to +4, osteopenia from -1 to -2.5, and osteoporosis ascribed values -2.5 and below.[81] In 2010, the United States Census reported a 43.9% prevalence for low bone mass and 10.3% prevalence for osteoporosis in the general population age 50 years and older.[82] In the orthopedic surgical literature, poor preoperative bone health is generally linked to poor functional recovery, higher fracture risk, and an increased need for secondary revision surgery.

Fortunately, there are options to help optimize bone health prior to spine-based procedures. In 2019, the International Society for Clinical Densitometry (ISCD) released a review of pertinent literature and guidelines for appropriate DEXA scanning indications.[83] The indications include all women age 65 and over and all men age 70 and over. Younger individuals should also undergo testing if one of the following is present: low body weight, prior fracture, high-risk medication use (e.g., glucocorticoids), disease associated with bone loss (e.g., vitamin D deficiency, rheumatoid arthritis, excessive alcohol consumption, chronic renal disease, hyperparathyroidism), and history of fragility fracture.

Interventions to improve bone health and density should be initiated as early as possible in the preoperative period, along with consultation with both rheumatology and endocrinology. The first step in treatment is optimizing nonpharmacologic measures, such as ensuring proper exercise and nutrition with adequate levels of calcium and vitamin D. Pharmacologic treatment, including antiresorptive drugs like bisphosphonates, estrogens, and calcitonin, can also be included for additional benefit, but they are only effective if the patient is vitamin D- and calcium-sufficient.[84] Of note, although it has found to have detrimental effects in animal studies, bisphosphonate therapy does not appear to delay human bone healing after acute fracture and can be safely administered in the postoperative period.[85,86]

Although improving bone health before pinning or fusion surgeries may be beneficial, recent studies suggest that bone mineral density may have no significant effect on the analgesic efficacy of vertebral bone augmentation.[87] Furthermore, based on a 2017 meta-analysis performed by Zhang et al., there was no increase in incidence of secondary vertebral compression fractures in patients undergoing vertebral augmentation versus conservative management.[88] However, these studies demonstrated that there is no benefit in delaying vertebral augmentation interventions in appropriate candidates with the intention of optimizing bone density.

Anatomical Variations

Prior Spine Surgery

Failed back syndrome (FBS) refers to a subset of patients who have new or persistent pain after undergoing at least one spinal surgery aiming to relieve back or leg pain. As spinal surgery increases in prevalence, pain specialists are more likely to encounter patients with histories of orthopedic surgical interventions. Recent studies estimate the prevalence of FBS from 10% to as high as 40%.[89,90] The causes of persistent or new pain can include infection, stenosis, fracture, instability, painful instrumentation, pseudarthrosis (the failure of bone formation due to improper healing), or adjacent segment pathology.[91] In patients with prior instrumentation, plain radiographs in dynamic views, including flexion, extension, and lateral flexion, should be attained to assess for spinal instability. CT without contrast should also be obtained to evaluate existing instrumentation and evidence of pseudarthrosis or fractures. MRI with gadolinium enhancement can also be used to identify neural compression or ongoing infection. Combinations of advanced imaging may be needed to help plan for the procedural approach.

Scoliosis

Adult scoliosis is defined as a 3-dimentional deformity of the spine with coronal deviation of > 10 degrees. Scoliosis in general has an estimated prevalence of up to 29% of the population, and the pathogenesis can be quite variable.[92] Some cases arise from hereditary causes and are categorized into congenital, neuromuscular, and adolescent idiopathic scoliosis, while others develop later in life as a result of degeneration and deformities elsewhere. Asymmetry at any spinal stabilization point (caused by, for example, degenerative disks or facet joints) may predispose an individual to development the condition. Patients with scoliosis are managed conservatively with physical therapy and epidural steroid injections; surgical interventions are reserved for rare severe cases. Patients with a history of early-onset scoliosis, however, may have undergone spinal fusion and instrumentation, which is generally reserved for the adolescent population and is seldom removed later in life.[93] As already mentioned, any history of instrumentation to the spine warrants preoperative imaging before spinal intervention.

Bertolotti's Syndrome

Bertolotti's syndrome, also known as lumbosacral transitional vertebrae, is a congenital spinal anomaly in which the transverse process of the last lumbar vertebra is enlarged and fuses with the cranial aspect of the first sacral vertebra, creating varying degrees of L5 "sacralization." The S1 segment can similarly exhibit "lumbarization," in which the first sacral vertebra is incompletely fused with the sacrum and appears as a sixth lumbar vertebra. Its prevalence is estimated to be from 4% to 30% in the general population, but it is largely underdiagnosed.[94] Diagnosis is typically achieved using standard AP radiographs, which demonstrate 76% to 84% sensitivity.

Nerve root identification and exiting trajectory are altered in Bertolotti's syndrome, which has significant implications in correlating functional symptoms with radiographic anatomy. The functional L5 nerve root always originates from the lowest mobile spinal level with a disk space. Therefore, in the case of S1 lumbarization, the functional L5 nerve root is located at the last mobile vertebral level at L6–S2. Conversely, in the sacralized L5 vertebrae, the functional L5 root corresponds to the anatomical L4 root.[95] When considering fluoroscopically guided specific nerve root interventions in this population, clinical correlation is imperative.

Lumbosacral transitional vertebrae can have varying degrees of severity, ranging from pseudo-articulation to complete fusion, and can be present unilaterally or bilaterally. The anatomical variations have important implications for any surgical procedures involving the lumbosacral region of the spine. For example, when considering pedicle access in the sacralized L5 vertebrae, proceduralists must note specific structural and dimensional differences, because the pedicle in the sacralized L5 vertebrae has been shown to have a significantly reduced transverse diameter, a shorter anterior diameter, and reduced pedicle height, but increased dorsal alar dimensions.[96] The angulation is also altered, in that the sacral ala show a steeper AP pedicle inclination at 45 degrees, compared to the 30-degree angulation seen in normal anatomy. Conversely, lumbarization of S1 creates more obtuse pedicles in the sagittal plane, with decreased AP inclination. Therefore, careful radiographic review of anatomical variation before any intervention accessing the sacral space is important.

These anatomical differences often lead to functional deficits and enhanced degeneration. According to cadaver studies, L5 fused sacra have significantly smaller height than normal sacra (if the fused L5 segment is excluded from measurement), a condition that reduces the load-bearing capacity by reducing SI joint surface area.[97] L5–S1 facets are altered; in the lumbosacral transitional vertebrae, the facets are smaller and more coronally oriented, predisposing the joint to quicker degeneration.[95] Degree and severity of spondylolysis in the setting of either type of transitional lumbar vertebrae is also increased.[98] S1 lumbarization has been implicated in S1 nerve root compression due to the increased mobility and ligamentous instability. The addition of a sixth mobile vertebra in the lumbosacral region predisposes patients to injury at adjacent levels. It is therefore highly likely to encounter a patient with Bertolotti's syndrome along the extended timeline of disease progression.

Baastrup's Disease

Baastrup's disease, also known as kissing spine disease or lumbar interspinous bursitis, is defined by contact between posterior spinous processes in the lumbar spine, a finding most readily revealed on dynamic flexion/extension lumbar plain films. A high prevalence—81.3%—has been reported in the geriatric population age 80 years or older, and the disease most commonly affects the L4–L5 level.[99] The pathology is theorized to arise from repetitive flexion and extension of the spine, resulting in eburnation and degeneration in the spinous processes. Ultimately, intraspinal cysts or adventitious interspinous bursa may form, leading to difficult spinal access at affected levels. High suspicion should be maintained in the lordotic and elderly patient with localized lumbar pain that is relieved with spine extension. When lumbar intervention like epidural steroid injection or stimulator lead placement is considered, the midline interspinous approach may be difficult and should be avoided, if possible, at affected levels.

Ligamentous Disease

Conditions that may affect the accessibility of the spinal anatomy include diseases of the spinal ligaments, such as diffuse idiopathic skeletal hyperostosis (DISH) and ossification of the posterior longitudinal ligament (OPLL). DISH is a form of spinal ankylosis resulting from multifactorial processes without a clearly identified etiology.[100] Diagnostic criteria for DISH described by Resnick and Niwayama include ossification of the anterior longitudinal ligament (ALL) over four adjoining vertebrae with sparing of the intervertebral disk spaces and non-involvement of the apophyseal and sacroiliac joints.[101] DISH most commonly affects the ALL of the thoracic spine but can be seen at other spinal levels. While calcification of the anterior ligament does not directly impede access to spinal structures via the posterior approach, the lack of articular range of motion may restrict optimal positioning for certain interventions.

OPLL is a multifactorial disease of ectopic bone formation caused by various environmental and genetic factors that results in degenerative changes leading to myelopathy or radiculopathy.[102] OPLL commonly affects the posterior longitudinal ligament of the cervical spine, as the name suggests. Calcification of the ligaments can readily be seen on lateral plain films, and many cases of OPLL are found and diagnosed incidentally. OPLL has a wide range of potential vertebral involvement, including continuous ligament involvement along several vertebrae, segmental interruption, or mixed.

Posterior needle access can be challenging in OPLL-affected areas when relying on tactile discrimination between tissue layers. DISH, however, presents different considerations. Therefore, reliance on intraoperative imaging is important for these patients in order to avoid complications and to maximize success, because access at the desired level may be difficult and the procedural approach may need to be altered to accommodate abnormal anatomy.

Positioning

Special attention should be given to patient positioning because variations can facilitate access to certain anatomical locations and improve procedural outcomes. The different patient positions also have unique physiologic advantages and disadvantages that should be manipulated to minimize adverse outcomes. Under general or sedation anesthesia, protective reflexes are often lost, and neurologic stretch injury can occur peripherally or centrally if continuous excessive tension is applied in high-risk areas. All OR staff should review proper and improper patient positioning methods to maximize safety and optimize surgical conditions. This section reviews the normal neutral anatomy in the most common surgical positions.

Supine Position

The supine position is the most common position for general surgery involving the abdomen or procedures requiring access to the anterior cervical spine. The patient is placed on their back with arms alongside their body or abducted to < 90 degrees on arm boards, with special care taken to maintain neutral positioning of the head, neck, and spine. Arm hyperabduction is avoided to minimize brachial plexus injury from humeral pressure in the axilla. Supination of the hands also provides protection against ulnar nerve injury by reducing external pressure across the medial elbow. Some variations of the supine position include the lawn chair position and frog-leg position. In lawn chair position, the hips and knees are flexed, which relieves pressure on the back and improves venous drainage from the legs to the heart. The frog-leg position entails flexion of the hips and knees, with the hips rotated externally and with lateral support of the knees to prevent excessive rotation and subsequent dislocation of the hips.

Lithotomy Position

The lithotomy position is a variation of the supine position in which the legs are abducted approximately 45 degrees from midline and are placed in support stirrups with the knees flexed. Peroneal nerve injury is the most common stretch/compression injury in this position and can be minimized by occasionally changing the position of the patient's legs and limiting the overall time spent in this position. The femoral nerve and lateral femoral cutaneous nerve can also be injured with excessive thigh abduction and external hip rotation. Both legs should be maneuvered in concert to prevent complications like muscular injury and spinal torsion. This position is commonly used in gynecologic, urologic, and rectal surgeries, but it is rarely utilized in interventional pain procedures.

Lateral Decubitus Position

The lateral decubitus position is most commonly required in kidney, hip, and various thoracic procedures. In this position, the patient lies on their side with the nonoperative side in the dependent/decubitus position. Once the patient is in the position, devices that support patient stability, such as an inflatable beanbag or hip bolster, may be used. A pillow can be placed between the bony prominences of the knees to reduce direct compression injury, and the legs are slightly flexed to avoid stretch of the lower extremity nerves. Arms should be positioned in front of the patient at less than 90-degree abduction, to avoid brachial plexus stretch injury, and an axillary roll can be placed inferior to the dependent axilla along the chest wall to prevent brachial plexus compression injury. The bony prominences of the upper extremities should be padded as well. The lateral decubitus position can be used for spinal cord stimulator implants if the generator is implanted into an abdominal site.

Prone Position

The prone position describes the patient lying in a face-down position, with the arms either tucked to their side or extended forward. This position is most commonly utilized in surgeries requiring access to the posterior fossa of the skull, posterior spine, buttocks, or perirectal area. This position is frequently used in the interventional spine practice, with either general anesthesia or MAC. An international panel of SCS implantation experts recommended that the prone position be utilized for most patients for patient comfort and ease of fluoroscopy, with the additional recommendation that an abdominal pillow be used to reduce natural lumbar lordosis and to spread spinous processes apart.[103] Specialized prone pillows help maintain neutrality of the head, neck, and spine without compressing vital structures of the face, including the eyes, nose, and chin. Direct compression of the eyes may result in postoperative vision loss (POVL) from occlusion of the central retinal artery. Although rare, ischemic optic neuropathy can also lead to POVL without any direct external pressure; the risk increases as the duration of surgery increases. Again, peripheral nerves at risk of stretch and compression injury include the ulnar nerve at the elbow or common peroneal nerve at or below the knees. In cases of arm abduction, the elbows and shoulders should have no greater than 90 degrees of angulation to prevent stretching of the nerves. A chest roll can be utilized to offload compression in the axilla and abdomen.

Operating Tables and the Prone Position

The general surgical table is the most common surgical table for most surgical subspecialties. This standard table comes with several adjustable features, including vertical height, craniocaudal sliding, right and left rotation or "airplaning," and flexion/retroflexion, as well as strategically located breaks in the bed allowing for adjustment of the head and legs. When combined with the proper adjuvant positioning equipment like the prone pillow, padding foam, and arm boards, this model allows for adequate surgical exposure and patient comfort for most interventional spine procedures. The general surgical table is also compatible with C-arm fluoroscopy, which further incentivizes its use.

However, four unique specialized OR tables specifically designed for surgical procedures in the prone position exist and have their advantages. Although these beds are seldom used for relatively short interventional spine procedures, their advantages and disadvantages are briefly described here. The models include the Allen/Jackson table, the Wilson frame, the Cambridge/Relton-Hall frame, and the Andrews frame. The Allen/Jackson table has two transverse support structures at the chest and hips that allow for the abdomen to remain pressure-free, which improves respiratory mechanics. This table also has built-in arm support and a facial support pillow, which obviates the need for additional accessories. The Wilson frame consists of two longitudinally convex support structures that distribute pressure across the patient's sides while the abdomen remains free of pressure. The convexity of the frame is designed to counteract natural lumbar lordosis, optimizing exposure of the lumbar spine. The Cambridge/Relton-Hall frame is a four-point supporting structure that can be either laid on top of a standard table or used as a free-standing device. The points of stabilization are located on either side of the chest wall and hips and are angled medially to prevent movement. The abdomen and anterior chest hang free and are free of pressure. Of note, all the specialized prone tables readily support use of C-arm fluoroscopy.

Perioperative Antibiotics

SSI is considered a preventable postoperative complication that can be reduced when proper intraoperative steps are taken. For example, the utilization of appropriate OR laminar airflow ventilation systems, discontinuation of immunosuppressive agents, and maintenance of body temperature and adequate circulation are additive in their risk-reduction effects.

However, the responsibility for ensuring proper administration and choice of antibiotics ultimately lies with the surgical team. In the landmark paper "Prophylactic Antibiotics in Surgery" published in 1993 by Ludwig et al, the core principles of antibiotic choice, indication, timing, dosing, and duration were outlined.[104] More recently, several surgical organizations collaborated in 2002 to create the SCIP and established an evidence-based set of guidelines and quality improvement measures to standardize perioperative antibiotic use.[105] The protocol called for seven main perioperative initiatives: (1) prophylactic antibiotics should be administered within 1 hour before surgical incision, (2) agents should be selected for activity against the most probable contaminants, (3) antibiotics should be discontinued within 24 hours after the surgery end-time, (4) euglycemia should be maintained, (5) hair at the surgical site should be removed with clippers, (6) urinary catheters should be removed within the first 2 postoperative days, and (7) normothermia should be maintained perioperatively. Using just the first three initiatives alone, Nguyen et al were able to demonstrate significant SSI incidence reduction in elective colorectal surgeries—from 21.7% in the control group to 3.4% in the implementation group.[106] Benefit of normothermic maintenance was also validated in a randomized controlled trial by Kurz et al, who demonstrated fewer SSIs in the group receiving active warming techniques than in the group receiving routine care (6% and 19%, respectively; $P = .009$).[107]

In 2013, the American Society of Health-system Pharmacists (ASHP) released the official Surgical Infection Society guidelines for surgical antibiotic prophylaxis and emphasized several additional key points. First, the guidelines define properties of the ideal antimicrobial agent: the antibiotic should prevent SSI and its morbidity/mortality, reduce the duration and cost of healthcare, produce no adverse effects, and have no adverse consequences for the microbial flora of the hospital. Cefazolin is the drug of choice for most surgical procedures because of its desirable duration of action, spectrum of activity against common skin flora (*S. aureus* and coagulase-negative staphylococci like *S. epidermidis*), reasonable safety profile, and low cost. If the patient has a beta-lactam allergy or history of MRSA infection, clindamycin (900 mg IV for adults, 10 mg/kg for pediatric patients) and vancomycin (15 mg/kg IV for both adults and pediatric patients) can be considered as the second- and third-line prophylaxis, respectively. The use of broad-spectrum antimicrobials for routine prophylaxis is discouraged due to their contribution to antibiotic resistance and increased side effects, with little evidence of additional benefit. The authors also acknowledge obesity as a risk factor for SSI and suggest weight-based dosing strategies. For example, 30 mg/kg IV cefazolin can be used in pediatric patients who weigh < 80 kg, 2 g IV for patients weighing more than 80 kg, and 3 g IV for patients weighing more than 120 kg. Specific dosing guidelines, duration of action, and redosing intervals of other perioperative antimicrobials are outside the scope of this text, but an exhaustive list may be referenced in the update to the previously published ASHP *Clinical Practice Guidelines for Antimicrobial Prophylaxis in Surgery*.[108]

Intraoperative Neuromonitoring

Induction of general anesthesia for minimally invasive pain interventions may be desirable in certain situations, as described in the section of this chapter called "Anesthetic Techniques."

However, when patient participation and awareness are impaired, quick neurophysiologic feedback is lost. In surgeries involving implantation of devices near high-risk structures, iatrogenic nerve injury or procedure failure secondary to direct surgical trauma and improper device placement may be increased. Intraoperative neuromonitoring methods, such as electromyography (EMG), somatosensory evoked potentials (SSEPs), and motor evoked potentials (MEPs), are well accepted and validated intraoperative techniques typically used to identify potential nerve injuries in the deeply anesthetized patient undergoing high-risk surgeries (e.g., craniotomy, laminectomy/fusion). The utility of neuromonitoring in common pain interventions is explored in this section.

Sacroiliac (SI) joint fusion has been performed via the traditional open approach for decades. With recent technical advancements, however, SI fusion can be performed with a minimally invasive approach under fluoroscopy. The recovery period is generally much shorter and is associated with a low risk of complications. However, pedicle screw placement under indirect visualization can be difficult, because the sacrum is much more anatomically complex than the lumbar vertebrae. In a retrospective analysis performed in 2014, Woods et al demonstrated the utility of neuromonitoring in minimally invasive SI (MIS) joint fusion surgery.[109] A total of 111 implants were successfully placed in 37 patients under general anesthesia with intraoperative EMG monitoring. The authors reported EMG had 80% sensitivity and 97% specificity in detecting neural injury surrounding the SI joint and asserted that EMG-guided placement of screws potentially avoided adverse neurologic sequelae in 7% of implants. Although further studies are needed to validate these findings, intraoperative EMG seems to show a promising safety profile in MIS under general anesthesia.

A commonly utilized protocol for neural surveillance during SCS lead placement is light sedation and real-time patient feedback. In some patients, this can be challenging due to agitation, disorientation, hearing deficits, or language barriers, and a general anesthetic technique is preferred. Because accurate placement of electrodes is critical for device efficacy, and although electrodes are largely anatomically placed, any patient feedback provides an extra level of insurance for proper posterior dorsal column lead placements. Furthermore, if tonic mapping is utilized, patient feedback is necessary for correct anatomical and physiologic dermatomal mapping. Several recent studies have shown that when neuromonitoring is adjunctively used with asleep placement, the technique has noninferiority to light sedation for SCS trial success. In a retrospective case series including 103 patients undergoing SCS lead placement under general anesthesia with EMG and SSEP monitoring, Schoen et al demonstrated an improved failure rate of 13.6% (14/103), as compared to an awake failure rate of ~20%.[110] Multiple other recent prospective and retrospective studies of intraoperative neuromonitoring found equivocal safety levels and failure rates requiring revision or removal when compared to the current rates reported in the literature.[111–113]

Postprocedural Concerns

Postoperative Antibiotics and SSI

SSI is defined as an infection occurring within 30 days after an operation if the infection involves skin and subcutaneous tissue, and within 1 year if a deep soft-tissue implant infection develops.[114] Many international professional societies have studied the use of routine postoperative antibiotics and have found no benefit in extending antimicrobial therapy beyond 24 hours postoperatively. In fact, Nguyen et al not only found lack of benefit to a lengthened course of prophylactic antibiotics beyond 24 hours, but also suggested harm from the increased risk of drug resistance and secondary infections, such as *Clostridium difficile*.[106] A 2018 overview of Cochrane Reviews, in which 7 trials and 1,484 patients undergoing colorectal surgery were examined, found no clear benefit to long-term antibiotic use (defined as at least a second intraoperative dose or a postoperative dose of antibiotic) compared with short-term use (defined as only a single preoperative antibiotic dose).[115] However, the reviews did not examine patients undergoing prosthetic device implant, which may serve as a potential nidus for infection.

Basavaraj et al examined 292 adult and pediatric patients undergoing cochlear implantation during a 15-year period and found an SSI rate of 4.1% (12/292), with 8 patients experiencing minor infection (e.g., hematoma, seroma, superficial cellulitis) and 4 patients experiencing major infection requiring admission for intravenous antibiotics, wound debridement, or ultimate explantation. Although the study had low power, no difference in infection rate was detected in patients who had long-term antibiotics (defined as a 5-day or 7-day course) verses short-term antibiotics (defined as a single preoperative dose). Another study aimed to investigate the efficacy of postoperative antibiotic use in 367 patients undergoing permanent pacemaker implantation or generator replacement found that 1/110 (0.9%) in the single preoperative antibiotic group and 4/257 (1.5%) in the pre- and postoperative antibiotic group developed device infection.[116] As mentioned above, a 2017 multicenter retrospective study by Hoelzer et al evaluating the infection rates and risk factors associated with spinal cord stimulator implants found that postoperative antibiotics did decrease the rate of infection,[76] although further studies are needed to fully explore the results from this study.

Interventional pain-specific data regarding device infection have recently been published. A retrospective study reviewing intrathecal drug delivery (IDD) device and SCS implants in a total of 142 cancer patients at MD Anderson Cancer Center found a 2.4% infection rate for IDD and a 3.4% infection rate for SCS.[117] The only significant risk factor in this population was mean surgical time, with the infection group averaging 215 minutes ± 93 minutes and the no infection group averaging 132 ± 52 minutes ($P = .02$). In a large multicenter retrospective analysis of 2,737 SCS implants, Bendel et al found an overall infection rate of 2.45%, with ultimate explantation in 77.6% of infections.[118] Median time to infection onset was 27 days, with the most common presenting symptom being localized incisional pain and the most common presenting sign being wound erythema and drainage. The vast majority of infected implant cases underwent laboratory testing, including a complete blood count, erythrocyte sedimentation rate, C-reactive peptide, and wound cultures. Of note, less than half (45.6%) of the diagnosed infections had a documented abnormal white blood cell count of $> 11.0 \times 10^9$/L. Another large retrospective study by Falowski et al analyzed 6,615 SCS implants in a United States payer database and found a 12-month device-related infection rate of 3.11%, with significant risk factors including peripheral vascular disease (OR, 1.784; $P = .0457$) and infection in the 12 months before implant (OR, 1.518; $P = .0386$).[119]

Delays in diagnosis and treatment may lead to serious complications, such as meningitis, epidural abscess, and osteomyelitis. The patient should be educated on signs and symptoms of infection and the surgical site should be examined regularly. If concerning signs/symptoms (e.g., surgical site pain or tenderness, erythema, heat, localized swelling, purulent drainage, incisional dehiscence) are reported, further investigation with diagnostic laboratory and imaging studies should be performed immediately. Ultrasonography can be utilized to identify fluid pockets or abscesses around the generator site, while CT is recommended for deeper infections. MRI may be useful when there is a higher degree of clinical suspicion for osteomyelitis or epidural abscess. If the patient exhibits signs of sepsis or hemodynamic compromise, initiation of empiric antibiotics with gram positive and negative coverage would be reasonable. While superficial infections may be treated with 7 to 10 days of first-generation cephalosporin therapy alone, deep implant infections require definitive treatment via irrigation, debridement, and device explantation.[120] Once source control is achieved and cultures are obtained, antibiotics tailored to causative organisms can be initiated for a course of 7 to 10 days.

Vertebral Augmentation Complications

Techniques for vertebral augmentation (VA) include vertebroplasty and kyphoplasty. Both procedures involve the injection of bone cement (polymethylmethacrylate [PMMA]) into the vertebral body, but kyphoplasty additionally aims to restore vertebral height with the use of an inflatable balloon catheter. Complications of the VA treatment of vertebral compression fracture are rare but can be devastating. Possible complications include hematoma formation, pedicle fracture, infection, and spinal cord injury, with the most common complication being bone cement leakage and migration.[121] Studies have shown an increased incidence of cement leakage in vertebroplasty versus kyphoplasty that is likely attributed to the lower viscosity of the bone cement used, the lack of cavity creation, and the higher-pressure environment required for augmentation.[122] Leakage is most often found to be asymptomatic but can rarely result in major events like pulmonary embolism or central cord compression. In efforts to minimize volume of injectate and thereby complications of its leakage, procedural limitations have been suggested, including treatment of 3 levels or less per session and longitudinal treatment for complex fractures over multiple sessions.

Patient factors may also be used to identify populations at risk for VA-related complications and can aid in proper patient selection. The 5-item Modified Frailty Index score (5i-mFI) is a comorbidity-based risk stratification tool that accounts for history of COPD, hypertension requiring medication, congestive heart failure, diabetes, and functional status.[123] This indexing system has been validated for adverse-event rate prediction in various surgeries, including spinal deformity correction, spinal fusion, and upper gastrointestinal tract surgery. A recent retrospective study by Segal et al has also shown that the 5i-mFI has promise for predicting 30-day postoperative complications after VA with the use of the that may aid in patient selection.[123] Although complications to VA are rare, significant morbidity and mortality may ensue and should be deliberately considered when offering this therapy.

Complications Associated with SI Joint Fusion

Specific complications associated with SI joint fusion include local injury to the pelvis, increased pain surrounding the SI joint, implant allergy or rejection, implant migration or failure, nerve impingement, and stress on surrounding bony structures. In a 2019 systematic review, 720 patients who underwent MIS joint fusion were examined; a total procedural complication rate of 11.11% and a device-related complication rate of 3.05% were found.[124] The most common reported procedural complications were wound infection, trochanteric bursitis, and hematoma formation, while the most common device-related complication was nerve impingement. A retrospective study performed by Schoell et al, however, found a higher overall complication rate of 16.4% at 6 months postop.[125] This study also reported that a significant 6.2% rate of novel lumbar pathology, such as disk displacement and stenosis, was found in the 6 months after SI fusion. In contrast, in the literature on lumbar interbody fusion surgery, studies cited up to 75% incidence of SI joint dysfunction within 5 years of lumbar surgeries.[126] The authors also noted a considerably higher postoperative infection rate of 4.1% relative to the approximate 1% infection rate cited by multiple systematic reviews on similar minimally invasive spinal procedures like discectomy, fusion, and foraminotomy. While MIS joint fusion has been proven to be superior to the open approach, the procedure is not without its own specific complications that must be weighed in the risk–benefit analysis. It should be noted that the percutaneous posterior SI joint fusion devices that have been recently popularized were not included in these studies. Further research is needed to compare their complication rates to those of traditional open and MIS joint fusion.

Mobilization and Activity Restrictions

In comparison to open techniques, minimally invasive procedures have the benefits of less blood loss, less postoperative pain, significantly reduced hospital stays, and earlier mobilization and recovery times. Although relative recovery is enhanced, general precautions should still be taken to minimize bleeding, maintain suture lines, and minimize procedural complications overall. Patients should generally be advised to refrain from strenuous activity for approximately 7 days after surgery. Complications specific to each procedure should also be considered. For example, the most common complication of SCS trial or implant is stimulator revision for lead repositioning. Several studies cite lack of efficacy or lead migration as the primary reason for failure.[127–129] Special precautions must be taken in the early phases of recovery to ensure lead fixation. According to an international panel of experts, patients may return to normal activities the day after implantation but must refrain from engaging in any extreme movements (e.g., golfing, strenuous workout, heavy lifting). Depending on the invasiveness of the procedure, physical therapy may be recommended at the 4-week mark. Ultimately, the activity restrictions following minimally invasive spine surgery are similar to those for general ambulatory surgery and should be clearly described to the patient and/or family before discharge.

Unanticipated Overnight Admission

Minimally invasive spine surgery has increased in popularity over the past decade, with surgeons citing safety levels similar to, and complication rates lower than, those for open surgery. Many procedures are now performed in ambulatory surgical centers that allow same-day discharge. Hospital admission after ambulatory surgery, however, does occur and increases unnecessary cost and healthcare burden. In a cohort study of 5,085 ambulatory orthopedic patients, Salas et al reported a 1.5% incidence of overnight admission, with the two most common causes being inadequate postoperative pain management and wound infection.[130] Risk factors included general anesthetic technique and increased length of surgery. Another study found an unanticipated admission rate of 2.67% in patients undergoing general ambulatory surgery and listed higher ASA class and advanced age as additional significant risk factors.[131] Caelenberg et al also identified surgery end-time between 12 and 3 PM (OR 1.73; 95% CI 1.05–2.86) and time of surgery past 3 PM (OR 6.52; 95% CI 4.11–10.34) as significant risk factors.[132] Therefore, unanticipated overnight hospital admission rates may be improved by identifying ASA 3–4 patients requiring a general anesthetic technique and scheduling this subgroup as OR first-case starts.

References

1. Dahlhamer J, Lucas J, Zelaya C, et al. Prevalence of chronic pain and high-impact chronic pain among adults—United States, 2016. *MMWR Morb Mortal Wkly Rep.* 2018;67(36):1001–1006.
2. National Institute for Health and Care Excellence (NICE). *National Institute for Health and Care Excellence Guidance.* 2013. https://www.nice.org.uk/about/what-we-do/our-programmes/nice-guidance/nice-guidelines.
3. Fleisher LA, Fleischmann KE, Auerbach AD, et al. 2014 ACC/AHA guideline on perioperative cardiovascular evaluation and management of patients undergoing noncardiac surgery: a report of the American College of Cardiology/American Heart Association Task Force on Practice Guidelines. *Circulation.* 2014;130(24):e278–e333.
4. *A.S.o.A. American Society of Anesthesiologists [ASA] Guidelines, Statements, Clinical Resources.* 2020; https://www.asahq.org/standards-and-guidelines.
5. Committee on Standard and Practice, P., Apfelbaum, J.L., et al., *Practice advisory for preanesthesia evaluation: an updated report by the American Society of Anesthesiologists Task Force on Preanesthesia Evaluation. Anesthesiology, 2012*; **116**(3): 522–538.
6. Johansson T, Fritsch G, Flamm M, et al. Effectiveness of non-cardiac preoperative testing in non-cardiac elective surgery: a systematic review. *Br J Anaesth.* 2013;110(6):926–939.
7. Das S, Ghosh S. Monitored anesthesia care: An overview. *J Anaesthesiol Clin Pharmacol.* 2015;31(1):27–29.
8. Sohn HM, Ryu JH. Monitored anesthesia care in and outside the operating room. *Korean J Anesthesiol.* 2016;69(4):319–326.
9. Kim SE, Kim E. Local anesthesia with monitored anesthesia care for patients undergoing thyroidectomy: a case series. *Korean J Anesthesiol.* 2016;69(6):635–639.
10. Furstein J, Patel M, Sadhasivam S, et al. Use of dexmedetomidine for monitored anesthesia care for diskography in adolescents. *AANA J.* 2011;79(5):421–425.
11. Sesay M, Tauzin-Fin P, Verdonck O, et al. Clinical evaluation of the Capnomask in the supine vs. prone position during monitored anaesthesia care. *Eur J Anaesthesiol.* 2008;25(9):769–771.
12. Sesay M, Tauzin-Fin P, Jeannin A, et al. Median effective infusion dose (ED50) of alfentanil for monitored anesthesia care of percutaneous vertebroplasty of osteoporotic fractures. *J Neurosurg Anesthesiol.* 2009;21(2):165–169.
13. Benjamin, Emelia J., et al. Heart disease and stroke statistics—2019 update: a report from the American Heart Association. *Circulation* 139.10 (2019); e56–e528.
14. Coffman J, Tran T, Quast T, et al. Cost conscious care: preoperative evaluation by a cardiologist prior to low-risk procedures. *BMJ Open Qual.* 2019;8(2):e000481.

15. O'Donnell FT. Preoperative evaluation of the surgical patient. *Mo Med.* 2016;113(3):196–201.
16. Okocha O, Gerlach RM, Sweitzer B. Preoperative evaluation for ambulatory anesthesia: what, when, and how? *Anesthesiol Clin.* 2019;37(2):195–213.
17. Goldman L, Caldera DL, Nussbaum SR, et al. Multifactorial index of cardiac risk in noncardiac surgical procedures. *N Engl J Med.* 1977;297(16):845–850.
18. Ford MK, Beattie WS, Wijeysundera DN. Systematic review: prediction of perioperative cardiac complications and mortality by the revised Cardiac Risk Index. *Ann Intern Med.* 2010;152(1):26–35.
19. Duceppe E, Parlow J, MacDonald P, et al. Canadian Cardiovascular Society guidelines on perioperative cardiac risk assessment and management for patients who undergo noncardiac surgery. *Can J Cardiol.* 2017;33(1):17–32.
20. American College of Surgeons. *American College of Surgeons National Surgical Quality Improvement Program Surgical Risk Calculator.* 2020. https://riskcalculator.facs.org/RiskCalculator/PatientInfo.jsp.
21. Bilimoria KY, Liu Y, Paruch JL, et al. Development and evaluation of the universal ACS NSQIP surgical risk calculator: a decision aid and informed consent tool for patients and surgeons. *J Am Coll Surg.* 2013;217(5):833–842, e831–e833.
22. Cohen ME, Liu Y, Ko CY, et al. An examination of American College of Surgeons NSQIP Surgical Risk Calculator accuracy. *J Am Coll Surg.* 2017;224(5):787–795, e781.
23. Fleisher LA, Beckman JA, Brown KA, et al. ACC/AHA 2007 guidelines on perioperative cardiovascular evaluation and care for noncardiac surgery: executive summary: a report of the American College of Cardiology/American Heart Association Task Force on Practice Guidelines (Writing Committee to Revise the 2002 Guidelines on Perioperative Cardiovascular Evaluation for Noncardiac Surgery) developed in collaboration with the American Society of Echocardiography, American Society of Nuclear Cardiology, Heart Rhythm Society, Society of Cardiovascular Anesthesiologists, Society for Cardiovascular Angiography and Interventions, Society for Vascular Medicine and Biology, and Society for Vascular Surgery. *J Am Coll Cardiol.* 2007;50(17):1707–1732.
24. Hlatky MA, Boineau RE, Higginbotham MB, et al. A brief self-administered questionnaire to determine functional capacity (the Duke Activity Status Index). *Am J Cardiol.* 1989;64(10):651–654.
25. Fletcher GF, Balady G, Froelicher VF, et al. Exercise standards. A statement for healthcare professionals from the American Heart Association Writing Group. *Circulation.* 1995;91(2):580–615.
26. Stone ME, Salter B, Fischer A. Perioperative management of patients with cardiac implantable electronic devices. *Br J Anaesth.* 2011;107(**suppl 1**):i16–i26.
27. Escarce JJ, Shea JA, Chen W, et al. Outcomes of open cholecystectomy in the elderly: a longitudinal analysis of 21,000 cases in the prelaparoscopic era. *Surgery.* 1995;117(2):156–164.
28. Rosen AK, Geraci JM, Ash AS, et al. Postoperative adverse events of common surgical procedures in the Medicare population. *Med Care.* 1992;30(9):753–765.
29. Thomas EJ, Goldman L, Mangione CM, et al. Body mass index as a correlate of postoperative complications and resource utilization. *Am J Med.* 1997;102(3):277–283.
30. Lawrence VA, Hilsenbeck SG, Noveck H, et al. Medical complications and outcomes after hip fracture repair. *Arch Intern Med.* 2002;162(18):2053–2057.
31. Smetana GW, Lawrence VA, Cornell JE, et al. Preoperative pulmonary risk stratification for noncardiothoracic surgery: systematic review for the American College of Physicians. *Ann Intern Med.* 2006;144(8):581–595.
32. De Oliveira GS Jr, Holl JL, Lindquist LA, et al. Older adults and unanticipated hospital admission within 30 days of ambulatory surgery: an analysis of 53,667 ambulatory surgical procedures. *J Am Geriatr Soc.* 2015;63(8):1679–1685.
33. Wong J, Lam DP, Abrishami A, et al. Short-term preoperative smoking cessation and postoperative complications: a systematic review and meta-analysis. *Can J Anaesth.* 2012;59(3):268–279.
34. Sorensen LT. Wound healing and infection in surgery: the pathophysiological impact of smoking, smoking cessation, and nicotine replacement therapy: a systematic review. *Ann Surg.* 2012;255(6):1069–1079.
35. Goertz O, Kapalschinski N, Skorzinski T, et al. [Wound healing complications in smokers, non-smokers and after abstinence from smoking]. *Chirurg.* 2012;83(7):652–656.
36. Shi Y, Warner DO. Surgery as a teachable moment for smoking cessation. *Anesthesiology.* 2010;112(1):102–107.

37. Chow CK, Devereaux PJ. The optimal timing of smoking cessation before surgery: comment on "Smoking cessation shortly before surgery and postoperative complications." *Arch Intern Med.* 2011;171(11):989–990.
38. Lankhorst MA. Smoking and chronic pain. *J Pain Palliat Care Pharmacother.* 2016;30(4):326–327.
39. American Spinal Injury Association and International Spinal Cord Society International Standards Committee. "The 2019 Revision of the International Standards for Neurological Classification of Spinal Cord Injury (ISNCSCI)—What's New?" *Spinal Cord.* 2019; 57(10): 815–817.
40. Schuld C, Franz S, Bruggemann K, et al. International standards for neurological classification of spinal cord injury: impact of the revised worksheet (revision 02/13) on classification performance. *J Spinal Cord Med.* 2016;39(5):504–512.
41. Williams M. Manual muscle testing, development and current use. *Phys Ther Rev.* 1956;36(12):797–805.
42. Kumar K, Rizvi S. Historical and present state of neuromodulation in chronic pain. *Curr Pain Headache Rep.* 2014;18(1):387.
43. Stanak M, Erdos J, Hawlik K, et al. Novel surgical treatments for gastroesophageal reflux disease: systematic review of magnetic sphincter augmentation and electric stimulation therapy. *Gastroenterology Res.* 2018;11(3):161–173.
44. Yeoh TY, Manninen P, Kalia SK, et al. Anesthesia considerations for patients with an implanted deep brain stimulator undergoing surgery: a review and update. *Can J Anaesth.* 2017;64(3):308–319.
45. Nutt JG, Anderson VC, Peacock JH, et al. DBS and diathermy interaction induces severe CNS damage. *Neurology.* 2001;56(10):1384–1386.
46. Ruggera PS, Witters DM, von Maltzahn G, et al. In vitro assessment of tissue heating near metallic medical implants by exposure to pulsed radio frequency diathermy. *Phys Med Biol.* 2003;48(17):2919–2928.
47. Hatton KW, McLarney JT, Pittman T, et al. Vagal nerve stimulation: overview and implications for anesthesiologists. *Anesth Analg.* 2006;103(5):1241–1249.
48. Cook TM, Woodall N, Harper J, et al. Major complications of airway management in the UK: results of the Fourth National Audit Project of the Royal College of Anaesthetists and the Difficult Airway Society. Part 2: intensive care and emergency departments. *Br J Anaesth.* 2011;106(5):632–642.
49. Practice guidelines for preoperative fasting and the use of pharmacologic agents to reduce the risk of pulmonary aspiration: application to healthy patients undergoing elective procedures: an updated report by the American Society of Anesthesiologists Task Force on Preoperative Fasting and the Use of Pharmacologic Agents to Reduce the Risk of Pulmonary Aspiration. *Anesthesiology.* 2017;126(3):376–393.
50. Glance LG, Blumberg N, Eaton MP, et al. Preoperative thrombocytopenia and postoperative outcomes after noncardiac surgery. *Anesthesiology.* 2014;120(1):62–75.
51. Qureshi AI, Zafar A, Miran MS, et al. Carotid endarterectomy in patients with thrombocytopenia: analysis of the National Surgical Quality Improvement Program Registry. *Oper Neurosurg.* 2017;13(1):150–156.
52. Kaufman RM, Djulbegovic B, Gernsheimer T, et al. Platelet transfusion: a clinical practice guideline from the AABB. *Ann Intern Med.* 2015;162(3):205–213.
53. Van Os EC, Kamath PS, Gostout CJ, et al. Gastroenterological procedures among patients with disorders of hemostasis: evaluation and management recommendations. *Gastrointest Endosc.* 1999;50(4):536–543.
54. Herman JA, Urits I, Kaye AD, et al. Thrombocytopenia and neuraxial anesthesia: are there platelet count thresholds? *J Clin Anesth.* 2020;63:109751.
55. van Veen JJ, Nokes TJ, Makris M. The risk of spinal haematoma following neuraxial anaesthesia or lumbar puncture in thrombocytopenic individuals. *Br J Haematol.* 2010;148(1):15–25.
56. Bailey LJ, Shehata N, De France B, et al. Obstetric neuraxial anesthesia at low platelet counts in the context of immune thrombocytopenia: a systematic review and meta-analysis. *Can J Anaesth.* 2019;66(11):1396–1414.
57. Domenicucci M, Mancarella C, Santoro G, et al. Spinal epidural hematomas: personal experience and literature review of more than 1000 cases. *J Neurosurg Spine.* 2017;27(2):198–208.
58. Narouze S, Benzon HT, Provenzano D, et al. Interventional spine and pain procedures in patients on antiplatelet and anticoagulant medications (second edition): guidelines from the American Society of

Regional Anesthesia and Pain Medicine, the European Society of Regional Anaesthesia and Pain Therapy, the American Academy of Pain Medicine, the International Neuromodulation Society, the North American Neuromodulation Society, and the World Institute of Pain. *Reg Anesth Pain Med.* 2018;43(3):225–262.

59. Douketis JD, Spyropoulos AC, Kaatz S, et al. Perioperative bridging anticoagulation in patients with atrial fibrillation. *N Engl J Med.* 2015;373(9):823–833.
60. Levine GN, Bates ER, Bittl JA, et al. 2016 ACC/AHA guideline focused update on duration of dual antiplatelet therapy in patients with coronary artery disease: a report of the American College of Cardiology/American Heart Association Task Force on Clinical Practice Guidelines: an update of the 2011 ACCF/AHA/SCAI guideline for percutaneous coronary intervention, 2011 ACCF/AHA guideline for coronary artery bypass graft surgery, 2012 ACC/AHA/ACP/AATS/PCNA/SCAI/STS guideline for the diagnosis and management of patients with stable ischemic heart disease, 2013 ACCF/AHA guideline for the management of ST-elevation myocardial infarction, 2014 AHA/ACC guideline for the management of patients with non-ST-elevation acute coronary syndromes, and 2014 ACC/AHA guideline on perioperative cardiovascular evaluation and management of patients undergoing noncardiac surgery. *Circulation.* 2016;134(10):e123–e155.
61. Jain A, Naniwadekar M. An etiological reappraisal of pancytopenia—largest series reported to date from a single tertiary care teaching hospital. *BMC Hematol.* 2013;13(1):10.
62. Gnanaraj J, Parnes A, Francis CW, et al. Approach to pancytopenia: diagnostic algorithm for clinical hematologists. *Blood Rev.* 2018;32(5):361–367.
63. Chiravuri S, De Jesus O. Pancytopenia, in *StatPearls.* 2020.
64. Huang J, McKenna N, Babins N. Utility of thromboelastography during neuraxial blockade in the parturient with thrombocytopenia. *AANA J.* 2014;82(2):127–130.
65. Artang R, Anderson M, Nielsen JD. Fully automated thromboelastograph TEG 6s to measure anticoagulant effects of direct oral anticoagulants in healthy male volunteers. *Res Pract Thromb Haemost.* 2019;3(3):391–396.
66. Solbeck S, Jensen AS, Maschmann C, et al. The anticoagulant effect of therapeutic levels of dabigatran in atrial fibrillation evaluated by thrombelastography (TEG®), Hemoclot Thrombin Inhibitor (HTI) assay and Ecarin Clotting Time (ECT). *Scand J Clin Lab Invest.* 2018;78(1–2):25–30.
67. Dunham CM, Rabel C, Hileman BM, et al. TEG® and RapidTEG® are unreliable for detecting warfarin-coagulopathy: a prospective cohort study. *Thromb J.* 2014;12(1):4.
68. Nascimento B, Al Mahoos M, Callum J, et al. Vitamin K-dependent coagulation factor deficiency in trauma: a comparative analysis between international normalized ratio and thromboelastography. *Transfusion.* 2012;52(1):7–13.
69. Hepner DL, Concepcion M, Bhavani-Shankar K. Coagulation status using thromboelastography in patients receiving warfarin prophylaxis and epidural analgesia. *J Clin Anesth.* 2002;14(6):405–410.
70. Lang T, von Depka M. [Possibilities and limitations of thrombelastometry/-graphy]. *Hamostaseologie.* 2006;26(3 suppl 1):S20–S29.
71. Routine preoperative tests for elective surgery. *BJU Int.* 2018;121(1):12–16.
72. Ead H. Glycemic control and surgery-optimizing outcomes for the patient with diabetes. *J Perianesth Nurs.* 2009;24(6):384–395.
73. Yang L, Sun Y, Li G, et al. Is hemoglobin A_{1c} and perioperative hyperglycemia predictive of periprosthetic joint infection following total joint arthroplasty? A systematic review and meta-analysis. *Medicine.* 2017;96(51):e8805.
74. Zerr KJ, Furnary AP, Grunkemeier GL, et al. Glucose control lowers the risk of wound infection in diabetics after open heart operations. *Ann Thorac Surg.* 1997;63(2):356–361.
75. McConnell YJ, Johnson PM, Porter GA. Surgical site infections following colorectal surgery in patients with diabetes: association with postoperative hyperglycemia. *J Gastrointest Surg.* 2009;13(3):508–515.
76. Hoelzer BC, Bendel MA, Deer TR, et al. Spinal cord stimulator implant infection rates and risk factors: a multicenter retrospective study. *Neuromodulation.* 2017;20(6):558–562.
77. Onyekwelu I, Yakkanti R, Protzer L, et al. Surgical wound classification and surgical site infections in the orthopaedic patient. *J Am Acad Orthop Surg Glob Res Rev.* 2017;1(3):e022.
78. Barrasa-Villar JI, Aibar-Remon C, Prieto-Andres P, et al. Impact on morbidity, mortality, and length of stay of hospital-acquired infections by resistant microorganisms. *Clin Infect Dis.* 2017;65(4):644–652.

79. Heuer A, Kossick MA, Riley J, et al. Update on guidelines for perioperative antibiotic selection and administration from the Surgical Care Improvement Project (SCIP) and American Society of Health-System Pharmacists. *AANA J.* 2017;85(4):293–299.
80. Wilson W, Taubert KA, Gewitz M, et al. Prevention of infective endocarditis: guidelines from the American Heart Association: a guideline from the American Heart Association Rheumatic Fever, Endocarditis, and Kawasaki Disease Committee, Council on Cardiovascular Disease in the Young, and the Council on Clinical Cardiology, Council on Cardiovascular Surgery and Anesthesia, and the Quality of Care and Outcomes Research Interdisciplinary Working Group. *Circulation.* 2007;116(15):1736–1754.
81. Faulkner KG. The tale of the T-score: review and perspective. *Osteoporos Int.* 2005;16(4):347–352.
82. Wright NC, Looker AC, Saag KG, et al. The recent prevalence of osteoporosis and low bone mass in the United States based on bone mineral density at the femoral neck or lumbar spine. *J Bone Miner Res.* 2014;29(11):2520–2526.
83. Anderson PA, Morgan SL, Krueger D, et al. Use of bone health evaluation in orthopedic surgery: 2019 ISCD official position. *J Clin Densitom.* 2019;22(4):517–543.
84. Karaguzel G, Holick MF. Diagnosis and treatment of osteopenia. *Rev Endocr Metab Disord.* 2010;11(4):237–251.
85. Kates SL, Ackert-Bicknell CL. How do bisphosphonates affect fracture healing? *Injury.* 2016;47(**suppl 1**):S65–S68.
86. Hak DJ. The biology of fracture healing in osteoporosis and in the presence of anti-osteoporotic drugs. *Injury.* 2018;49(8):1461–1465.
87. Liu J, Liu Z, Luo J, et al. Influence of vertebral bone mineral density on total dispersion volume of bone cement in vertebroplasty. *Medicine.* 2019;98(12):e14941.
88. Zhang H, Xu C, Zhang T, et al. Does percutaneous vertebroplasty or balloon kyphoplasty for osteoporotic vertebral compression fractures increase the incidence of new vertebral fractures? A meta-analysis. *Pain Physician.* 2017;20(1):E13–E28.
89. Inoue S, Kamiya M, Nishihara M, et al. Prevalence, characteristics, and burden of failed back surgery syndrome: the influence of various residual symptoms on patient satisfaction and quality of life as assessed by a nationwide Internet survey in Japan. *J Pain Res.* 2017;10:811–823.
90. Sebaaly A, Lahoud MJ, Rizkallah M, et al. Etiology, evaluation, and treatment of failed back surgery syndrome. *Asian Spine J.* 2018;12(3):574–585.
91. Bederman SS, Le VH, Pahlavan S. An approach to lumbar revision spine surgery in adults. *J Am Acad Orthop Surg.* 2016;24(7):433–442.
92. Wong E, Altaf F, Oh LJ, et al. Adult degenerative lumbar scoliosis. *Orthopedics.* 2017;40(6):e930–e939.
93. El-Hawary R, Chukwunyerenwa C. Update on evaluation and treatment of scoliosis. *Pediatr Clin North Am.* 2014;61(6):1223–1241.
94. Alonzo F, Cobar A, Cahueque M, et al. Bertolotti's syndrome: an underdiagnosed cause for lower back pain. *J Surg Case Rep.* 2018;2018(10):rjy276.
95. Jancuska JM, Spivak JM, Bendo JA. A review of symptomatic lumbosacral transitional vertebrae: Bertolotti's syndrome. *Int J Spine Surg.* 2015;9:42.
96. Mahato NK. Pedicular anatomy of the first sacral segment in transitional variations of the lumbo-sacral junction. *Spine.* 2011;36(18):E1187–E1192.
97. Mahato NK. Morphological traits in sacra associated with complete and partial lumbarization of first sacral segment. *Spine J.* 2010;10(10):910–915.
98. Kim NH, Suk KS. The role of transitional vertebrae in spondylolysis and spondylolytic spondylolisthesis. *Bull Hosp Joint Dis.* 1997;56(3):161–166.
99. Kwong Y, Rao N, Latief K. MDCT findings in Baastrup disease: disease or normal feature of the aging spine? *AJR Am J Roentgenol.* 2011;196(5):1156–1159.
100. Hiyama A, Katoh H, Sakai D, et al. Prevalence of diffuse idiopathic skeletal hyperostosis (DISH) assessed with whole-spine computed tomography in 1479 subjects. *BMC Musculoskelet Disord.* 2018;19(1):178.
101. Resnick D, Niwayama G. Radiographic and pathologic features of spinal involvement in diffuse idiopathic skeletal hyperostosis (DISH). *Radiology.* 1976;119(3):559–568.

102. Tetreault L, Nakashima H, Kato S, et al. A systematic review of classification systems for cervical ossification of the posterior longitudinal ligament. *Global Spine J.* 2019;9(1):85–103.
103. Kumar K, Buchser E, Linderoth B, et al. Avoiding complications from spinal cord stimulation: practical recommendations from an international panel of experts. *Neuromodulation.* 2007;10(1):24–33.
104. Ludwig KA, Carlson MA, Condon RE. Prophylactic antibiotics in surgery. *Annu Rev Med.* 1993;44:385–393.
105. Rosenberger LH, Politano AD, Sawyer RG. The surgical care improvement project and prevention of post-operative infection, including surgical site infection. *Surg Infect.* 2011;12(3):163–168.
106. Nguyen N, Yegiyants S, Kaloostian C, et al. The Surgical Care Improvement Project (SCIP) initiative to reduce infection in elective colorectal surgery: which performance measures affect outcome? *Am Surg.* 2008;74(10):1012–1016.
107. Kurz A, Sessler DI, Lenhardt R. Perioperative normothermia to reduce the incidence of surgical-wound infection and shorten hospitalization. Study of Wound Infection and Temperature Group. *N Engl J Med.* 1996;334(19):1209–1215.
108. Bratzler DW, Dellinger EP, Olsen KM, et al. Clinical practice guidelines for antimicrobial prophylaxis in surgery. *Surg Infect.* 2013;14(1):73–156.
109. Woods, Michael, et al. Utility of intraoperative neuromonitoring during minimally invasive fusion of the sacroiliac joint. *Advances in Orthopedics.* 2014; 154041.
110. Schoen N, Chieng LO, Madhavan K, et al. The use of intraoperative electromyogram during spinal cord stimulator placement surgery: a case series. *World Neurosurg.* 2017;**100**:74–84.
111. Hwang R, Field N, Kumar V, et al. Intraoperative neuromonitoring in percutaneous spinal cord stimulator placement. *Neuromodulation.* 2019;22(3):341–346.
112. Tamkus AA, Scott AF, Khan FR. Neurophysiological monitoring during spinal cord stimulator placement surgery. *Neuromodulation.* 2015;18(6):460–464; discussion 464.
113. Mammis A, Mogilner AY. The use of intraoperative electrophysiology for the placement of spinal cord stimulator paddle leads under general anesthesia. *Neurosurgery.* 2012;70(2 suppl operative):230–236.
114. Mangram AJ, Horan TC, Pearson ML, et al. Guideline for prevention of surgical site infection, 1999. Centers for Disease Control and Prevention (CDC) Hospital Infection Control Practices Advisory Committee. *Am J Infect Control.* 1999;27(2):97–132; quiz 133–134; discussion 196.
115. Liu Z, Dumville JC, Norman G, et al. Intraoperative interventions for preventing surgical site infection: an overview of Cochrane Reviews. *Cochrane Database Syst Rev.* 2018;2:CD012653.
116. Lee WH, Huang TC, Lin LJ, et al. Efficacy of postoperative prophylactic antibiotics in reducing permanent pacemaker infections. *Clin Cardiol.* 2017;40(8):559–565.
117. Engle MP, Vinh BP, Harun N, et al. Infectious complications related to intrathecal drug delivery system and spinal cord stimulator system implantations at a comprehensive cancer pain center. *Pain Physician.* 2013;16(3):251–257.
118. Bendel MA, O'Brien T, Hoelzer BC, et al. Spinal cord stimulator related infections: findings from a multicenter retrospective analysis of 2737 implants. *Neuromodulation*, 2017. **20**(6): 553–557.
119. Falowski, S.M., Provenzano, D.A., Xia, Y., et al. Spinal cord stimulation infection rate and risk factors: results from a United States payer database. *Neuromodulation.* 2019;22(2):179–189.
120. Esquer Garrigos Z, Farid S, Bendel MA, et al. Spinal cord stimulator infection: approach to diagnosis, management, and prevention. *Clin Infect Dis.* 2020;70(12):2727–2735.
121. Health Quality Ontario. Vertebral augmentation involving vertebroplasty or kyphoplasty for cancer-related vertebral compression fractures: a systematic review. *Ontario health technology assessment series.* 2016;16(11):1–202.
122. Taylor RS, Taylor RJ, Fritzell P. Balloon kyphoplasty and vertebroplasty for vertebral compression fractures: a comparative systematic review of efficacy and safety. *Spine.* 2006;31(23):2747–2755.
123. Segal DN, Wilson JM, Staley C, et al. The 5-item Modified Frailty Index is predictive of 30-day postoperative complications in patients undergoing kyphoplasty vertebral augmentation. *World Neurosurg.* 2018;116:e225–e231.
124. Shamrock AG, Patel A, Alam M, et al. The safety profile of percutaneous minimally invasive sacroiliac joint fusion. *Global Spine J.* 2019;9(8):874–880.
125. Schoell K, Buser Z, Jakoi A, et al. Postoperative complications in patients undergoing minimally invasive sacroiliac fusion. *Spine J.* 2016;16(11):1324–1332.

126. Ha KY, Lee JS, Kim KW. Degeneration of sacroiliac joint after instrumented lumbar or lumbosacral fusion: a prospective cohort study over five-year follow-up. *Spine.* 2008;33(11):1192–1198.
127. Patel, Smruti K., et al. Spinal cord stimulation failure: evaluation of factors underlying hardware explantation. *Journal of Neurosurgery: Spine.* 2019; 21(1): 133–138.
128. Dupre DA, Tomycz N, Whiting D, et al. Spinal cord stimulator explantation: motives for removal of surgically placed paddle systems. *Pain Pract.* 2018;18(4):500–504.
129. Mekhail NA, Mathews M, Nageeb F, et al. Retrospective review of 707 cases of spinal cord stimulation: indications and complications. *Pain Pract.* 2011;11(2):148–153.
130. Jimenez Salas B, Ruiz Frontera M, Seral Garcia B, et al. Causes of unplanned admission after orthopedic procedures in ambulatory surgery. *Rev Esp Cir Orthop Traumatol.* 2020;64(1):50–56.
131. Whippey A, Kostandoff G, Paul J, et al. Predictors of unanticipated admission following ambulatory surgery: a retrospective case-control study. *Can J Anaesth.* 2013;60(7):675–683.
132. Van Caelenberg E, De Regge M, Eeckloo K, et al. Analysis of failed discharge after ambulatory surgery: unanticipated admission. *Acta Chir Belg.* 2019;119(3):139–145.

5

Spinal Diagnostics for Interventional Pain and Surgery

Jeffrey D. Petersohn

Diagnosis—The Nexus of Art and Science

In 1677, the philosopher Spinoza wrote in *The Ethics* that, "The endeavor to understand is the first and only basis of virtue." Physicians in training frequently hear rounding physicians intone, "Each patient deserves the dignity of a diagnosis," and R. Shane Tubbs cited J. Patrick Johnson's observation, "Surgery is simple—it requires only anatomy with hemostasis," but it is clear that correct and timely diagnosis underlies all medical and surgical interventions and this is truly the art of understanding not just structure, but the science of why.[1] Because the goal of interventional and surgical pain practice is to improve or resolve pain and its functional deficits, the process begins with an understanding of the anatomy and pathophysiology of pain.

Regrettably, little has been written to guide physicians comprehensively in the art of diagnosis that is specific to the diagnostic process required to understand spinal pain. It has been assumed, without evidence, that if a student learns anatomy and pathophysiology, a miraculous stroke of lightning will occur somewhere between the third year of medical school and completion of fellowship to turn mere mortals into superb clinical diagnosticians. If only this were true!

This chapter aims to provide an introduction to spinal diagnostics, and more broadly to teach an approach to the diagnosis of spinal pain that can be applied in a coherent, sequential, and thoughtful fashion. Limited literature references are cited, not because there is a complete paucity of literature, but because most of the current literature promotes the premise that the patients studied had only one clinical pain problem at time. While the presence of a single painful disorder may be a reasonable surmise in addressing a patient population with acute disk herniation for which an accurate diagnosis can be made promptly, this is not the level of diagnostic challenge that regularly presents to consultants in interventional pain, neurosurgery, or orthopedics, in which a variety of coexisting diagnoses must be considered, weighed, evaluated, and excluded in order to plan competent treatment.

In *The Ethics*, Spinoza also wrote, "I do not know how to teach philosophy without disturbing established religion." And so it is with interventional pain: In reviewing the diagnostic utility of facet joint palpation, for example, the published literature is nearly deadlocked between articles supporting the practice and those condemning it. How can this be so? A review of the "Methods" sections of over 20 research articles on this very topic revealed that not a single article on facet palpation explicitly excluded patients with radiculopathy by active evaluation for radiculopathy (instead, researchers made a default assumption that the lack of extremity pain was sufficient for this purpose) and no article explicitly excluded orthopedic disorders of shoulder, hip, knee, or sacroiliac joint in the patient selection criteria. Clinically, some—but not all—radiculopathies may be accompanied by facet tenderness, and it may be present at none, one, several, or many joint levels. Patients with diffuse cervical facet tenderness often have pain for which the ipsilateral shoulder is ultimately demonstrated to be the true source of pain and the facet joint is an innocent bystander that has no role in pain production. The presence of even 10% to 15% of patients with these coexisting diagnoses in a typical study of facet pain so alters the statistical result that in a typical study of 40 to 80 patients, the introduced noise buries the signal, that is to say, the truth. Only a very few articles detailed the clinical criteria or techniques used for accurate enumeration of facet joints based upon palpation[2] or ultrasound.[3] Similarly, articles on diagnosis of sacroiliac joint pain do not routinely use active examination to exclude patients with facet pain or lumbar radiculopathy; again, the signal of truth is buried in the noise of coexisting diagnoses.

In clinical practice, EMG may report "chronic L5–S1 radiculopathy" that upon diligent evaluation is revealed to be not radiculopathy, but sacroiliac joint pain. Similarly, patients with "carpal tunnel syndrome" may have a normal carpal tunnel and median nerve but a symptomatic C5–C6 disk herniation or radiculopathy due to foraminal stenosis. The diagnostic system must be refashioned to resolve these errors and controversies so that patients can be confident in our approach to their care.

This chapter begins by considering the two broad categories of pain origination, neuropathic and nociceptive, and then proceeds to introduce a model of lumbosacral spinal pain that divides spinal disorders into diagnostic subsets for strategizing the overall process of spinal diagnosis. The model is unique in that it considers and allows for multiple coexisting painful disorders that may evolve or change over time during the course of the patient's treatment. After briefly noting clinically common dyads and triads of pain that often confront physicians in interventional spine and surgical practice, the discussion proceeds to outline a recursive, algorithmic, process-based clinical approach to diagnosis, with reference to specific components of the physical examination that generate information necessary to define the relevant anatomical and pathophysiologic subsets that require integration with the results of radiographic and advanced imaging studies. Last, the chapter presents guidelines for the selection of, indications for, and notable technical nuances in artful deployment of, several commonly used modalities for interventional spinal diagnostics.

Pain originating within, or due to primary involvement of, neural structures is termed *neuropathic pain*. Mechanisms that create neuropathic pain may involve neural compression or traction by bone, disk, hypertrophic ligaments, adipose tissue, adhesions, or scar, but other common mechanisms include neural ischemia, metabolic disorders, toxic conditions, and genetic disorders, as well as tumors that compress or infiltrate neural structures. While a host of neuropathic pain disorders may produce "back pain"—for example, sodium or potassium channel abnormalities; autoimmune disorders targeting myelin (multiple sclerosis), aquaporin-4 (neuromyelitis optica), and AMPA or NMDA receptors; neural involvement in diabetes mellitus or liver disease; adverse effects of taxols, vinca alkaloids, or other medications; endocrine or metabolic disorders, such as hyperparathyroidism—because these disorders do not necessarily target only the spine, a fuller exploration of their mechanisms of pain production and their treatment exceeds this chapter's remit.

What is termed *nociceptive* pain is produced by articular, vascular, or visceral structures that have some form of innervation communicating along a peripheral afferent pathway, including somatic, sympathetic and vagal systems, where information flows toward the central nervous system (CNS), where the neural signals are processed, modified, and often, but not always, somatotopically organized. In the CNS, the signals are processed through complex neural circuitry, ramifying to various cerebellar and subcortical centers, including the limbic system, thalamus, and eventually the cerebral cortex, where the complex sensory and emotional responses identified and experienced as pain manifest. Several higher centers in the brain provide descending modulation of more distal afferent traffic, and modification of the attentional thalamic pathways may reduce the perceived severity, or the angst, of the pain experience. Unfortunately, precise correlation of anatomical pain production with the localization of pain reported by the patient is generally lacking, and axial spinal pain may be experienced regionally, with multiple causes of pain producing symptoms that are not differentiable by the patient. It is here that the process of spinal diagnosis begins.

In the diagnosis of pain, it is fair to warn the reader to avoid the lure of Occam's razor, the thinking that a single process with the simplest explanation will regularly yield an understanding of an individual's clinical pain. Regrettably, this approach is often unsuccessful. Instead, an algorithmic approach is fruitful in spinal diagnostics. While the approach may initially appear laborious and complex, the algorithm considers the pathophysiology and anatomy of pain production by division into anatomical subsets and then approaches the issues clinically in a hierarchical and recursive fashion, so that even complex pain disorders can be analyzed, unraveled, and understood. The reader is assured that this process yields success in freeing most patients from the bitter grip of pain.

Spinal diagnostic procedures are designed to identify the structures and pathways that produce or transmit pain. Some diagnostic procedures, such as steroid injections, may also provide primary and possibly definitive treatment for pain, while in other circumstances, the lack of durability of response to injection should prompt a search for another cause of clinically recurrent or coexisting pain or a plan for definitive minimally invasive or surgical treatment. While some patients present with only a primary cause of pain, often by the time consultation is arranged with a pain physician, significant neural and orthopedic compensation has occurred, such that a very different clinical presentation is offered.

Modification of the musculoskeletal kinetic chain is a strategy frequently adopted by patients in minimizing their pain. Unfortunately, this typically unintentional functional acquisition (or adaptation) often produces a new pain process, with the resulting disturbance of gait or stance often more severe and functionally limiting than the primary pain process. A patient presenting with hip pain and antalgic gait may subsequently be determined to have symptomatic underlying lumbar spinal stenosis and lumbar facet pain that, when diagnosed and treated, not only may resolve the original complaint of hip pain, but also may improve functional walking and standing tolerance as well as improve the patient's interrupted pattern of sleep. However, it is important to point out that radiculopathies from L2 to L4 frequently produce referred hip pain, as do symptomatic lumbar facet pain processes. Similarly, sacroiliac joint tenderness can be produced by foraminal stenosis, disk herniation, or osseous stenosis affecting any nerve roots from T11 to S2. Because a FABER maneuver is often positive in these cases, if it is the only test performed, it will mislead the physician. These pain processes are frequently considered to be examples of referred pain, a product of the spinal neural processing scheme that misassigns pain to an uninvolved structure. However, when review of a hip MRI reveals a normal glenohumeral joint space, with only gluteus minimis tendinosis noted, it will become abundantly clear that this pain is not likely to be referred, and instead that an underlying pain process is probably causing a gait abnormality. Clearly, the complexity of pain diagnosis requires an orderly approach to understanding and dissecting the clinical presentations and using tools of physical examination and appropriate imaging to determine the root cause of pain and the modalities required for resolution.

For example, while we typically think of spinal stenosis as a pain process that improves when the patient is sitting, a patient complaining of severe buttock pain and inability to sit might ultimately be found to have severe lumbar spinal stenosis with compensatory lumbar flexed gait that is producing hamstring tendinosis with severe focal tenderness at the insertion of the biceps femoris on the ischia. This condition is frequently mistaken for ischiogluteal bursitis, but it is more correctly a painful gait-related enthesiopathy, and MRI of the pelvis or thigh will show the elevated T2 signal in the myotendinous junction and muscle. This condition may be notable on ultrasound evaluation as well.

While both patients are diagnosed as having spinal stenosis, the substantially differing clinical presentations show plainly that for diagnosis, the devil is in the details. Just as the epidemiologic detritus that is ICD-10 coding lacks clinical relevance because it omits tools to coherently link pathophysiology and anatomy, we can neither consider sensibly nor plan spinal diagnostics articulately without understanding these linked pain processes. Addressing only the most severe presenting complaint that is the result of several concurrent painful processes often misleads the physician, who must learn to solve the Rubik's cube in sequence. Hence, haphazard "What you see is what you treat" or "one-off" approaches to diagnosis are seldom optimal and an algorithmic approach is far superior.

It is helpful when planning spinal diagnosis to be able to broadly classify painful disorders based on the clinical and structural origin of pain. While the International Association for the Study of Pain classifications for pain and headache span many pages, the busy clinician needs a simpler, more rugged approach. Just as Swan and Ganz revolutionized cardiology by dividing categories of heart failure so as to be able to manage each subgroup more optimally, the model presented here also subdivides pain into categories with implications for diagnosis and management.[4]

Overlapping Lumbosacral Pathoanatomical Subsets–A Clinical Model

An operational model of lumbosacral pain is presented in Figure 5.1 to allow categorization of the various mechanisms of pain production for common sources of pain in the lumbosacral (L/S) spine. (The model was developed for the L/S spine because L/S pain is the most common pain complaint seen, but with some modification, similar models could be produced for cervical or thoracic pain.) Also, progressive transitions are allowed to occur between quadrants, when, for example, progressive stenosis or disk herniation produces radiculopathy or when injury to the facet joints leads to instability and injury to the

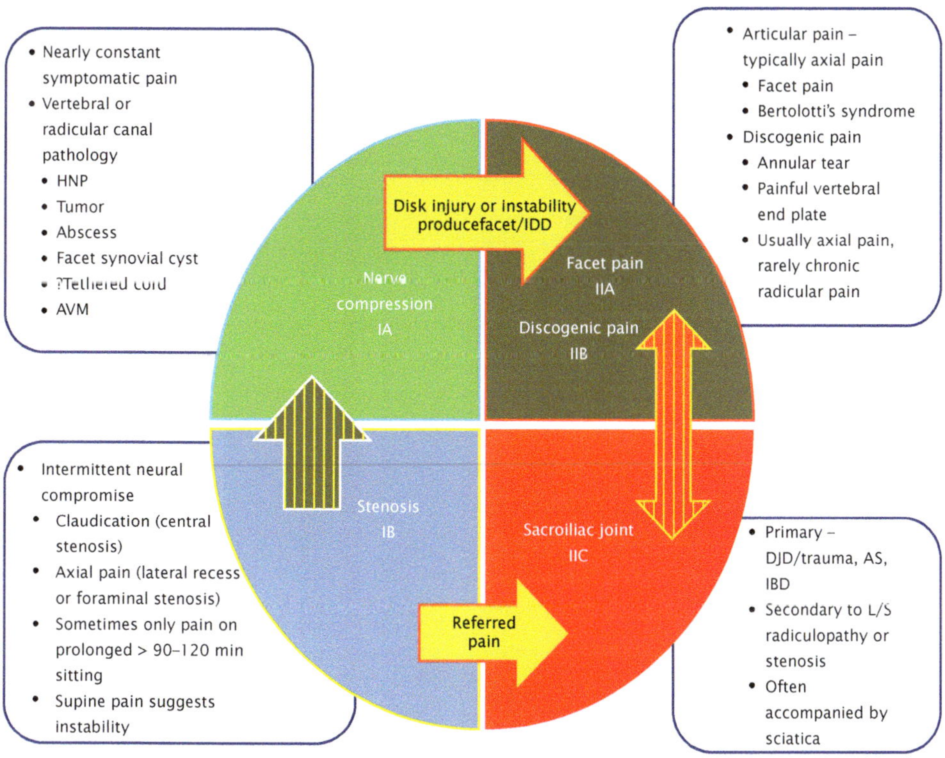

FIGURE 5.1. Model of lumbar spine pain grouped into overlapping pathoanatomical subsets and showing examples of possible coexisting pain disorders with pathophysiologic/clinical transitions. Copyright J. D. Petersohn, MD. 2018. Used with permission of the author.

intervertebral disk, resulting in facet hypertrophy, mechanical overload, loss of disk height, proliferation of hypertrophic facet capsule, and progressive foraminal and lateral recess stenosis. Changes in the mechanics of the lumbar spine alter sacral loading and sagittal balance, producing sacroiliac joint (SIJ) pain. Thus, alteration in one subset (or compartment) may produce change in the function of another subset. Multiple causes of pain can coexist in this model, and transitions or progressions of pain can be artfully considered. The advantages of using this model are that it provides a classification system that is functionally helpful to the interventional physician in the development of a differential diagnosis and that it guides the intelligent selection of spinal diagnostic targets that allow the physician to fully understand the structures producing pain. In cases where surgery is not clearly indicated, when a patient returns to the office after a diagnostic or therapeutic procedure and the physician has no idea what structures to evaluate or where to seek the likely cause of residual pain, this model provides a path and a cognitive framework for understanding the other causes of pain that should be considered.

The model divides painful disorders of the spine and spinal nerves clinically into two general groups. Group I is composed of processes that compromise spinal neural function, producing predominantly neuropathic pain, and Group II is composed of processes with pain due to disorders of the mechanical function and articular elements of the spine and related structures. Group I is further subdivided into Group IA, disorders involving constant compromise of neural function, and Group IB, disorders with intermittent compromise of neural function. Group II's painful disorders are subdivided by the primary spinal articular structures: Group IIA, the intervertebral disk; Group IIB, the zygapophysial, atlantoaxial, and atlanto-occipital joints; and Group IIC, the sacroiliac joints as well as other extraspinal articular structures.

This model is deliberately constructed to allow painful spinal disorders to involve more than one group. For example, disk herniation might be classified as IA or IB, or a facet synovial cyst might be considered IIB, but the pain produced is typically radicular and intermittent, by compression of a spinal nerve root, making it a IB pain disorder, or, if the pain is constant, IA. Similarly, epidural scarring or multiple sclerosis would be considered to belong in Group IA.

With the focus on the pathophysiology of pain, space-occupying lesions, whether hypertrophic facet, ligamentum flavum thickening, facet synovial cyst, or disk herniation, have similar mass effects or restriction of neural movement that produces neural pain, but to approach the diagnosis, we must consider the specific structure that is producing the pain.

Mechanical microinstability can be a source for transition between facet and intervertebral disk pain processes (as well as for production of facet synovial cysts). Injuries can produce coexisting disorders in several subclasses. Facet pain often accompanies spinal stenosis and sacroiliac joint pain often accompanies facet pain.

The schema establishes rules for transitions between the diagnostic subset quadrants based upon known pathophysiology—and only three possible transitions apply in the example above.

The model allows for L/S radicular pain to be "referred" to the SIJ complex.

While all extraspinal articular sources of L/S pain could fall into class IIIC, only SIJ pain is relevant to this chapter.

To use the model, the clinical pain disorders are first divided into Group I disorders, involving myelopathy, radiculopathy, or neuropathic pain, and Group II, mechanical disorders. A differential diagnosis of disorders in Group I is pursued first, based on history, physical examination, imaging, and occasionally electrodiagnostics. If clinical myelopathy is evidenced, no spinal diagnostic injection procedures are usually necessary, although there are autoimmune, toxic, endocrine, and metabolic disorders producing clinical findings that mimic myelopathy. Specifically, with evidence of symptomatic spinal cord compression, spinal diagnostic injections should be avoided, because they could worsen the condition by increasing, even transiently, local pressure upon the compressed area of the spinal cord.

In circumstances where compression of the spinal cord is reported on MRI imaging, however, the study should be carefully reviewed for evidence of myelomalacia in the area of reported compression, and if there is no myelomalacia and no long-tract neurologic abnormalities are found on examination, low-volume nerve root injections, as described below, may be considered to evaluate or treat radiculopathy.

This model addresses the sequencing of the process of spinal diagnostics: Processes in Group IA are addressed first, and those in Group IB second. Group II disorders are then addressed in the sequence of facet disorders, SIJ disorders and discogenic pain, based upon the incidence of these disorders and the greater complexity and risks associated with evaluation of primary discogenic pain using provocative diskography. Radicular pain due to a disk herniation is a Group I disorder, and diagnostic provocative diskography is rarely required for affirmative diagnosis, although the author has seen several patients with small annular tears of the intervertebral disk adjacent to the dorsal root ganglion producing radicular pain without obvious compression of the ganglion or exiting nerve root.

As already mentioned, similar models can be constructed for cervical and thoracic spinal pain, but they are not delineated here.

The Confounders

Many pain processes or complaints do not present in isolation. Common confounders, pairs (dyads) or triads of clinical pain presentation, include:

- Headache, shoulder, and cervical pain of zygapophysial joint and/or radicular origin
- Cervical radiculopathy and shoulder pain
- Neurocompressive peripheral pain thought to be due to ulnar or median nerve disorders with cervical pain due to HNP (herniated nucleus pulposus) or stenosis
- Meralgia paresthetica due to compression or traction of the lateral femoral cutaneous nerve at the inguinal ligament (this seldom results from more proximal putative sites of neural compromise)
- Cervical radiculopathy due to traction of the lower cervical nerve roots or the brachial plexus in flexion-extension (whiplash) injuries
- Cervicalgia due to lumbar or thoracolumbar zygaphophysial (facet) pain

- Cervical radiculopathy and referred dorsal medial scapular, thoracic, or anterior pectoral pain
- Extra-articular hip pain due to compensatory gait with primary lumbar spine pain, including radiculopathy, facet pain, or SIJ pain
- Pain in the thigh, perineum, or testicle due to gait alteration, especially with adductor weakness or lumbar radiculopathy
- SIJ pain manifesting after treatment of lumbar facet pain or lumbar fusion surgery
- Subacute presentation of spinal facet pain adjacent to levels after spinal fusion.
- Painful abnormal gait (anterior glide syndrome) with gluteus medius, adductor longus, medial gastrocnemius, and tibialis anterior tenosynovitis and/or motor deficits due to SIJ pain.
- Sacroiliac and hip pain co-presenting
- Severe abdominal pain due to ACNES (abdominal cutaneous nerve entrapment syndrome) pain and thoracic facet pain
- Coexisting cervical or lumbar radiculopathy due to disk herniation or stenosis, with coexisting cervical or lumbar zygapophysial joint pain.
- Lumbar radiculopathy and referred SIJ pain
- Dorsal thigh pain and lumbar radiculopathy due to spinal stenosis with ischiogluteal bursitis and/or proximal biceps femoris tendinosis

This list is not designed to be exhaustive, only to be illustrative of common overlapping clinical presentations that must be routinely discerned, scrutinized, discriminated, and treated by clinicians. Moreover, it is a warning to readers that there are few original clinical presentations of pain, and many clinical presentations are resolvable if an algorithmic approach is followed.

The ultimate purpose of this model of spinal pain processes is to facilitate the next step, an intellectually rigorous formulation of a sequential recursive diagnostic algorithm for each subset of pain, or if the reader prefers, a clinical rubric for diagnosis, stepping sequentially through the categories of pain production based on their identified anatomical subsets.

As a general hierarchy of concerns, the algorithmic model seeks to affirm and treat Group I disorders first; after exclusion of myelopathy on clinical and imaging grounds, radiculopathies are evaluated because they are common, generally have localized determinants identifiable on examination that can be correlated with imaging studies, and typically are responsive to treatment. Only after radiculopathies are addressed does the algorithm consider common axial pain syndromes, including zygapophysial facet pain, and last, it addresses the nociceptive roles of SIJ and discogenic or vertebrogenic pain.

It is fundamentally important for the reader to keep in mind that some diagnostic procedures also provide substantial therapeutic utility; for example, addressing a symptomatic radiculopathy with a diagnostic selective nerve root injection not only affirms the diagnosis but also resolves an identified radiculopathy. However, meaningful improvement in an identified radiculopathy may produce sufficient alteration in posture or increased range of motion of the adjacent spinal segments so as to elicit new radiculopathic findings at an adjacent nerve level that were clearly not present clinically at the time of initial evaluation. This phenomenon is neither a poor outcome nor a complication. Far more common that one might expect, this phenomenon may account for almost a third of overall "failed" responses to injections, based on the author's experience. In a clinical context, the patient returns for followup after a nerve root injection, grievingly noting that they are clinically unimproved or worsened, and grimly bearing the assumption that the diagnosis was wrong, or the intervention was ineffective. In the worst case, the patient erroneously concludes that injury was caused by a diagnostic procedure. Physical examination should be performed to document resolution or residual of the previously treated radiculopathy, including motor deficits, and it may demonstrate new physical findings that recommend additional targets to be addressed for precise diagnosis and successful treatment of the patient.

A similar phenomenon can occur after surgery, where a coexisting but unrecognized cause of pain precipitates a "poor" surgical result. Surgeons are blamed, patients are frustrated, and insurers redouble their efforts to avoid paying for surgical procedures due to the perceived unsatisfactory outcomes. Unfortunately, most of the pain and surgical literature reporting treatment outcomes seldom dives deep enough to identify patients who have enjoyed successful improvement in pain produced by the index structure that was addressed, but whose pain now originates elsewhere. The notion common in clinical practice that a diagnosis made at one point in time is applicable forever is clearly rubbish. We often fail to consider that the patient continues to lack complete pain relief due to exposure or identification of other sources of pain. Often, the collateral source of pain may not require the surgeon's skills for treatment, but absent timely reexamination and referral for spinal diagnostics, the patient remains miserable, and the surgeon, culpable.

Following successful treatment of a facet pain process with radiofrequency (RF) lesioning, it is not at all uncommon that an adjacent facet joint level or the SIJ is found to become symptomatic, necessitating a return to the diagnostic algorithm to determine the anatomical cause and to plan additional treatment. Professional humility and diagnostic curiosity are required, and the infallible physician or surgeon is soon brought to task.

While our internal medicine colleagues have no apparent difficulty conceiving that a patient can have multiple coexisting diagnoses, such as heart failure, hypertension, diabetes, and hypothyroidism, when I forwarded this observation to a hardened physician employed to guard against inappropriate utilization of resources by other physicians on the behalf a major insurance company, I was told that the comparison was unfair. I submit that the only unfairness is to the patient, when we do not appreciate the limiting parallels of our own reasoning processes.

While experienced physicians often skip steps in an algorithm, the habit of accurate diagnosis is only acquired by repetition of simple steps, and cautionary rigor is merited.

The Diagnostic Algorithm

While it is not that only rubric that might be followed, this diagnostic algorithm has been crafted and molded over three decades by the author and countless residents, fellows, and colleagues. It may be viewed as a dynamic plan, and it will be subject to modification over time. There are six basic steps:

1. History and physical examination
2. Optional conservative care
3. Advanced imaging and formulation of the differential diagnosis of pain
4. Achieving clinical coherence using focused reexamination to refine the diagnosis
5. Planning and execution of spinal diagnostic/therapeutic interventions
6. Reevaluation, reexamination, and reconsideration, with return to Step 3 or 4, as necessary.

Step 1: Thorough History and Meticulous Physical Examination

The components of the medical history need not be enumerated here. As for the physical examination, it need not be exhaustive, but it should be meticulous. The following recommendations are offered as a guideline and should not be considered to be a standard of care:

The neurological examination includes observation of stance, gait, abnormal seated posture, and facility in arising to stand or in changing positions on an exam table.

Motor power should be examined with specific consideration of the neural origin of muscular innervation:

C4 = rhomboid
C5 = shoulder abduction
C6 = biceps or pincer grasp
C7 = triceps, resisted forearm pronation
C8 = digit span
T1 = hand intrinsics
L1, L2 = hip flexors
L3= thigh adduction
L4 = quadriceps
L5 = ankle dorsiflexion
S1 = EHL (extensor hallucis longus) or knee flexors

In evaluation of motor power, the resistance offered by the examiner should not be minimal and time must be taken for each muscle group to be tested, with more than several seconds required while the examiner provides progressively graduated resistance to the patient's voluntarily generated and increasing muscle power. While it is well understood that many muscles have innervation from multiple spinal nerve roots, these maneuvers generally provide adequate differentiation to allow addressing one or perhaps two specific nerve roots. In examination of the biceps or triceps, it is important to place the elbow adjacent to the flank and for it to remain there during these maneuvers. Patients usually want to please the examiner, but for diagnosis, it is important to avoid the patient's succeeding by rotation of the forearm at the elbow as this recruits muscle groups with disparate innervation and reduces the anatomical specificity of the examination maneuver. Similar to the maximal force EMG, this clinical examination technique is sensitive for radiculopathy and is the very efficient bedside clinical equivalent.

The effective use of these maneuvers can virtually eliminate the need for EMG; it has done so in the author's practice. The key is in the provision of adequate and gradually increased resistance. Maximal resistance in upper extremity examination may be offered at approximately 10 to 15 lbs in pincer grasp, but it may be 20 to 40 lbs in biceps or triceps resistance. In the lower extremities, resistance offered may be typically 25 to 60 lbs. The resistance provided should be adjusted depending on the specific muscle group examined, muscle bulk, and fitness of the individual. The examiner should be aware of the examinee's hand dominance, but clinical experience and familiarity are required to judge how much weakness constitutes expectable asymmetry due to handedness when assessing a motor deficit. Caution, gentleness, and reduced force are sensible when examining frail or osteoporotic patients or sites of recent fracture or injury. Repeated motor power maneuvers may demonstrate fade in cases of symptomatic radiculopathy where the initial examination of motor power suggests only an equivocal finding.

Sensory examination may use a pin or toothpick, but a Wartenburg pinwheel is useful. Routine two-point sensory discrimination testing is not generally necessary.

Cranial nerve examination is generally unnecessary, except if there is concern about primary intracranial disorders.

Nerve compression and tension tests including Spurling's, straight leg raise, Bakody, and femoral stretch (reverse nerve tension tests) as well as lumbar lateral bending; these should be performed as necessary.

A search for pathologic Hoffman or Babinski reflex, ankle clonus, or abnormal tandem gait may be employed if clinical myelopathy is suspected.

For orthopedic examination of affected regions, whether spinal or peripheral joints, in addition to range of motion, visual inspection, joint palpation, and usual orthopedic tests appropriate for the painful structure, at least one joint both more proximal and distal to the painful structure merits examination, if possible. Description of the maneuvers may be found in major textbooks.

In the spine, palpation of dorsal spinous processes and facets as well as the paraspinal muscles is useful. In the thorax, palpation of the ribs with medially directed pressure on individual ribs in the midaxillary line may be helpful in identification and localization of a thoracic radiculopathy, with tenderness also notable in some circumstance not only at the interspace but at individual sternocostal joints. Finding of crepitance, give way, shift, or step-off can be recorded.

Palpation should be performed in a systematic fashion, with uniform pressure over one spinal or peripheral joint, interspace, dorsal spinous process, or rib at a time or as may be required, then sequentially over the entire length of the joint, and this process should not be "unduly hurried. The examiner should attempt to enumerate the areas of tenderness and specifically note whether the tenderness is focal or diffuse. In enumerating cervical facet joints, the patient examined with the head placed in anatomical position with the physician standing to the patient's side. A horizontal line is drawn extending posteriorly from the retromandibular angle and a vertical line is drawn descending from the mastoid process, with the point of intersection overlying the C2–C3 facet. Subsequent facet joints can be roughly enumerated at subsequent thumb's breadth distally.

The SIJ should be examined using multiple maneuvers,[5,6] but a recent article reported a lack of correlation of SIJ pain determined using multiple maneuvers with the results of SIJ injection.[7] This circumstance occurs clinically, and in some circumstances, performance of diagnostic lateral sacral branch is affirmative. Falowski et al published a useful review of techniques.[8]

The examination may be extended to other organ systems at the examiner's discretion.

It is at this point that the physician must decide if there is a reasonable likelihood of the presence of a radicular pain process. It is important to remember that radicular pain processes often produce axial pain, including headache and axial low back pain. The notion that a diagnosis of radiculopathy requires pain in the extremity or in the distal distribution of the dermatome is incorrect. Similarly, the term *sciatica* has been appropriated to mean any pain at or distal to the hip, losing its original meaning in the process.

Step 2: Conservative Care versus Diagnostic Imaging

Depending upon the clinical severity and magnitude of both physical findings and functional impact of pain, a course of conservative care may be elected prior to advanced imaging. Insurer medical protocols routinely deny payment for imaging other than plain radiographs upon initial presentation absent a patient presenting *in extremis*, but it seems uniquely odd that radiologists with limited postgraduate bedside experience act as the arbiters of appropriate timing for advanced imaging.

In the presence of severe pain, marked functional weakness that renders an individual functionally limited in activities of self-care, or in individuals in whom weakness substantially limits ambulation or poses significant risk of tripping or falling, delay for conservative care strategies is often inappropriate. Rehabilitation can be addressed following more expeditious advanced diagnosis and treatment steps in these patients.

Patients exhibiting a clinical picture consistent with serious systemic illness, infection, acute vascular conditions, endocrine disorders, neurologic events, fracture, or malignancy, among other disorders, should urgently bypass the rationing protocols and be promptly imaged or emergently routed to appropriate colleagues for further evaluation. Parturients merit special concern and should generally be comanaged with the obstetrician.

When conservative care is elected, D. J. Kennedy, Chair of Physical Medicine and Rehabilitation at Vanderbilt University, researched extensively the basis for determining 6 weeks to be the adequate or optimal duration for conservative, noninterventional, and nonoperative care, and found no actual research to substantiate this common protocol. In the absence of robust data, recommendations for conservative care as embodied in textbooks and in policies from CMMS and insurers may simply promulgate wasteful historical practice patterns. For pathologies like facet pain or sacroiliac joint pain, there exists only an abyss of evidence for the clinical success of conservative care, such as physiotherapy, chiropractic, or NSAID administration.

It must be acknowledged that routine advanced imaging and speedy evaluation of all patients by a limited number of interventional physicians would be burdensome, not to mention professionally exhausting. Unfortunately, early identification of patients unlikely to benefit from conservative efforts remains challenging, and decisions to escalate care are typically based upon a default gestalt of clinical urgency, progression of symptoms, or lack of progress with a conservative regimen. There is low quality evidence supporting selection strategies that require patients to demonstrate failure to improve with multiple classes of medications or with multiple conservative modalities.

Step 3: Advanced Diagnostic Imaging

The preferred imaging modality of choice for spinal pain or headache is MRI after plain radiographs. Period.

While this author favors ordering cervical or lumbar x-rays with flexion and extension studies performed upon initial examination, dynamic views can be initially deferred and are sometimes only completed as a predicate to surgery. The diagnostic yield of dynamic x-rays remains modest, but the findings can significantly alter treatment and they should certainly not be forgotten. When reviewing dynamic x-rays, a search must be made for both translational instability and angular instability; the latter is more common in the lower lumbar spine and may merit anterior column stabilization. In the lumbar spine, the addition of a Ferguson view (AP beam angled cephalad by 15°–20°) is useful for identifying transitional L/S anatomy, a common source of pathology in patients with low back pain, but unfortunately, this view is not at all useful for understanding SIJ pathology, the rationale originally given for its use.[9]

Protocols used for MRI vary by institution, differing significantly in the specific imaging planes scanned and in the orientation of image slices. The algorithm described herein uses a coronal T1 scout for spine imaging and insists that axial images be oriented strictly orthogonal to the T1 scout image axis, with adjacent slice thickness of no more than 2.5 mm, and with imaging from each vertebral endplate across each disk space to the adjacent vertebral endplate. T2 images better reflect differences in tissue composition and make visualization of nerve structures easier to review than on T1 images. While some physicians prefer stacked axial images, these become difficult to interpret in spinal regions with significant kyphosis or lordosis, due the increased angulation between the plane of imaging and the axial plane of the disk space. Sagittal slice thickness is often defaulted to 4 mm or greater, obscuring the detail of the nerve roots adjacent to the cervical uncovertebral joints and proximal foramen in the cervical spine and in the lumbar spine, defeating attempts to view the lateral recesses, foramen or far lateral regions where focal neural impingement is common and also in the neural foramen just distal to the dorsal root ganglion. A 3-mm sagittal slice thickness is recommended with both T1 and T2 sequences. T1 images may be more useful when evaluating foraminal apertures. For patients with lumbar spinal stenosis, the pillow used to elevate the knees for patient comfort may be eliminated, as the resulting lumbar flexion likely enlarges the AP dimension of the vertebral canal, providing a false reassurance of the narrowed vertebral canal volume.

The literature reports discrepancies of 30% or more between initial radiology reading and radiologists rereading MRI studies or when neurosurgeons or orthopedic surgeons review studies after radiology interpretation.[10] Many radiologic findings specifically relevant to surgical and interventional planning, including Tarlov cysts, facet synovial cysts, hypertrophic facet joint capsules, deviations of normal nerve root position within the neural foramen, far lateral disk herniations, or vascular abnormalities, such as vertebral artery loops, are not routinely included in official radiology reports and interventional physicians and surgeons should strongly consider routine reading of all their patient's imaging studies.

Specific indications for performance of MRI sequences using a gadolinium-based contrast agent include a differential diagnosis of epidural scar or tumor, but with recent information regarding potential gadolinium toxicity with accumulation of the element in brain tissue, especially in patients with renal disease, discretion in the use of gadolinium-containing MRI contrast agents should be exercised. Free gadolinium is a competitive inhibitor of Ca^{2+}, so that the element binds to organic structures and can interfere with normal biological processes. Two general structural classes of gadolinium contrast are commercially available, linear and macrocyclic, with the former associated with significant deposition of gadolinium in the dentate nucleus; hence, linear agents should be avoided in pain imaging except where allergy or intolerance is demonstrated.[11] If a malignant process is considered, PET scanning may be considered.

Patients having implanted devices, including pacemakers and spinal cord stimulators, or those with retained fragments of ferrous metals, may have significant risk of unwanted thermal heating or theoretical electrical current induction within the strong magnetic and rapidly alternating radiofrequency fields of the MRI unit, hazards that can contraindicate MRI scanning. In these patients, CT scanning is generally useful. Certain FDA-conditional approvals for MRI imaging of patients with implanted devices require special software for imaging that may not be widely available, and again, CT is an alternative. Sagittal CT sections with both bone and soft tissue windows are usually required for the spine. When considering a diagnosis of cervical spondylosis or stenosis, use of a reduced 10-cm window size with thin 1-mm thick serial cuts in 45° left and right anterior oblique planes will easily demonstrate focal foraminal stenosis or uncovertebral pathology less apparent on conventional sagittal or axial planes, especially if thick or poorly aligned slices are used.

When selecting imaging parameters, keep in mind that traditional sagittal, axial, and coronal planes are artifacts of standard anatomy that may be less relevant to the articular structures to be examined and consider using nonstandard imaging planes that may be more helpful for diagnosis. This is especially relevant in patients with scoliosis.

While reformatted CT images can be expeditiously generated on a workstation using the acquired CT data set, use of additional oblique or nonstandard MRI imaging planes will increase total MRI scan time somewhat. However, the added value of precise anatomical information to the surgical specialist and interventionalist may be quite significant. In evaluation of cervical spondylitic stenosis, reformatted images in 45° anterior oblique planes that are approximately orthogonal to the radicular canal make visualization of the anatomy easier than in review of the typical coronal/sagittal/axial views.

When viewing the SIJ, oblique coronal plane views are helpful because the auricular joint form is not easily visualized in coronal or sagittal planes.

In reviewing the imaging studies, the interventional physician should take a systematic and sequential approach to make certain that all aspects of the imaging study are considered, but symptomatic pathologies in the lateral recess and neural foramina, including disk protrusions, ligamentum flavum hypertrophy, and facet hypertrophy, are sometimes missed on axial images, and neural impingement of clinical relevance is frequently noted on sagittal views. Far lateral disk herniations are very frequently missed on axial views, but many are not symptomatic. Regarding all radiographic studies, Tim Maus of the Department of Radiology at the Mayo Clinic fondly admonishes, "Do not fall in love with the lesion," reminding us to diligently look at all aspects of the study, in order to avoid overlooking serious conditions, such as a bone marrow finding consistent with multiple myeloma or prostate cancer, when pursuing a more obvious focal disk herniation.

While "Bristol" and "ship shape" describe maritime seaworthiness, radiology reports seldom include reassuring quality metrics. Despite the North American Spine Society's calling for removal of 0.3T MRI units from clinical practice over a decade ago, these machines remain in clinical use, despite their poor image quality. Unfortunately, radiology facilities apply no uniform standard to describe the diagnostic quality of each clinical imaging study in routine practice, and facility accreditation standards largely reflect safety concerns, not the clinical usefulness of studies. While large radiology groups often agree on the descriptive terminology that will be used for spinal imaging, compliance among individual radiologists varies. Images obtained on open 0.6T MRI units may be adequate in younger patients, but they tend to be less detailed than 1.5 or 3.0T closed-unit studies, and often the 0.6T studies are of lesser diagnostic utility in older patients with degenerative or spondylitic anatomy. Many centers do not routinely redo defective or technically inadequate studies automatically; however, most conscientious facilities will recall the patient for additional imaging sequences when requested by the ordering physician. Radiology interpretations seldom point out what may be obscured in poor-quality studies except where concerns for malignancy or occult pathology motivates the recommendation for additional or follow-up imaging. Facilities or radiologists routinely reporting disk pathology at many levels or compression of the thecal sac at many levels in patients without grossly stenotic findings or obviously short pedicles should be flagged for careful scrutiny by the reviewing physician. A consulting diagnostic radiologist should be chosen as carefully as one would choose an associate to hire.

Traditionally, the imaging of spinal nerves is based upon visualized water content of anatomical structures immediately adjacent to a nerve, such as disk, fat, or CSF. MRI neurography provides high-resolution images of the spinal nerves based upon the intraneural water flow of the nerve itself.[12,13] The mathematical algorithms used are similar to those developed for tractography and diffusion tensor imaging used in brain imaging. Of course, the techniques are familiar to anyone who has completed at least three semesters of calculus and two semesters of differential equations and has a passing familiarity with fast Fourier transforms, Runge-Kutta methods, and Poisson's equation. While MRI neurography is used in evaluation of peripheral nerve and plexus disorders, it is an emerging technology that may prove diagnostically useful for spinal disorders because it may be helpful in identifying focal areas of neural compromise or inflammation that are simply "invisible" to the typically used MRI protocols. This modality typically requires an expensive supplemental special software package. While plexus imaging may be performed with a 1.5T unit, a 3.0T MRI unit would be more appropriate for spinal nerve imaging. The availability of this technique is limited, but it may be found in larger research university practices.

CT myelogram can be useful if instability, symptomatic pseudobulging, or radiculopathy is suspected or for surgical planning, especially where spondylolysis is present or calcifications of ligaments, tumors, or disk structures are considered. Extensive aortoiliac calcification may indicate needed preoperative cardiovascular evaluation due to the substantial epidemiologic association of cardiac and peripheral vascular disorders.

Last, for visualization of peripheral nerves or large joints, there is an expanding role for use of ultrasound imaging, which may be advantageous in allowing dynamic imaging of multiple structures that may inform diagnosis. Unfortunately, bone reflects ultrasound, so that peripheral causes of spinal pain may be artfully evaluated with ultrasound, but ultrasound is seldom useful for spinal diagnosis. Not all institutions have individuals skilled in diagnostic musculoskeletal or peripheral nerve ultrasound examination, but this modality is likely to become increasingly useful in the future. Ideally, the trend toward incorporation of ultrasound-guided injection techniques will improve the utilization and sophistication of diagnostic ultrasound as well.

At this point, the first step of our cognitive diagnostic process occurs, the assembly of a lengthy differential diagnosis for possible causes of pain compatible with 1) the clinical complaint, 2) the clinical history, and 3) potential causes of neural pathology. The list should routinely include disk herniation or stenotic pathology identified in the central canal, lateral recess, foramina, or far lateral spaces. Potential causes for pain of radicular origin are also considered, including causes of compression of the spinal cord or nerve roots as well as instability or spinal deformity.

In the absence of a primary neurologic process, such as radiculopathy of any origin, including symptomatic spinal stenosis, postlaminectomy epidural scarring, disk herniation, or the diagnosis of a focal peripheral neuropathy, including so-called tunnel syndromes identified on imaging, a differential diagnosis of primary orthopedic causes of pain originating in the facet joints, shoulder, hip, knee, or SIJ can be formulated.

Step 4: Testing the Differential Diagnosis

At this point, after the formulation of a first pass at a differential diagnosis based upon, and consistent with, the clinical history and the anatomy as demonstrated by the MRI or CT images, the patient can be artfully examined. A very specific and directed physical examination is performed to assess the patient for the focal orthopedic and neurologic findings that support or exclude items on the differential diagnosis. The examination includes detailed neurologic examination and the focal neurologic or regional orthopedic maneuvers relevant to affirm or rule out each diagnosis.

It is at this stage, for example, that a small C5–C6 disk herniation lacking affirmative correlative motor or sensory deficits and a negative Spurling's maneuver is pushed lower on the differential diagnosis as a potential source of pain. When painless weakness of resisted shoulder abduction is demonstrated, absent biceps or pincer grip weakness, the imaging may be reexamined. While the search for pathology affecting the C5 nerve root on the imaging study is appropriate, the sensitivity of imaging is limited such that, and a physician who is confident in their examination shoulder consider proceeding to address the putative C5 pathology. With negative Jobe's, Neer, O'Brien, or drop-arm maneuvers arguing against a primary orthopedic shoulder articular pathology, the negative findings support a concern for radiculopathy. While there is a possibility of an aberrant C5 spinal cord rootlet emerging within the C6 nerve root sleeve, a common anatomical variation that is not found on routine imaging, but only at autopsy, the interventional physician might reasonably choose to address both the C5 and C6 nerve roots.

Isolated ankle dorsiflexion weakness represents a special case in the setting of SIJ tenderness, and sacroiliac provocative maneuvers are often helpful in discriminating L5 radiculopathy from a true SIJ pain process. As an aside, it is my frequent finding that a FABER maneuver is often positive in L5 radiculopathies, but when additional confirmatory SIJ tests are negative, it is my practice to address the sacroiliac joint first.

Step 5: Planning the Intervention

Interventional diagnostic techniques are selected based upon the identified pathology.

Radicular pain of any cause is addressed with selective nerve root block.

With peripheral nerve pain due to neural compression or traction, while traditional regional anesthesia techniques can be considered, they often require very large volumes of injected local anesthetic and consideration should be given to ultrasound-guided nerve block.

Facet pain—most typically at one or two levels only, not infrequently bilateral—can be addressed with diagnostic medial branch block using local anesthetic only. Only infrequently does facet pain present clinically at more than two adjacent levels, although it may present at the junctional levels both above and below areas of surgically or congenitally fused (non-segmented or transitional) spinal anatomy.

With large-joint articular pain, consideration can be given to intraarticular joint injection, typically with local anesthetic and steroid. Given the paucity of nerve fibers within articular cartilage and vastly predominant sensory innervation of the joint capsule, approaches anesthetizing specific articular nerves containing the afferent sensory nerve branches may be considered for diagnostic purposes.

The intervertebral disk is addressed with diagnostic diskography. While vertebral endplate pathology seen as Modic I or II changes on MRI has been shown to indicate vertebrogenic origin of pain, there is extensive dissenting literature regarding the clinical relevance of Modic changes. Readers are advised to follow the emerging literature.

Pressure-controlled diagnostic lumbar provocative diskography can be considered for identification of symptomatic "discogenic" pain. Post-discogram CT study may be quite helpful in revealing additional pathology, including focal HNP or spondylosis that produces radicular but not purely discogenic pain. There may be substantial overlap between discogenic and vertebrogenic pain and innervation; this remains an area for further investigation.

Step 5 concludes with performance of the planned diagnostic or therapeutic intervention.

Step 6: Clinical Reevaluation

A patient with substantially or completely resolved pain may be considered for entry into a functional rehabilitation program at the physician's discretion.

Clinical reevaluation after intervention is de rigeur and should never be omitted in patients with residual or recurrent pain.

If the patient is unimproved or incompletely improved, review of the operative report, the pattern of contrast dispersal, or the neurogram may evidence satisfactory procedural technique or identify suboptimal technique that merits repetition or even a modified approach.

If the anatomy underlying the pain process is determined at this point to be intractable or reprobate, surgical or minimally invasive options may be discussed, or appropriate referrals can be made, depending upon the training, skill set, and experience of the physician. Among the remaining unimproved or partially improved patients, the reexamined patient reenters the algorithm at Step 3, where a search is made first for new or residual radicular findings. It is appropriate to consider pain pathologies that may exist concurrently and those demonstrating interrelated pathophysiology so that the physical reexamination deliberately seeks these findings. The list of common dyads and triads in clinical pain may be of help. If no evidence for radiculopathy is present, zygapophysial joint etiologies are considered, and thereafter attention turns to SIJ pain and ultimately discogenic and vertebrogenic pain in accord with the model of pathoanatomical subsets. In patients with atypical anatomy, including scoliosis or transitional anatomy, additional steps to address these structures with diagnostic injections may be considered.

Repeat imaging studies are useful if a substantial time interval has elapsed, if surgery or minimally invasive procedures have been performed, or if significant interval trauma has occurred over the interval.

Rereading the original MRI/CT imaging study in Step 3 may identify abnormalities missed by the clinician (or the radiologist) on earlier review.

This concludes the six-step algorithm for diagnosis and the discussion turns to specific techniques used for spinal diagnosis.

Specific Spinal Diagnostic Injection Techniques

There are three general classes of diagnostic injection techniques to be considered for evaluation of spinal pain:

1. Epidural injections—typically transforaminal technique
2. Diagnostic medial branch blocks
3. Specialized articular injections, including intraarticular steroid, local anesthetic, or contrast, as well as diagnostic provocative diskography

A fourth category of more obscure and technically demanding injections, including atlantoaxial and atlanto-occipital joint and C2 ventral plexus blocks, are not detailed here.

Epidural Injections

Epidural injections are among the most common interventions performed by interventional pain physicians; however, there is vast variation in the technique, the drugs used, and the volume of injection. It should be apparent that any diagnostic technique should have a substantial degree of both face validity and construct validity. It goes without saying that spinal diagnostic procedures must be performed under imaging guidance, typically fluoroscopy, to be anatomically validated with injection of a contrast agent documenting the approximate spread of a precisely measured volume of injectate. Fluoroscopic images should be retained for good documentation practice as well as for reimbursement. Furman's text may be a useful guide for mastering these techniques.[14]

Steroids provide short-term suppression of the focal hyperexcitability of the neural membrane. Period.

Controversies remain about whether steroid injections are appropriate for diagnosis or treatment of facet pain, for discogenic pain, or for postlaminectomy pain syndrome. Arguments based on data offer no more than weak support, although a vast body of meta-analysis and ample literature of questionable rigor can be plumbed to support such arguments.

For epidural injections to be clinically useful, anatomical specificity must prevail. To this end, injection of a liquid medication into the dorsal epidural space will typically flow cephalad and less often caudad, with the specific delivery of medication to the nerve root of interest depending upon the injection pressure and the intrinsic resistance to flow produced by tissues within the epidural space, including the presence of the dorsal median raphe. The flow resistance is highly variable and even with injection into the lumbar dorsal lateral recess, perfect confinement to a single nerve level is highly unlikely. For this reason, it is unreasonable to suggest that dorsal interlaminar epidural steroid injection or caudal epidural injection provides the necessary anatomical specificity for diagnosis.

The commonly preferred route that routinely provides focal targeting of injectate is the transforaminal technique, although a catheter introduced into the epidural space can be steered into to a single nerve root sleeve for injection. Somewhat more difficult to master than interlaminar techniques, the use of an oblique radiographic approach to place a needle at the inferior margin of the pedicle immediately above the nerve root of interest is now largely routine. In the circumstance especially common at the L5–S1 interspace, where the height and/or width of the intertransverse space is compromised, use of a double-needle technique with a slightly angled introducer and curved center-set needle can be required, and these sets are commercially available in both 18/20 and 20/25 gauge sets. Double-needle technique can also be useful where the L5–S1 facet is markedly hypertrophic and there is insufficient space lateral to the facet for the needle to follow a curvilinear path to the anatomical target. The specific needle-tip placement can be further optimized to deliver medication to the lateral recess, dorsal root ganglion, far lateral space, or the lateral recess at the level either above (most common) or below the interspace of injection. While some argue that the posterior foramen is a safer region to target than the anterior foramen, due to a lower likelihood of inadvertently injecting transforaminal arteries in the posterior foramen, most injections of contrast in the posterior foramen fail to provide the necessary anatomical specificity with a well-defined contrast flow pattern seen under fluoroscopy that confirms single-nerve anatomical targeting. A lack of precise targeting entirely defeats any rationale for a diagnostic injection procedure, and posterior epidural space injections are discouraged. If the physician elects to inject steroid, it is recommended that use of the nonparticulate steroid dexamethasone and subsequent meticulous removal of air from all syringes and tubing prior to injection is the best option.

Transforaminal epidural injections are also called selective nerve root injections, but, as discussed, the degree of selectivity demonstrated on contrast injection is imperfect and is affected by precise needle placement and both the volume and speed of injection. The benefit of using the term *selective nerve root injection* derives from the semantic advantage of linking the precise nerve that is the putative source of the pain with the same anatomical identifier for an anatomically specific procedure. Furthermore, epidural injections are usually labeled by the vertebral body above and below the foramen; hence, C5–C6 is at the neural foramen through which the C6 nerve passes. Reducing the nominative of the injected level to a single letter and one or two digits reduces the likelihood of a typographical error on a scheduling list omitting one or the other, such that the wrong neural foramen and injection of the incorrect nerve would be avoided. Last, since there are 8 pairs of cervical nerves, such that each nerve exits above the named pedicle, except for C8 which emerges between C7 and T1, all other nerves exit below the named pedicle; this facilitates correlation of the nerve injected with the expected neurologic picture not only for diagnosis, but subsequently when the patient is reevaluated after treatment, in the event of residual or recurrent pain.

The sensitivity and specificity of selective nerve root blocks vary with the operator's technique, and it may be useful to use contrast injected under continuous fluoroscopy to guide the volume of steroid and local anesthetic mixture to avoid a lack of specificity. In 2008, Yeom et al calculated, based upon 70% pain relief as indicative of satisfactory outcome, a 57% sensitivity, 86% specificity, positive predictive value of 77%, and negative predictive value of 71%, with lumbar selective nerve root block.[15] False positives were associated with contrast flow into the epidural space, and false negatives were due to insufficient volume, insufficient flow of the injectate, and epineural injection. While a more recent systematic review concluded there is limited evidence to support the use of selective nerve root block for surgical planning, this was primarily due to the paucity of published literature.[15] However, the utility of selective nerve root block as a diagnostic technique when it entirely resolves the patient's problem entirely may be far greater.

The contrast pain pattern seen under fluoroscopy is instructive, with vascular injection generally seen easily on continuous injection under live fluoroscopy or with digital subtraction (angiography). The extent of contrast spread achievable with a fixed volume of injection can be defined and documented at each nerve level using a calibrated syringe, with subsequent low-volume injection of local anesthetic with or without steroid. This volume is routinely less than 2 mL and may often be as little as 0.5 mL or less in the thoracic or cervical regions.

The physician should routinely obtain and retain fluoroscopic images in both AP and lateral views. Often, in the lumbar spine, 30° medial or lateral oblique images show the contrast filling in the medial or subpedicular nerve segment to advantage, with notation of filling deficits that are otherwise not observable. In the cervical spine, use of AP and oblique views is sufficient, and often focal filling defects are noted on these injections that affirm neural filling defects seen on other imaging studies, including HNP, severe foraminal stenosis, or uncovertebral spondylosis. Because CT myelography often does not deliver contrast to the neural foramen, the neurogram images may be useful for surgical planning, especially where foraminotomy is considered.

Before going further, it is worth warning the reader that the one scenario that cannot be artfully delineated by selective nerve root block is when a nerve is compromised both proximally in the lateral recess and distally in the neural foramen. Selective nerve root injection is very good at narrowing painful anatomy to a single nerve root, but it does not appear to discriminate where within a single spinal nerve root pain originates, and anatomical imaging must be carefully scrutinized to plan care in this circumstance.

Interpretation of single selective nerve root injection results for surgical planning where there is evidence of anatomical compromise at the injected nerve level on imaging, physical examination, or both, varies:

- When no contrast appears in the targeted anatomical region, unless severe compression is seen on MRI/CT or there is complete obstruction to contrast flow, the result is not further interpretable. The possibility of impalement of the needle tip in a fibrous structure or epineurium, a syringe swap, or a labeling error should also be considered.
- When there is no reduction in pain, with contrast demonstrating technically adequate placement, the level is considered to be non-nociceptive. In occasional cases of severe neural foraminal compression, this result may be a false negative.
- With a 1- to 2-day reduction in pain as an affirmative response to local anesthetic alone, the brevity of response demonstrates nonresponsiveness to steroid and suggests a structural basis for recurring radiculopathy, such as severe compression or impingement.
- A 2- to 3-day reduction in pain may suggest a partial response at an adjacent nerve level, and indicates there should be repeat low-volume injection for confirmation. It often suggests a limited effect with symptoms originating at an adjacent nerve level.
- Five to ten days of affirmative response, with limited duration of the affirmative response to injection, suggest a role for surgical decompression by open or endoscopic technique.
- For patients experiencing more than 10 days of clinically substantial pain relief, it is the author's practice to offer one repeat injection if the pain returns in less than 6 weeks, but if durable improvement exceeding 4 to 6 months cannot be obtained, full consideration of other sources of pain is made using the algorithm. If no other source of pain is identified and in the presence of a persisting or repeatedly inducible neurologic defect, surgical intervention, typically decompression by direct open surgical or endoscopic technique or by indirect means with use of an

intervertebral spacer device, is offered. Evidence of present or incipient instability, including scoliosis, may recommend consideration for fusion.
- When affirmative response to steroid-containing injection exceeds 10 days, the durability of response should dictate the next steps, if any.

Medial Branch Blocks

We are fortunate to benefit from the 2020 "Consensus Practice Guidelines on Interventions for Lumbar Facet Joint Pain from a Multispecialty, International Working Group" and its discussion of medial branch blocks by Cohen et al.[16] Except for research studies, the recommendations affirmed use of single, anatomically targeted, low-volume local anesthetic nerve blocks for routine practice. While the addition of steroid to the local anesthetic was not prohibited, facet pain is not known to be a neuropraxic or primary neurologic disorder, and the rationale for consideration of the addition of steroid was not specified, but it may reflect the variability of practice patterns and may not be the product of any underlying science.

In 2020, Manchikanti et al published "Comprehensive Evidence-Based Guidelines for Facet Joint Interventions in the Management of Chronic Spinal Pain: American Society of Interventional Pain Physicians (ASIPP) Guidelines."[17] While this lengthy article affirmed moderate or strong evidence for the success of facet interventions, the extensive meta-analysis instructively catalogs a wide range of outcomes and wide variation in the calculated positive predictive values for these interventions. No reviewed source papers comprehensively reevaluated the specific causes of the false-positive diagnosis or the limited outcome success of RF lesioning. In some outcome studies, very small gauge RF needles (22 gauge) were used, likely resulting in the targeted nerve's being incompletely or entirely untreated by the RF thermal lesioning offered. There is some variability in the precise path of travel of the medial branch nerve (or the equivalent L5 dorsal primary ramus), so that anticipated anatomical drug delivery is hampered. As for RF outcomes, variability in nerve course or other technical reasons, including small needle gauge, inadequate technique, or calcified mammillo-accessory ligament, prevented a satisfactory therapeutic response to RF lesioning. In humility, one must also consider the strong possibility that the original diagnosis of pain may be incomplete, due to multiple structural causes of pain, or it may be incorrect, and reflecting a false-positive diagnostic result.

Diagnostic medial branch block has been demonstrated to be efficacious in multiple publications, and several cautions are noted:

1. At the C2 nerve level, there are several medial branches, with the most cephalad of the branches providing innervation to the muscular rotators of the skull base. The middle and upper C2 medial branches should be avoided, with meticulous imaging and precise targeting of the anatomy necessary to avoid head drop.
2. Cervical medial branches cross the lateral masses at varying levels seen on lateral images, as described by Bogduk,[18] and these branches are usually located on a contralateral oblique view just posterior and inferior to the neural foramen.

3. The eighth cervical medial branch crosses the first rib, and all named thoracic and lumbar medial branches cross over the named transverse process one level below (e.g. L3 branch crosses L4 transverse process).
4. The C8–T11 medial branches travel laterally from the neural foramen in the intertransverse space, turning posteriorly just medial to the lateral costotransverse joint to cross the transverse process, traveling from deep to superficial before finally turning medial and inferiorly to ramify in the multifidus.[19] With the superior aspect of each vertebral body at a subject transverse process level flattened radiographically on C-arm, the medial branch nerves usually cross on the superior aspect of the transverse process just medial to the lateral costotransverse joint, and the medial branch can usually be targeted on the superior aspect of the transverse process. Needle depth must never exceed the anterior aspect of its transverse process, to avoid pneumothorax. However, when the superior vertebral body endplate is squared, but the rib head appears elevated cephalad relative to the transverse process, the medial branch is also displaced cephalad into the intertransverse space approximately or slightly less than the distance that the rib head rises cephalad above the superior aspect of the transverse process. In this latter case, where the medial branch crosses cephalad to the transverse process the target point for both neural blockade and RF at these levels remains medial to its lateral costotransverse joint capsule and elevated cephalad above the transverse process at approximately the same distance as the rib head appears cephalad to the transverse process. Needle depth control is critical, and the needle must never pass deeper to the transverse process as seen on lateral radiographic view. At these levels, easy unguarded entry into the pleural space can produce pneumothorax. A variety of steeply declined or inferolateral superior techniques passing the needle on the superficial aspect of the rib have been described.
5. Too large a volume of local anesthetic will produce false-negative responses on medial branch block. With precise needle placement, injected volumes of 0.2 mL are often sufficient to produce neural blockade of the lumbar or cervical medial branch, but in no case should more than 0.5 mL be used.
6. When performing lumbar medial branch block, it is well to maintain the needle just lateral to the superior articular process and in a lateral view, dorsal to the midpoint of the superior articular process at L3 and above to minimize the risk of dysesthesia from inadvertent RF lesioning of the sensory afferents of the superior cluneal nerve.
7. After completion of satisfactory RF lesioning in the thoracic spine, evidence of thoracic facet pain at one or two levels subjacent to the prior treated levels may be noted and must be addressed with diagnostic medial branch block and RF lesioning at the adjacent nerve levels.
8. In patients with "normal" MRI anatomy without evidence for, or following successful treatment of, radiculopathy from adjacent structures or adjacent articular structures, including shoulder, hip, or SIJ, according to Baye's theorem, the pretest probability of facet pain rises substantially, and the likelihood of a false-negative diagnostic block (e.g., missing the diagnosis of facet pain) also rises dramatically.

Interpretation of Results of Low-Volume Diagnostic Medial Branch Blocks

Some authorities insist on >80% relief of pain to consider a result to be affirmative, others suggest a >50% threshold, and the data from Cohen suggest that the acceptable diagnostic threshold percentage of pain improvement to advance to RF lesioning may be as low as 37%. Some authors recommend adding criteria for short-term functional improvement, but consensus has not been achieved on this point. It is the author's preference to incorporate functional testing routinely in patients who do not have constant pain where interruption of pain can clearly be affirmed after the diagnostic block. While use of a pain diary has been traditional, the outcome decision is binary, and it is unclear that this merits the time and effort for completion of a formal hourly diary as was recommended in the 1980s.

- Unimproved pain, a negative response, suggests either no evidence for pain, or that the procedure was not technically adequate (false negative), or that pain originates at other levels or within other structures.
- Three to 12 hours of improvement is an affirmative response to diagnostic block.
- With more than 18 hours of improvement, it is a likely false-positive response, and the physician should consider repetition of the diagnostic block.
- Thirty-six hours of improvement is a true negative, implying a non-facet cause of pain.

Some readers may view this discussion as academic, since the perceived risk of an enduring adverse outcome with RF lesioning using modern equipment and with meticulous attention to anatomical technique is extremely low, and the effective adverse outcome of a failed RF lesioning procedure is simply failure to obtain resolution of pain. With the dramatic and steady decline in professional reimbursement over 30 to 40 years, RF lesioning is now offered at nearly de minimis cost, and the aggregate costs of diagnostic blocks are not significantly less than the cost of RF lesioning alone, such that in patients with nonradicular pain absent clinical findings of SIJ pain, it may be economically rational to avoid the medial branch block entirely and to perform only the RF lesioning procedure.

After RF lesioning, changes in stance and gait occur with resolution of pain and spasm, and after successful lumbar RF lesioning, approximately 25% of patients have new SIJ findings and as many as 40% of patients demonstrate recurrence of previously symptomatic SIJ pain or spinal stenosis and clinical re-examination of patients is mandatory to determine the cause of residual pain.

When reviewing outcome literature on lumbar RF lesioning, it is important to realize that there are only one published paper and one published research abstract reporting on SIJ pain after RF lesioning. All other papers reporting that patients did not have substantial resolution of all pain complaints adhere to the trope that the outcomes represent false-positive diagnostic blocks. However, the facts support an alternative explanation: a second (or even third) cause of pain has been revealed after resolution of facet pain. Additional studies of this topic are clearly merited!

Intraarticular Injections and Diagnostic Diskography

While intraarticular injection is presumed to be anatomically specific, substantial questions have been raised about the anatomical specificity of such injections, especially as many circumstances are known where the hip capsule is contiguous with the iliopectineal bursa and it is unclear where the anesthetic or steroid is having (or is failing to have) effect. In the SIJ, where there is no formal joint capsule and the anterior and posterior ligaments bridging the joint do not limit either the flow of contrast or the diagnostic local anesthetic or steroid injected, it may not be possible to artfully separate intraarticular from extraarticular pain mechanisms.

In the case of the SIJ, it may not be technically possible to place a needle into the inferior recess of the joint due to osteophytes. Defects in the contiguity of the anterior or posterior ligaments may provide a low-pressure runoff for injectate, such that the cephalad or middle aspects of the joint cannot be with filled with injected contrast, local anesthetic, and/or steroid. In some of these cases, alternative techniques entering the upper or middle portion of the joint directly may achieve clinical success.[20]

While some patients enjoy long-term resolution of pain from a single SIJ injection, others experience brief improvement consistent only with the duration of local anesthetic used. In many patients, the appearance of multiple chondral erosions in the ilial or sacral SIJ surfaces on arthrogram is associated with intractability to intraarticular injection, yet other patients will obtain months or years of pain relief. It is likely that there are both intra- and extraarticular sources of pain, but the overall ligamentous stability and other factors, including pelvic incidence, sacral slope, and pelvic tilt affecting sagittal alignment and alterations of the dynamic transfer of forces to the femoral heads and sacrum, may be important in better understanding the basis for SIJ pain.

Even more curiously, patients demonstrating intractability to technically adequate intraarticular SIJ injection and subsequently undergoing RF lesioning of the dorsal sacroiliac lateral branch innervation often do well for varying periods of time. With recurrence of pain 6 or more months after successful RF lesioning, some of the same patients respond to repeat intraarticular injection. Clearly, there are some aspects of sacroiliac pain production that we do not understand.

When considering lateral sacral diagnostic nerve blocks, the total volume of local anesthetic administered at multiple locations makes the overall anatomical specificity of anesthetization uncertain. Also, it is unclear if diagnostic lateral sacral block or SIJ injection will improve SIJ pain referred from other locations; hence, dependence upon pain relief to indicate an affirmative outcome may not be anatomically specific.[21]

For patients who have undergone an initial successful RF lesioning of the lateral sacral branches, those with recurrent pain following clinically successful RF lesioning are now being offered surgical approaches using transiliac cortical screw fixation, posterolateral intra-articular devices or posterior SIJ fusion using "box-cutter" and slightly oversized rectangular or tapered bone graft systems, with excellent outcomes. While unilateral fusion in situ of one SIJ is not uncommonly seen on CT of the lumbar spine, these patients do not appear to have grossly increased incidence of hip disease. Given the role of the sacroiliac ligaments in facilitating vaginal birth, however, the author recommends thoughtful professional judgment, typically avoiding offering SIJ fusion to women of childbearing age or younger.

Provocative Diskography

Nothing will divide a room of surgeons so quickly as a discussion of the utility of diskography in clinical care of spinal pain. With a near-religious zeal, proponents urge this diagnostic test to be used as a basis for subsequent disk resection, thermal annuloplasty, thermal disk resection, basivertebral RF lesioning, or discectomies and fusion. Opponents dismiss the concept of discogenic pain as nonsense, providing counterarguments that discogenic pain is misdiagnosed pain from other causes. This controversy has been going on for a half century, and resolution is not yet at hand.

Provocative diskography is a diagnostic procedure with absolutely no proven intrinsic therapeutic benefits in which the intervertebral disk nucleus is cannulated and subsequently injected with a mixture of radiographic contrast under pressure in an awake patient.[22] The pressure is slowly increased to a pressure threshold equivalent to lifting 25 to 50 lbs, with the examiner observing for the presence of anatomical defects in the nuclear retention of injected contrast or contrast filling of an annular defect while also observing for simultaneous reproduction of the typical pain of severity 6/10 VNAS or greater. The procedure should be performed in an operating room suite with aseptic technique using intradiscal manometry to monitor injection pressure and to avoid overpressurization and structural damage to the disk. With the use of 25-gauge needles with a distal curve, needles advance from a posterolateral site in oblique fluoroscopic view to enter the disk nucleus. Non-ionic contrast, typically iohexol or iopamidol, is usually diluted to 150 to 225 mg/mL iodine to avoid beam-hardening artifact on the subsequent CT scan. An intradiscal antibiotic, usually gentamicin 2 mg/mL or clindamycin 10 mg/mL, is added for antibiotic prophylaxis. The pressure at which contrast flows initially into the disk nucleus is called the "opening pressure." If there is no severe pain produced at 50 PSI above the opening pressure, the disk is considered to be non-nociceptive. At least one disk adjacent, or two, if possible, are also studied as control disks. Reproduction of concordant pain at low injection pressure is considered diagnostic for discogenic pain. Specific parameters for injection protocols and pressure thresholds can be found in the IPSIS (formerly the Spinal Intervention Society, now the International Pain & Spine Intervention Society) guidelines and are widely reprinted in many texts. False-positive rates using SIS/IPSIS guidelines for interpretation are below 5%.[23] Repetitive provocation can be helpful in reducing false-positive findings, as 20% of positive disks in a pilot retrospective study of over 200 "positive" disks did not evidence consistent reproduction of pain within 10 PSI above the initial injection pressure.

Following instillation of contrast in the intervertebral disk, postdiskogram CT scanning with soft tissue windows is used to assess the extent of annular disruption. Patients usually experience 3 to 5 days of worsened low back pain. Infection is the dreaded complication of diskography, and the infection risk is addressed with intradiscal antibiotics and meticulous aseptic technique. If discitis is suspected, CBC with differential and ESR can be drawn, but MRI with gadolinium contrast is usually definitive, showing diffuse inflammatory response extending across the disk space and including the vertebral endplate regions.

Treatment for discitis requires IV antibiotics, but expeditious use of a spinal endoscopy for intradiscal irrigation and debridement may produce more prompt and possibly superior outcomes.

Bogduk et al showed the innervation of the intervertebral disk to include branches of the sinuvertebral nerves, the rami communicans, ventral ramus and grey ramus. Anterior innervation originates from the lumbar sympathetic chain.[24] The basivertebral nerve originates from both sympathetic ganglia and somatic nerve roots. Discogenic pain, per Coppes et al[25] and Adams et al,[26] is assumed to arise in the defective posterior annulus after injury or partial delamination, with initiation of pathologic neovascularization and neo-innervation responses such that the posterior annulus effectively becomes a newly nociceptive end organ after injury. Annular injury appears to initiate complex catabolic changes in the disk nucleus with degradation of glycosaminoglycans, but this view may be unduly nearsighted, because the possibility of coincident endplate injury must be considered. There is no supporting evidence for the use of any specific regimen of conservative care in discogenic pain. Patients with annular injury and discogenic pain noted outcomes not dissimilar from outcomes of discectomy and fusion with use of biacuplasty, per Desai et al.[27] Lotz et al studied lumbar vertebral endplate injuries, finding endplate microfractures, altered chemistry, and increased endplate permeability in the pathogenesis of injury and noting that this leads to alterations in both the biology and mechanical function of the adjacent intervertebral disk. Additionally, Lotz and colleagues observed that the endplate changes correlate with the previously described Modic I and II changes. Other authors disagreed about the clinical importance and diagnostic utility of Modic changes. Thus, it may be that basivertebral and discogenic pain are closed related in structure, function, mechanics, and innervation but represent a spectrum of pain-producing modalities of injury. It is not yet known if treating basivertebral afferent nerve pain with intraosseous RF lesioning is routinely indicated in patients with annular pain reproduced on diskography in the absence of endplate fractures or Modic changes. With this newer biologic research, clinical trials of intraosseous catheter RF lesioning of the basivertebral nerve have produced surprisingly good outcomes for pain relief and function in this group that was once subjected to an intellectual tug of war,[28] being either avoided by surgical colleagues or subjected to instrumented discectomy and fusion or else a variety of nonsurgical interventions, including biacuplasty and Disc-FX. While enthusiasts of basivertebral RF lesioning declare that provocative lumbar diskography is unnecessary, there is only very limited clinical research demonstrating the substantial diagnostic equivalency of observed Modic changes and provocative (or analgesic) diskography. It is also important to point out that many patients undergoing diagnostic diskography have evidence on the postdiskogram CT of focal disk herniations, especially small foraminal disk herniations, foraminal stenosis, and lateral recess stenosis. In the absence of the presentation of radicular pain in an extremity, it is possible that the pain was neither correctly diagnosed nor treated. More worryingly, it is clear that we need to take a broader view of the pathogenesis of lumbar spine pain to correctly classify patients. Use of an algorithm, as described at the beginning of this chapter, should reduce or prevent the early diskogram studies that inappropriately classified patients as having discogenic pain just because the treating physician did not consider the possibility of a radicular pain process as causing non-extremity axial only pain or in cases where multiple sources of pain existed but were not more thoroughly evaluated.

By addition of minimally invasive modalities, such as endoscopic discectomy, foraminotomy by interlaminar or transforaminal technique, and mechanical stabilization procedures, including posterior interspinous fusion and SIJ fusion, the broad scope and bright future of interventional care offer the power to accurately understand the anatomy and the pathophysiology of an individual's pain and provide the broad skill set needed in both diagnostic and therapeutic contexts. Patients can be assured that we understand more than ever before the cause of their pain and suffering and, therefore, that they are offered a better opportunity for improvement tomorrow.

The practitioner's skill originates with knowledge of anatomy, neurology and orthopedics combined with precise and practiced clinical examination skills and the ability to personally read MRI and CT imaging studies; all remain critical to improving patient outcomes. Resolving one presenting cause of pain can initiate changes in posture, stance, and gait with alteration in segmental lordosis aggravating foraminal narrowing to produce new radiculopathies or by changing mechanical spinal loading, may unveil facet or sacroiliac joint pain. When a seemingly unimproved patient returns to the office, 21st century medicine must robustly identify these new causes of pain by diligent re-examination of the patient.

It is hoped that the reader will glean a few useful insights from this chapter and return to see their patients with fresh eyes and know these circumstances differently, as if for the first time.

References

1. Tubbs RS. "Surgery is simple—it requires only anatomy and hemostasis." *Clin Anat.* 2015;28(7):281.
2. Cohen SP, Williams KA, Nguyen C, et al. Multicenter, randomized, comparative cost-effectiveness study comparing 0, 1, and 2 diagnostic medial branch (facet joint nerve) block treatment paradigms before lumbar facet radiofrequency denervation. *Anesthesiology.* 2010;113(2):395–405.
3. Siegenthaler A, Eichenberger U, Schmidlin K, et al. What does local tenderness say about the origin of pain? An investigation of cervical zygapophysial pain. *Anesth Analg.* 2010;110(3):923–927.
4. Swan HJ, Ganz W, Forrester J, Marcus H, Diamond G, Chonette D. Catheterization of the heart in man with the use of a flow-directed balloon-tipped catheter. *N Engl J Med.* 1970;283:447–451.
5. Laslett M, Aprill C, McDonald B, et al. Diagnosis of sacroiliac joint pain: validity of individual provocation tests and combinations of tests. *Manual Ther.* 2003;10(3):207–218.
6. Telli H, Telli S, Topol M. The validity and reliability of sacroiliac joint provocation tests. *Pain Physician.* 2018;21;E367–E376.
7. Schneider BJ, Ehsanian R, Rosati R, et al. Validity of physical exam maneuvers in the diagnosis of sacroiliac joint pain. *Pain Med.* 2020;21(2);255–260.
8. Falowski S, Sayed D, Pope J, et al. A review and algorithm in diagnosis and treatment of sacroiliac joint pain. *J Pain Res.* 2020;13:3337–3348.
9. Illeez GI, Atici A, Ulger EB, et al. The transitional vertebrae and sacroiliac joint dysfunction. *Eur Spine J.* 2018;27:187–193.
10. Speciale AC, Pietrobon R, Urban CW, et al. Observer variability in assessing lumbar spinal stenosis severity on magnetic resonance imaging and its relation to cross-sectional spinal canal area. *Spine.* 2002;27(10):1081–1086.
11. Karabulut N. Gadolinium deposition in the brain: another concern regarding gadolinium-based contrast agents. *Diagn Intervent Radiol.* 2015;21(4):269–270.

12. Chhabra A, Andriesek G, Soldatos T, et al. MRI neurography: past, present, future. *Am J Radiol.* 2011;187:583–591.
13. Du R, Auguste KI, Chin CT, et al. Magnetic resonance neurography for the evaluation of peripheral nerve, brachial plexus and nerve root disorders. *J Neurosurg.* 2010;112(2):362–371.
14. Furman M, Berkwits L, Cohen I, et al. *Atlas of Image-Guided Spinal Procedures.* 2nd ed. Elsevier; 2017.
15. Yeom JS, Lee JW, Park KW, et al. *Am J Neuroradiol.* 2008;29(5):1017–1023.
16. Datta S, Manchikanti L, Falco FJ, et al. Diagnostic utility of selective nerve root blocks in the diagnosis of lumbosacral radicular pain: a systematic review and update of current evidence. *Pain Physician.* 2013;16(2 suppl);97–124.
17. Cohen SP, Bhaskar A, Bhatia A, et al. Consensus practice guidelines on interventions for lumbar facet joint pain from a multispecialty international working group. *Reg Anesth Pain Med.* 2020;45:424–467.
18. Manchikanti L, Kaye AD, Soin A, et al. Comprehensive evidence-based guidelines for facet joint interventions in the management of chronic spinal pain: American Society of Interventional Pain Physicians (ASIPP) guidelines. *Pain Physician.* 2020;23:S1–S127.
19. Bogduk N. The clinical anatomy of the cervical dorsal rami. *Spine.* 1982;7(4):319–330.
20. Chua WH, Bogduk N. The surgical anatomy of thoracic facet denervation. *Acta Neurochir.* 1995;136:140–144.
21. Dreyfuss P, Cole AJ, Pauza K. Sacroiliac joint injection techniques. *Phys Med Rehab Clin North Am.* 1995;6(4):785–813.
22. King W, Ahmed SU, Baisden J, et al. Diagnosis and treatment of posterior sacroiliac complex pain: a systematic review with comprehensive analysis of the published data. *Pain Med.* 2015;16(2):257–265.
23. Bogduk N, Aprill C, Derby R. Lumbar discogenic pain: state-of-the-art review. *Pain Med.* 2013;14(6);813–836.
24. Wolfer LR, Derby R, Lee JE, et al. Systematic review of lumbar provocation discography in asymptomatic subjects with a meta-analysis of false-positive rates. *Pain Physician.* 2008;11(4):513–538.
25. Bogduk N, Tynan W, Wilson AS. The nerve supply to the human lumbar intervertebral discs. *J Anat.* 1981;132:39–56.
26. Coppes MH, Marani E, Thomeer RT, et al. Innervation of "painful" lumbar discs. *Spine.* 1997;22(20):2342–2349.
27. Desai, MJ, Kapural L, Petersohn JD, Vallejo R, Menzies R, Creamer M, Gofeld M. A prospective, randomized, multi-center open-label clinical trial comparing intra-discal biacuplasty to conventional medical management for discogenic lumbar back pain. *Spine.* 2016: 41(13);1065–1074.
28. Adams MA, Stefanakis M, Dolan P. Healing of a painful intervertebral disc should not be confused with reversing disc degeneration: implications for physical therapies for discogenic back pain. *Clin Biomechanics.* 2010;25(10):961–971.
29. Lotz AC, Fields AJ, Liebenberg EC. The role of the vertebral endplate in low back pain. *Global Spine J.* 2013;3(3):153–163.
30. Conger A, Schuster NM, Cheng DS, et al. The effectiveness of intraosseous basivertebral nerve radiofrequency neurotomy for the treatment of chronic low back pain in patients with Modic changes: a systematic review. *Pain Med.* 2021: 22(5);1039–1054.

PART 2

Decompressive Procedures

6

Minimally Invasive Lumbar Decompression

Sameer Jain and Navdeep Singh Jassal

Introduction

Lumbar spinal stenosis (LSS) is a degenerative spinal condition that is a common cause of disability in the elderly. The North American Spine Society defines LSS as "a condition in which there is diminished space available for the neural and vascular elements in the lumbar spine secondary to degenerative changes in the spinal canal."[1] It has been reported that at least 10% of the population develops symptoms related to LSS by the age of 70.[2] The most common clinical presentation of LSS is neurogenic claudication. Neurogenic claudication is a constellation of symptoms that includes pain in the buttocks and legs, accompanied by paresthesias and numbness/weakness, and it is worsened with prolonged standing or walking and is alleviated with sitting down or lumbar flexion.[3] The most common causes of LSS are disk degeneration (anterior to the spinal canal) and facet and ligamentum flavum hypertrophy (LFH; posterior to the spinal canal).[4]

Conservative management of LSS is challenging. The use of conservative measures, including physical therapy, NSAIDs, and other pharmacologic therapies, has shown limited benefit.[5] Interventional pain management procedures like epidural steroid injection (ESI) have been shown to provide only a short duration of pain relief.[6,7] Hence, traditionally, the treatment of LSS has been limited to extensive spine surgery, which demands a lengthy recovery period, exposes the patient to an increased number of potential complications, and imposes an extensive economic burden on the healthcare infrastructure. However, during the last decade, we have seen the advent of new, minimally invasive, percutaneous image-guided lumbar decompression (PILD) procedures that have proven safety and efficacy in the treatment of LSS and are supported by several randomized controlled clinical trials.

This chapter focuses on the only commercially available PILD treatment option for stenosis secondary to LFH—minimally invasive lumbar decompression (MILD®; Vertos Medical, Aliso Viejo, CA, USA).

Indications

The MILD procedure is currently only indicated for symptomatic LSS (central or foraminal) secondary to LFH. Patients usually present with pain, numbness, and heaviness or tingling in the back, legs, or buttocks when standing or walking. Patients often have limited mobility and spend time sitting to avoid pain. Forward flexion or sitting aids in decompression and is a hallmark of improvement of symptoms corresponding to neurogenic claudication. Patients ambulate in a flexed/stooped posture, which opens the central canal to provide temporary relief of their low back and lower extremity neurogenic claudication symptoms. They also use an assistive device, such as a cane or walking aid (rolling walker), and sleep in the fetal position.

Once candidates for MILD exhibit features of symptomatic LSS with neurogenic claudication, they must also meet the following criteria:

1. LFH ≥ 2.5 mm, confirmed by imaging
2. Spinal stability ≤ Grade II
3. Central canal stenosis, including in patients with comorbid conditions, such as foraminal stenosis, lateral stenosis, facet hypertrophy, or disk bulge

Evidence

The efficacy and safety of the MILD procedure have been demonstrated in several level 1 studies. Table 6.1 summarizes the eight major prospective clinical trials and one meta-analysis that showed the efficacy and safety of the MILD procedure in the treatment of LSS secondary to LFH. All initial studies showed improvement in primary and secondary endpoints through the follow-up period. The first multicenter randomized controlled trial (MIDAS I) compared the effectiveness of the MILD procedure to the efficacy of lumbar ESI for the treatment of LSS.[8] In this study, 302 patients were randomized to either the MILD or the ESI treatment arm and were followed for 1 year. ODI, ZCQ, and NPRS were the measured criteria for improvement. At 1 year, patients who underwent the MILD procedure showed significant improvement in all domains. This study was followed by MIDAS II, a randomized, controlled, multicenter trial,[9] which enrolled 143 patients who were followed up at 6 months, 1 year, and 2 years. ODI, NPRS, and ZCQ were the criteria measured for improvement. Patients who underwent the MILD procedure showed long-term improvement in all the domains when followed over a period of 2 years.

TABLE 6.1.

Study	Study Type	Inclusion Criteria	Number of Patients (*N*)/ Follow-up period	Control/ Active Intervention	Outcome Measures Analyzed	Results	Conclusion
Chopko et al[10]	Prospective clinical study	Symptomatic LSS, failed conservative therapy	78/6 weeks	—/MILD	At baseline: VAS, ODI, ZCQ, SF-12v2® Health Survey	At baseline: VAS = 7.3 (3–10) ODI = 47.4 (16–84). At 6-week follow-up: VAS = 3.7 (0–10) ($P < .0001$) ODI = 29.5 (0–72) ($P < .0001$). SF-12v2 showed statistically significant (95% CI) improvement for all but the GH survey scale. There were no major device- or procedure-related complications reported.	MILD procedure showed promising results in treating LSS.
Chopko et al[11]	Prospective clinical study	Symptomatic LSS, failed conservative therapy	14/23.5weeks	—/MILD	VAS, ODI	Preoperative VAS = 7.61, ± 2.0, vs. postoperative VAS = 3.61 ± 2.9 ($P = .05$). Preoperative ODI = 50% vs. postoperative ODI = 43.9% ($P > .05$). No complications reported.	MILD was efficacious in decreasing pain secondary to LSS.
Schomer et al[12]	Meta-analysis	Symptomatic LSS, failed conservative therapy	107/12 weeks	—/MILD	VAS, ODI	Baseline: VAS = 7.4(-), ODI = 48. 3 months: VAS= 3.9(-) ($P < .0001$) ODI = 30.9 ($P < .0001$). Statistically significant improvements seen in both outcome measures.	MILD is safe and effective in treating LSS.
Basu et al[13]	Prospective clinical study	Symptomatic LSS, failed conservative therapy	27/6 months	—/MILD	VAS, ODI, ZCQ	Baseline: VAS = 9.1 (95% CI ± 0.59) ODI = 55.1 (95% CI ± 6.34). 6 months: VAS = 3.9 (95% CI ± 2.25; $P < .0001$) ODI = 31.1 (95% CI ± 9.29; $P < .0004$). ZCQ showed significant improvement in all domains. No device- or procedure-related complications were reported.	MILD procedure showed promising results in treating LSS but further clinical trials were indicated.

(continued)

TABLE 6.1. Continued

Study	Study Type	Inclusion Criteria	Number of Patients (N)/ Follow-up period	Control/ Active Intervention	Outcome Measures Analyzed	Results	Conclusion
Deer et al[14]	Prospective clinical study	Symptomatic LSS, failed conservative therapy	46/12 months	—/MILD	VAS, ODI, ZCQ	Baseline: VAS = 6.9 (95% CI ± 0.6) ODI = 49.4 (95% CI ± 2.5). 12-month follow-up: VAS = 4.0 (95% CI ± 1.0; $P < .0001$) ODI = 32.0 (95% CI ± 5.8; $P < .0001$). Statistically significant improvements were achieved in all ZCQ domains, including symptom severity, both symptom severity subdomains (pain and neuro-ischemic) and physical function (paired *t*-test; $P < .0001$).	MILD procedure provided significant improvement in pain and functional disability in patients with LSS.
Brown et al[15]	Prospective randomized clinical trial	Symptomatic LSS, failed conservative therapy	38/6 and 12 weeks	ESI/MILD	VAS, ODI, ZCQ	*MILD treatment group*: Baseline: VAS = 6.3 (95% CI ± 0.7) ODI = 38.8 (95% CI ± 4.2). 6 weeks: VAS = 3.8 (95% CI ± 1.3) ODI = 27.4 (95% CI ± 7.0). 12 weeks: VAS = 3.4 ODI = 18.6. The change in VAS from baseline to week 6 and baseline to week 12 was significant ($P < .01$), but the change from week 6 to week 12 was not significant. The change from baseline to 6 weeks post MILD and baseline to 12 weeks post MILD was significant ($P < .05$), but the change from 6 weeks to 12 weeks was not significant ($P > .05$). *ESI treatment group:* Baseline: VAS = 6.4 (95% CI ± 1.0) ODI = 40.5 (95% CI ± 5.9). 6 weeks: VAS = 6.3 (95% CI ± 1.4; $P > .05$) ODI = 34.8 (95% CI ± 8.2; $P > .05$). ZCQ score showed significant improvement at 6 and 12 weeks for MILD treatment group.	MILD procedure is more effective than ESI in providing symptomatic relief for patients with LSS.

Chopko et al[16]	Prospective clinical study	Symptomatic LSS, failed conservative therapy	45/2 years	—/MILD	VAS, ODI, ZCQ	Baseline: VAS = 7.2 (95% CI ± 0.6) ODI = 48.4 (95% CI ± 4.4). 2 years: VAS = 4.8 (95% CI ± 0.8; $P < .0001$) ODI = 39.8 (95% CI ± 5.6; $P < .0001$). All ZCQ domains showed statistically significant improvement at 2-year follow-up. No major adverse events were reported.	MILD procedure is efficacious in treating neurogenic claudication secondary to LSS.
Benyamin et al[8]	Prospective, multicenter, randomized controlled clinical study	Symptomatic LSS, failed conservative therapy	302/6 months and 1 year	ESI/MILD	ODI, NPRS, ZCQ	Mean improvement in the MILD group from baseline to 1-year follow-up: ODI = 16.2 ± 1.6 NPRS = 2.8 ± 0.3 ZCQ = 0.5 ± 0.1 ($P < .001$). At 1 year, MILD procedure showed significant improvement over the active control (i.e., ESI) in all domains.	MILD procedure is more effective than ESI in treating symptoms secondary to LSS.
Staats et al[9]	Prospective, multicenter, randomized controlled clinical study	Symptomatic LSS, failed conservative therapy	143/6 months 1 year, and 2 years	—/MILD	ODI, NPRS, ZCQ	At 2 years: ODI improved by 22.7 points (95% CI, 18.5–26.9), NPRS improved by 3.6 points (95% CI, 3.1–4.2), and ZCQ symptom severity and physical function domains improved by 1.0 (95% CI, 0.8–1.2) and 0.8 points (95% CI, 0.6–0.9), respectively. Improvements in all domains were statistically significant. There were no serious device-related adverse events.	MILD procedure is effective in providing long-term symptomatic relief to patients suffering from neurogenic claudication secondary to LSS.

Patient Selection and Contraindications

Before being deemed a candidate for MILD, a patient must meet the following criteria:

1. LSS must be symptomatic (i.e., presence of neurogenic claudication).
2. Spine imaging must demonstrate spinal stenosis and presence of LFH.
3. LFH must be ≥ 2.5 mm (see Figure 6.1).
4. Spinal stability must be ≤ Grade II (as per Meyerding classification, which divides the superior endplate of the vertebra below into 4 quarters, so that the grade depends on the location of the posteroinferior corner of the vertebra above: Grade I, 0%–25%; Grade II, 26%–50%).

Absolute contraindications to the MILD procedure are prior spine surgery at the level considered for treatment and local infection at the site considered for treatment. Relative contraindications to the procedure are presence of systemic infection and presence of a bleeding diathesis or a coagulation disorder.

Perioperative Management

Preoperative testing may include basic labs, including coagulation profile and an electrocardiogram. Preoperative antibiotic prophylaxis is defined as antibiotic administration prior to surgery to help decrease the risk of postoperative infections. Although the MILD procedure

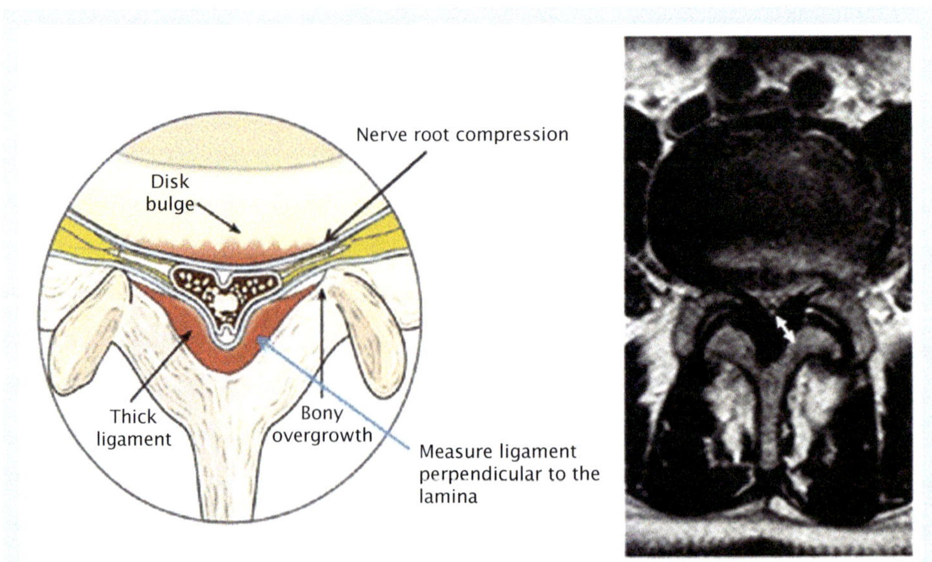

FIGURE 6.1. Ligamentum flavum thickness is measured perpendicular to the border of the lamina (shown by white double-sided arrow on the T2 axial MRI image on the right). Ligamentum flavum hypertrophy is shown on the left in pink. Notice nerve root compression caused by the hypertrophied ligamentum flavum that can cause symptoms of neurogenic claudication.

involves no implant, causes minimal blood loss, and requires minimal dissection, it is generally standard practice to give a single dose of preoperative IV antibiotic. Cefazolin 2 g (3 g for weight >120 kg) is used most often for surgical prophylaxis in patients with no history of beta-lactam allergy or a history of MRSA infection. Clindamycin can be used in instances of penicillin allergy. Anticoagulation generally follows the Neurostimulation Appropriateness Consensus Committee (NACC) recommendations.[15] The NACC review summarizes the literature and provides evidence-based guidelines for anticoagulation during neurostimulation procedures. There is good evidence for the perioperative discontinuation of anticoagulant therapy to avoid complications like bleeding and epidural hematoma.

Generally, the MILD procedure is performed with monitored anesthesia care (MAC) in an outpatient surgery center or hospital setting. Neuromonitoring is not required, as the procedure is completed using direct visualization under fluoroscopy and posterior from the epidurogram or the ventral interlaminar line (VILL). The patient can be discharged safely to home on the day of the procedure.

Equipment

The procedure utilizes a standard epidural injection tray, a scalpel, and the MILD tool kit (Figure 6.2). The MILD toolkit includes:

- Portal (5.1-mm portal minimizes tissue disruption)
- Trocar and handle

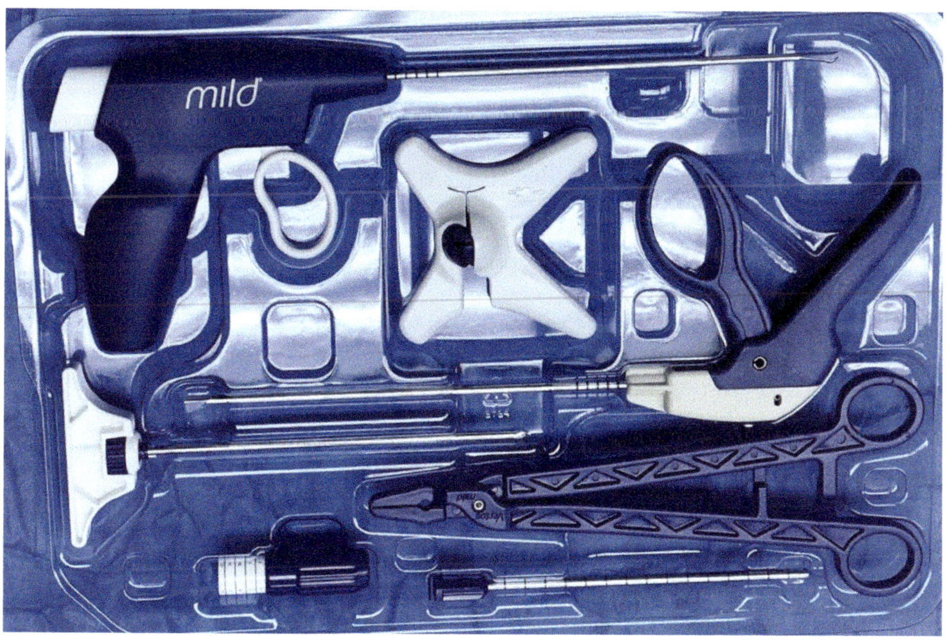

FIGURE 6.2. MILD toolkit.

- Portal stabilizer (minimizes medial and lateral movement)
- Depth guide (ensures depth of cutting device)
- Bone rongeur (allows removal of chips of inferior and superior lamina)
- Tissue sculptor (allows resection and retraction of ligamentous tissue)

Standard Technique

Positioning

The patient is placed in the prone position, with pillows under the abdomen. It is important to reduce the lumbar lordosis in order to facilitate the remaining steps in the procedure.

Fluoroscopy and Epidurogram

Fluoroscopy guidance is important for the epidurogram and trajectory. The midline spinous processes are marked, as well as the medial pedicular lines at the intended level of the decompression. These markings are used for trajectory and orientation of the instruments (to prevent crossing over the midline).

An epidural needle is then placed and accessed using the technique of choice (loss of resistance technique, hanging drop, or visualization/fluoroscopic guidance). It is placed close to the midline and ipsilateral to the treatment side and level (or adjacent level; Figure 6.3).

Access is confirmed using a small amount of non-ionized contrast in the contralateral oblique fluoroscopic view (40°–45°) with extension tubing. This is necessary to ensure the safety of the technique (Figure 6.4).

Trajectory

Skin entry is usually started one and a half levels below and 15° off the midline of the ipsilateral side to be treated. A 22-gauge 5-inch spinal needle can be used under fluoroscopic guidance to assist with angle of trajectory and with anesthetizing to the inferior lamina. Anteroposterior view is used to determine the medial and lateral trajectory. The contralateral oblique view is used to visualize the depth of the needle.

Trocar-Portal Unit

A stab incision is made with a No. 15 blade. The assembled trocar-portal unit (MILD tissue access device) is advanced under contralateral oblique fluoroscopic view along the predetermined trajectory. It is advanced until the device touches the superior surface of the inferior lamina. The trocar can be removed after releasing the locking screw on the handle. The portal stabilizer should then snap into place to stabilize the cannula.

Depth Guide

For safety and to limit the depth of instrument insertion into the portal, a depth gauge is attached to the distal end of the portal. The depth gauge can be adjusted to allow the

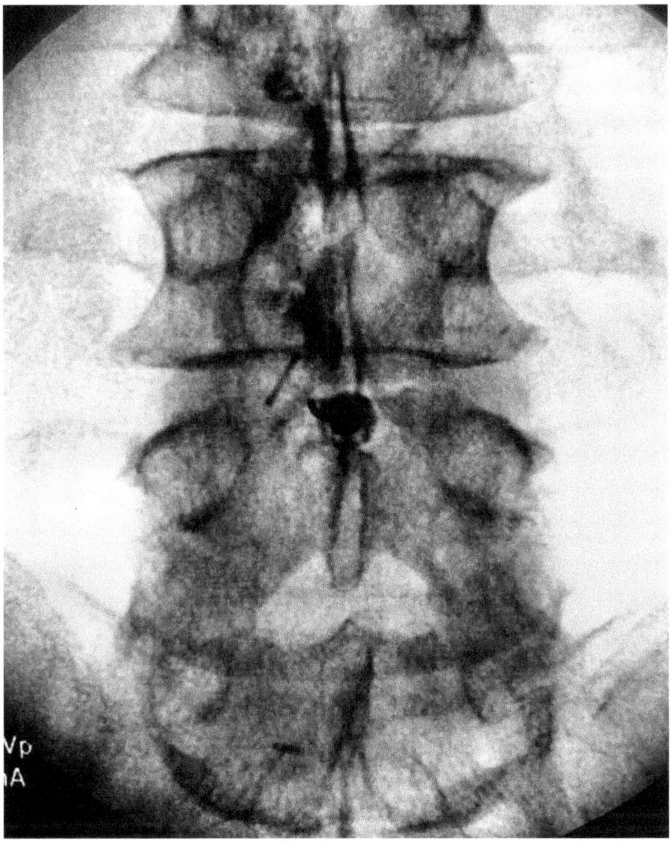

FIGURE 6.3. Ideally, the epidurogram is created by placing the epidural needle at the superior aspect, on the ipsilateral side and level being decompressed. If anatomy does not allow this, the epidural needle can be placed at an alternate level and create a similar visual barrier.

instruments to advance in 5-mm increments (from the tip of the port) into the working area (Figure 6.5).

Then, the bone rongeur can be rotated 180° and is used to work at the superior lamina in the same fashion (medial to lateral end; see Figure 6.7).

Debulking

The tissue sculptor is used by scooping in an upward motion from an inferior to superior direction and activating the trigger. This provides a means of cutting the ligamentous tissue. This is also done in a medial to lateral fashion in the working interlaminar space. The sculptor can be used to take multiple bites and is withdrawn from the port to dislodge tissue and to avoid overfilling. Live fluoroscopic guidance must be used to visualize the epidurogram throughout the procedure and to ensure that instruments remain posterior to the level of the epidurogram (see Figure 6.8).

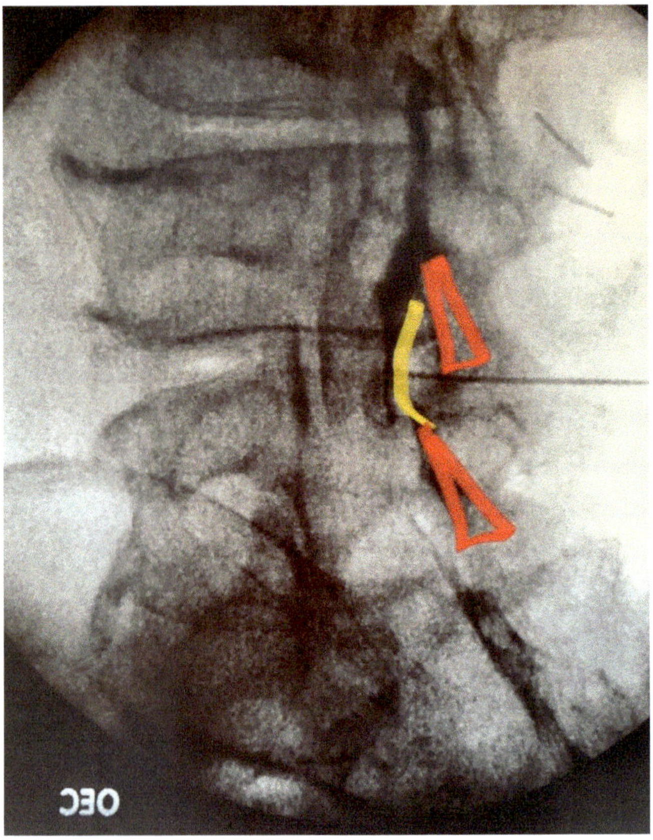

FIGURE 6.4. CLO view at 45° can allow visualization of lamina (shown in red) at the L4–L5 interlaminar space. The epidural needle is placed at the most superior aspect (ideally). Notice that the needle is deeper than normal, as the L4–L5 level has ligamentum flavum hypertrophy. This creates a visual barrier of the anterior-most aspect (shown in yellow) of the ligamentum flavum. As decompression occurs, this yellow line will begin to flatten out.

Procedure Completion

The procedure is completed when there is a dramatic reduction of available resectable tissue at the debulked level. The access portal is removed, and the incision is closed and dressed (after hemostasis). The procedural steps are done in a similar fashion on the contralateral side of the same level and at other levels, if clinically necessary.

Procedural Evolution—Streamlined Technique

With over 30,000 MILD procedures performed to date, the standard technique has evolved into the streamlined technique, based on experience and continuous improvement. The streamlined technique was organically devised by Dr. Brent Chafin, who has been offering MILD to his patients since 2010 and has himself treated over 1,500 patients. After treating hundreds of patients, Dr. Chafin developed efficiencies in his approach to MILD, and he partnered with leading MILD physicians from all over the country to leverage group

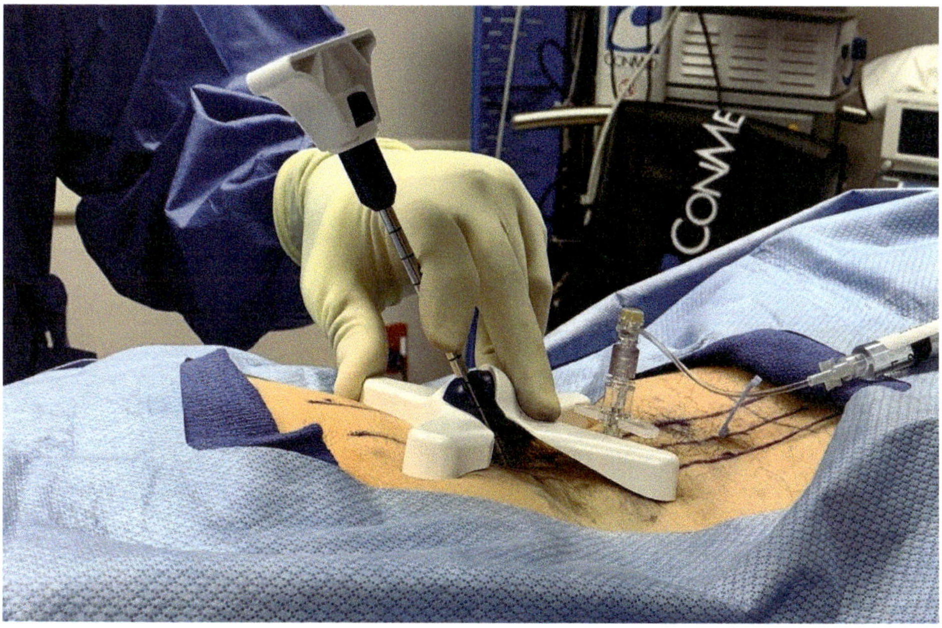

FIGURE 6.5. The nondominant hand holds the portal. The portal stabilizer eliminates medial and lateral movement. The epidural needle is above at the target level being decompressed. Skin markings (seen in blue) are used for trajectory and orientation of the instruments (to prevent crossing over the midline). Chips of the inferior lamina are removed by inserting the bone rongeur through to the port. The bone rongeur is advanced over the lamina lip before bites are taken to ensure that adequate material removal is achieved. The bone rongeur should be removed after each pass to remove the lamina chips. Starting from the medial surface of the inferior lamina and progressing toward the lateral end is recommended.

experience and expertise in an effort to further refine the approach. The physicians who contributed to the effort included Dr. Navdeep Jassal, Dr. Tim Deer, Dr. Dawood Sayed, Dr. Peter Pryzblykowski, Dr. Mark Coleman, Dr. Anjum Bux, Dr. Alex Escobar, Dr. Harry Sukumaran, and Dr. Stanley Golovac.

The streamlined technique allows physicians to increase procedural efficiency by using a single midline incision and single midline epidurogram to effectively and safely access multiple treatment zones. Thus, the MILD procedure affords flexibility in responding to patients' anatomical variations, and the physician performing the procedure can choose either the standard technique (multiple incisions) or the streamlined technique (single midline incision). For either technique, the physician can use epidurography (multiple epidurograms for the standard technique or a single midline epidurogram for the streamlined technique) or the VILL to visualize the safety barrier (without contrast).

In the streamlined technique's approach to decompression, there is general guidance to use the "rule of threes."

- Three bites on the superior lamina with the bone rongeur
- Three bites on the inferior lamina with the bone rongeur
- Three sets of three scoops with the tissue sculptor to detach and debulk the hypertrophic ligament

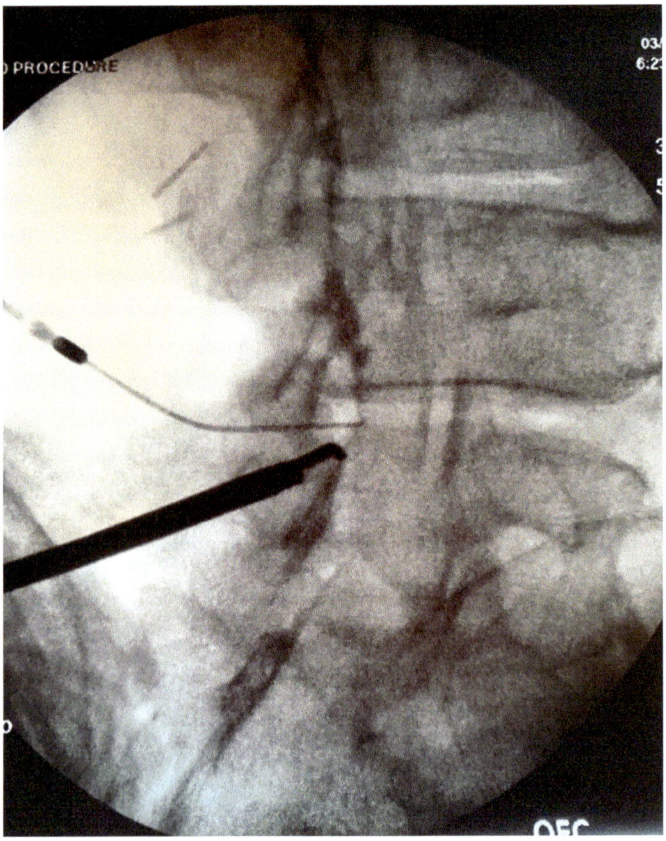

FIGURE 6.6. Bone rongeur is being used to allow for ease of entry of tissue sculptor at the target level being decompressed. Notice the distal end of the bone rongeur over the lip of the inferior lamina.

Because the streamlined technique uses one midline incision, the procedure involves pulling back the MILD portal to the subcutaneous tissue to change the level or side of treatment. This is done by using the degree of elasticity of the skin and tissue, sometimes referred to as turgor.

The use of contrast at the end of the procedure has been abandoned in both the standard and the streamlined technique. Current practice involves decompression until there are diminishing returns with the bone rongeur and tissue sculptor, following the rule of threes.

Once all levels have been treated, the devices are removed as a unit and a Steri-Strip is applied to close the incision.

Postoperative Management and Follow-up

There are some general considerations after a MILD procedure.

1. Following treatment with the MILD procedure, patients can resume normal activity within 24 hours with no restrictions. Patients can start a home exercise program

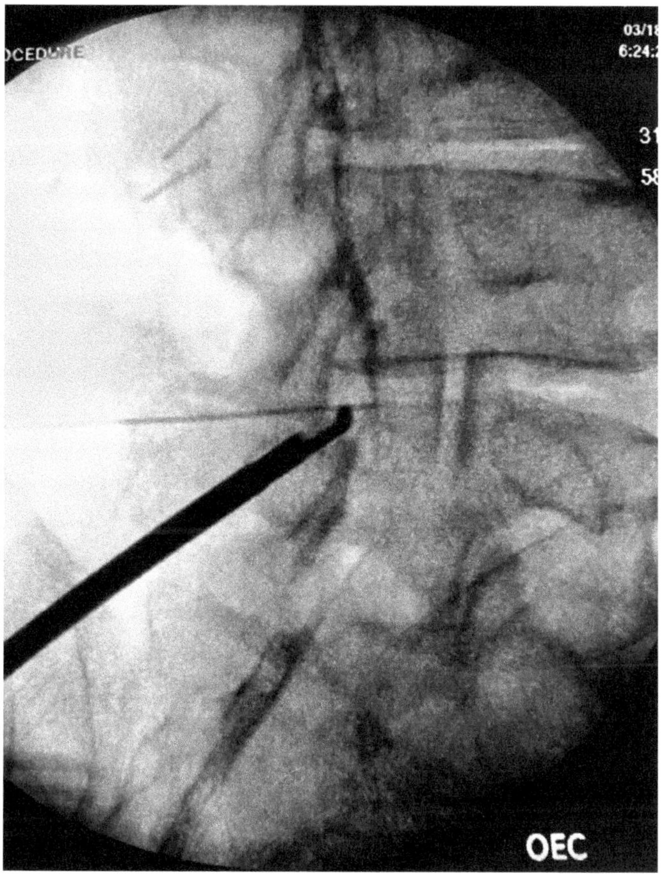

FIGURE 6.7. Bone rongeur is being used to allow for ease of entry of tissue sculptor at the target level being decompressed. Notice the distal end of the bone rongeur over the lip of the superior lamina. The bone rongeur is rotated 180° after being used on the inferior lamina.

immediately that involves walking and core strengthening. The walking program starts from the patient's own baseline effort and slowly progresses in distance over the next 6 weeks. Core strengthening can be continued with simple stretches. Examples of such stretches are pelvic tilt, knee to chest, and lower trunk rotation. Patients should be encouraged by improvement of walking and standing over the next 3 months, and it is important to establish patient's expectations of improvement with time and with continued postprocedure reconditioning.[16]

2. Postoperative dressing can be removed in 48 hours, as there are typically only one or more small puncture incisions from the 5.1-mm portal. Standard follow-up generally includes a visit 2 weeks after the procedure. If the patient can benefit from continued structured functional conditioning, a 4- to 6-week formal physical therapy regimen specifically for LSS with neurogenic claudication may be prescribed.
3. Standing time, walking distance, and patient satisfaction are typical assessments that can be followed to determine patient outcome and success. Pain relief is only one aspect of determining success from the procedure.

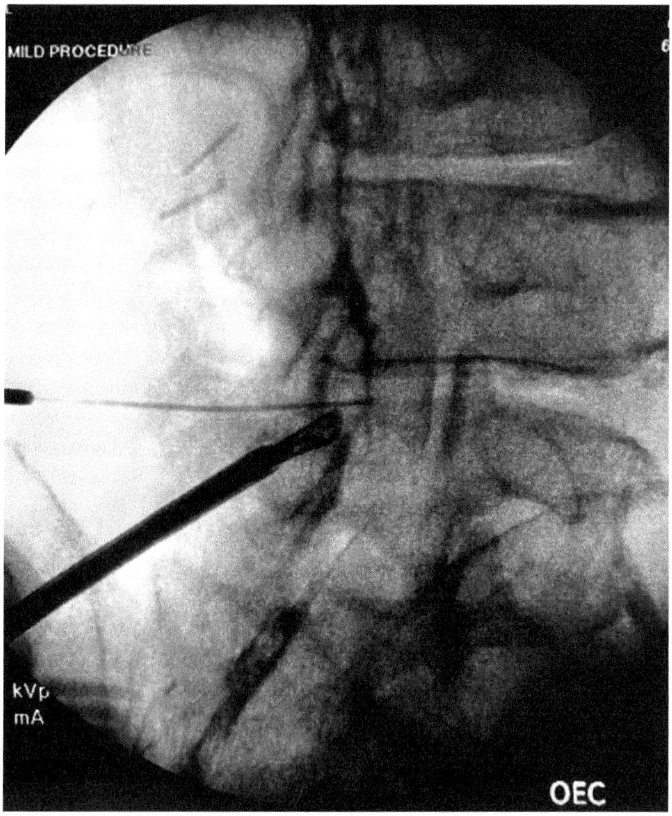

FIGURE 6.8. Tissue sculptor used in an inferior to superior motion trajectory to allow ligamentum flavum to fill the tool.

4. A follow-up with the physician is typically conducted at 4 to 6 weeks after the MILD procedure, and then monthly for the next 2 months.
5. In the event the patient is continuing to experience discomfort from other pain generators (such as facet-mediated pain or myofascial pain), it is recommended to wait 10 to

TABLE 6.2. Safety Comparison through 2-Year Follow-Up (MiDAS ENCORE Study)

Reoperation	**5.6%** Eight patients underwent a subsequent surgical procedure at the index level
Device- and procedure-related adverse events (AEs)	**1.3%** Two patients were described: 1. Intraoperative oozing observed at treatment site. Gelfoam was administered. Patient was discharged on the same day with no complications. 2. Patient experienced postoperative pain, possibly related to MILD, that resolved within 3 days of the index procedure.
Device- and procedure-related serious AEs	**0%**
Lumbar spine fractures	**0%**
Removal of hardware	**0%** (There are no implants with the MILD procedure.)

12 weeks before proceeding with additional treatment, to allow for further MILD procedural benefit.

Complications and Management

Potential complications are similar to those with any spinal procedure, including bleeding, infection, and nerve injury. Dural tear is a potential complication, although it is extremely rare. Procedural safety has been well studied in MiDAS ENCORE, a prospective, multicenter, randomized controlled clinical study. The 2-year results of MiDAS ENCORE showed that the safety of the MILD procedure is comparable to that of a lumbar ESI.[14]

The bone rongeur and tissue sculptor have both been carefully developed with safety in mind. Of note, the tissue sculptor has a smooth scooping surface on the distal end and should never be rotated 180° during use. This, coupled with direct visualization in the contralateral oblique view, allows for exceptional procedural safety, as indicated above.

Conclusion

LSS is a common degenerative process of the spine that not only is painful, but also affects functional mobility. Patients present with symptoms of neurogenic claudication, and the MILD procedure treats the root cause by safely debulking the ligamentum flavum. The MILD technique does not involve the use of implants, making it currently the safest option with durable outcomes. Thirteen peer-reviewed studies have shown that MILD has a safety profile comparable to that of ESI. With safety and efficacy in mind, MILD should be considered the first-line intervention after conservative treatment options have failed in patients with LSS and neurogenic claudication.[17,18]

References

1. North American Spine Society. *Evidence Based Clinical Guidelines for Multidisciplinary Spine Care: Diagnosis and Treatment of Degenerative Lumbar Spinal Stenosis*. Burr Ridge, IL: North American Spine Society; 2007.
2. Ishimoto Y, Yoshimura N, Muraki S, et al. Prevalence of symptomatic lumbar spinal stenosis and its association with physical performance in a population-based cohort in Japan: the Wakayama Spine Study. *Osteoarthritis Cartilage*. 2012;20(10):1103–1108.
3. Mekhail N, Costandi S, Abraham B, Samuel SW. Functional and patient-reported outcomes in symptomatic lumbar spinal stenosis following percutaneous decompression. *Pain Pract*. 2012;12(6):417–425.
4. Hansson T, Suzuki N, Hebelka H, Gaulitz A. The narrowing of the lumbar spinal canal during loaded MRI: the effects of the disc and ligamentum flavum. *Eur Spine J*. 2009;18(5):679–686.
5. Ammendolia C, Stuber KJ, Rok E, et al. Nonoperative treatment for lumbar spinal stenosis with neurogenic claudication. *Cochrane Database Syst Rev*. 2013(8):CD010712.
6. Manchikanti L, Knezevic NN, Boswell MV, Kaye AD, Hirsch JA. Epidural injections for lumbar radiculopathy and spinal stenosis: a comparative systematic review and meta-analysis. *Pain Physician*. 2016;19(3):E365–E410.
7. Fukusaki M, Kobayashi I, Hara T, Sumikawa K. Symptoms of spinal stenosis do not improve after epidural steroid injection. *Clin J Pain*. 1998;14(2):148–151.

8. Benyamin RM, Staats PS, MiDAS ENCORE Investigators. MILD® is an effective treatment for lumbar spinal stenosis with neurogenic claudication: MiDAS ENCORE randomized controlled trial. *Pain Physician.* 2016;19(4):229–242.
9. Staats PS, Chafin TB, Golovac S, et al. Long-term safety and efficacy of minimally invasive lumbar decompression procedure for the treatment of lumbar spinal stenosis with neurogenic claudication: 2-year results of MiDAS ENCORE. *Reg Anesth Pain Med.* 2018;43(7):789–794.
10. Chopko B, Caraway DL. MiDAS I (MILD Decompression Alternative to Open Surgery): a preliminary report of a prospective, multi-center clinical study. *Pain Physician.* 2010;13(4):369–378.
11. Chopko BW. A novel method for treatment of lumbar spinal stenosis in high-risk surgical candidates: pilot study experience with percutaneous remodeling of ligamentum flavum and lamina. *J Neurosurg Spine.* 2011;14(1):46–50.
12. Schomer DF, Solsberg D, Wong W, Chopko BW. MILD® lumbar decompression for the treatment of lumbar spinal stenosis. *Neuroradiol J.* 2011;24(4):620–626.
13. Basu S. MILD procedure: single-site prospective IRB study. *Clin J Pain.* 2012;28(3):254–258.
14. Deer TR, Kim CK, Bowman RG 2nd, Ranson MT, Yee BS. Study of percutaneous lumbar decompression and treatment algorithm for patients suffering from neurogenic claudication. *Pain Physician.* 2012;15(6):451–460.
15. Brown LL. A double-blind, randomized, prospective study of epidural steroid injection vs. the MILD® procedure in patients with symptomatic lumbar spinal stenosis. *Pain Pract.* 2012;12(5):333–341.
16. Chopko BW. Long-term results of percutaneous lumbar decompression for LSS: two-year outcomes. *Clin J Pain.* 2013;29(11):939–943.
15. Deer TR, Narouze S, Provenzano DA, et al. The Neurostimulation Appropriateness Consensus Committee (NACC): recommendations on bleeding and coagulation management in neurostimulation devices. *Neuromodulation.* 2017;20(1):51–62. doi:10.1111/ner.12542. Erratum in *Neuromodulation.* 2017;20(4):407. PMID: 28042905.
16. Mekhail N, Costandi S, Abraham B, Samuel SW. Functional and patient-reported outcomes in symptomatic lumbar spinal stenosis following percutaneous decompression. *Pain Pract.* 2012;12(6):417–425. doi:10.1111/j.1533-2500.2012.00565.x.
17. Jain S, Deer T, Sayed D, et al. Minimally invasive lumbar decompression: a review of indications, techniques, efficacy and safety. *Pain Manag.* 2020;10(5):331–348. doi:10.2217/pmt-2020-0037. PMID: 32609052.
18. Deer TR, Grider JS, Pope JE, et al. The MIST guidelines: The Lumbar Spinal Stenosis Consensus Group guidelines for minimally invasive spine treatment. *Pain Pract.* 2019;19(3):250–274. doi:10.1111/papr.12744. PMID: 30369003.

7

Endoscopic Discectomy

Jeffrey D. Petersohn, Mayank Gupta, and Umar M. Syed

Introduction

The traditional model of surgical treatment of spine disease often requires sizable incisions with division of, and/or stripping of, paraspinal muscle and resection of bone to allow access to the vertebral canal and foramina for decompression of neural structures. When the postsurgical anatomic integrity of the residual spinal elements is judged structurally inadequate, surgical stabilization of the spine is effected with fusion of spinal segments with a variety of anterior, posterior, and 360° techniques using morcellated or cortical bone graft, osteoinductive putty, or growth factors, such as BMP. Internal fixation systems using interbody cages and pedicle or lateral mass screws with cross-linked rod systems have become commonplace. Plates and screws may also be used. Unfortunately, the consequences of the surgical disruption of posterior elements and postsurgical compromise of the extensor muscular compartment frequently results in disturbed biomechanics of the postsurgical spine and poor late surgical outcomes. These changes include adjacent segment compromise with facet pain or facet hypertrophy, junctional disk herniations, postsurgical kyphosis, hypolordosis, pelvic imbalance, and the consequences of perineural scarring. These problems have prompted the development of minimally invasive techniques that produce less blood loss, require less disruption of the adjacent anatomy, with less postoperative structural compromise, and allow more rapid patient recovery from surgery. Technological advances in instrumentation and developments in surgical technique have allowed for proliferation of a panoply of minimally invasive techniques. Some apply the term *endoscopic* to describe use of a system of progressive tubular dilators that allow a 12-mm or larger channel through which conventional instruments are passed, producing modest reduction of incision size and a reduced extent of disruption of overlying muscle and connective tissue relative to conventional surgery. True endoscopic spine surgery uses a system of sequential dilators passed over a guidewire to expand a small cutaneofascial incision and to allow placement of a cylindrical working sleeve in a transmuscular opening approximately 7 to 8.5 mm in diameter, through which is inserted a full-video endoscope providing digital magnification of the image at the distal tip of the instrument. A typical endoscope contains two fiberoptic bundles, allowing illumination by an external light source and transmission of a high-quality video image using a 20° to 30° distally angled lens on a digital camera. The endoscope also contains channels for irrigation, suction, and passage of working instrumentation.

Curiously, few surgical specialties prize large incisions and disruption of normal anatomy to unnecessary advantage except when diminishing the performance of full-video endoscopy as "percutaneous," implying that a less destructive access route to surgically relevant anatomy is somehow inferior. Considering that in teaching hospitals, surgical access to the spine and closure of the incision are often deferred to the lowly medical student or intern, the incision is not the relevant issue. Clearly, and without regard to surgical approach technique, the most respected skills require similar dexterity, judgment, and facility to accomplish specific anatomic modification of structures within, and adjacent to, the vertebral canal. With the spinal endoscopist's use of magnified images, sophisticated instrumentation allows precise tissue resection, neural decompression, and superior hemostasis using flexible bipolar radiofrequency (RF) cautery with resection of the disk and ligamentous and osseous structures. Spinal endoscopy may use intralaminar, transforaminal, or extraforaminal approaches, as dictated by the anatomy of the pain process and planned surgical treatment. Unlike shoulder or knee arthroscopy, where openings between structures are present and allow navigation within the native joint, spinal endoscopy requires continuous irrigation under pressure to distend the interstructural relationships, providing a fluid-filled working volume that allows anatomic visualization. With the use of continuous irrigation, typically containing antibiotics, the postoperative infection rate is at least 40% less than for lumbar microdiscectomy, and with the meticulous hemostasis provided by use of flexible bipolar RF cautery, there is far less perineural and postoperative scarring than with conventional surgical approaches and has shown to be highly efficacious through numerous RCTs and meta-analyses. The rate of dural tears compares favorably with the rate for microdiscectomy, with less than 1% incidence with

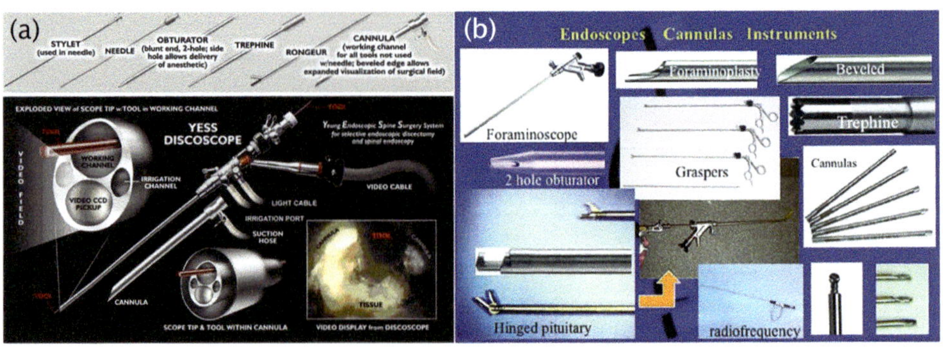

FIGURE 7.1. Commonly used instruments in endoscopic spine surgeries.[4]

transforaminal approaches and 1% to 3% in interlaminar approaches, and with reduced incidence seen with more experienced physicians.

The learning curve for acquiring skills for the performance of endoscopic spine surgery is lengthier than with open procedures. The challenges of orientation, structural identification, and the specifics of use of endoscopically adapted instrumentation, reamers, drills, and burrs recommend both classroom didactic, cadaveric experience and a period of supervised training; this quality of instruction may not be widely available in all venues. There are at least four major manufacturers of a full-range of endoscopic instrumentation, each of whom offers workshop training programs, lectures, and instructional videos for interested physicians.

This chapter introduces the current evidence, indications, and optimal technique for the minimally invasive endoscopic treatment of disk herniations.

Indications

Surgical endoscopic procedures are indicated for the treatment of pain and/or neurologic deficits caused by structural neural compromise, including, but not limited to, that produced by disk herniations, spondylosis, facet synovial cysts, hypertrophic ligamentum flavum, or hypertrophic facet joints.

As for any spinal surgery, patients should have first participated in a temporally circumscribed program of nonsurgical management, including physical therapy or its equivalent, and, as appropriate, diagnostic or therapeutic spinal injections following diagnostic imaging using x-rays and one or more of MRI, CT, or CT/myelography.

Spinal endoscopic techniques are not limited to use in the lumbar spine, and they have been shown useful for cervical and thoracic pathologies in case studies and published series. While lumbar spinal endoscopic procedures are performed safely by physicians trained in a variety of primary specialties, completion of fellowship training in cervical and thoracic spinal surgery would be a reasonable preparation before venturing into these regions of the spine.

Evidence

The therapeutic benefit and safety of endoscopic discectomies have been established in numerous randomized controlled trials and retrospective meta-analyses. Efficacy and complications were similar when compared to open discectomy or microdiscectomy. Outcomes were measured by ODI and VAS scores. Additional measures included postoperative pain, length of hospital stay, and recovery time, which were all significantly decreased when endoscopic procedures were compared to alterative procedures. Table 7.1 is a summary of the relevant studies.

In comparisons of relative outcomes of endoscopic spinal decompression versus microdiscectomy (MLD), central disk HNP outcomes were superior for MLD, with equivalent outcomes for lateral recess and foraminal decompression. The endoscopic technique is substantially superior for far-lateral or extraforaminal pathology, including HNP.

TABLE 7.1.

Study	Study Type	Inclusion Criteria	Patients (*N*)/ Follow-up Period	Control/ Active Intervention	Outcome Measures Analyzed	Results	Conclusion
Chen et al[5]	Randomized controlled trial	Patients with imaging-confirmed LDH with persistent signs and symptoms of radiculopathy	$N = 153$	MED/PTED	ODI	Patients in the MED group at 3, 6, and 12 months: Those in the far-lateral herniation group had significantly less improvement in ODI scores than those in the paramedian group. Patients in the PTED group: Those in the median herniation group had less improvement in ODI scores than those in the paramedian group.	PTED appeared to be better for treatment of far-lateral herniations, while MED was more suited for median disk herniations. PTED did not show better clinical outcomes or safety than MED.
Gadjradj et al[6]	Prospective case series	Patients who underwent PTED for LDH	$N = 166$	—/PTED	VAS, QBPDS	Baseline: VAS = 82.5 ± 17.3 QBPDS = 60 ± 18.4. 6 weeks: VAS = 28.8 ± 24.5 QBPDS = 26.7 ± 20.6. Significant reduction at 6 weeks and a further reduction at 52 weeks.	PTED is a safe and effective treatment for LDH and shows similar outcomes to open MD.
Liu et al[7]	Clinical outcome comparison study	Patients with symptomatic LDH at L3–L4 and L4–L5 treated with PTED, MED, and MD	$N = 192$/2 years PTED: $n = 60$ MED: $n = 63$ MD: $n = 69$	PTED/MED/MD	VAS, ODI	Incision length, operation duration, blood loss, length of hospital stay, and postoperative incision pain were best in the PTED group ($P < .05$). VAS score of low back pain was significantly better ($P < .05$) at the last follow-up than in the other groups. All groups had significantly improved postoperative VAS and ODI scores when compared to preoperative groups.	Patients who underwent PTED have less low back pain over 2 years and have more rapid recoveries than patients who underwent MED or MD. PTED, MED, and MD are all effective techniques for treatment of LDH.
Ohya et al[8]	Retrospec-tive propensity score matched analysis	Patients admitted between July 2010 and March 2013 who underwent MED and OD	$N = 26{,}612$ OD: $n = 20{,}190$ MED: $n = 6{,}422$	OD/MED	Major complications, hospital stay, in-hospital mortality	Significant decrease in major complications for patients undergoing MED when compared to OD (0.8% vs. 1.3%; $P = .01$). Significant decrease in hospital stay in the MED group (11 vs. 15 days; $P < .001$). No significant difference in the in-hospital mortality between the two groups.	MED was associated with a significantly decreased rate of major complications and length of hospital stay in comparison to OD.

Gibson et al[9]	Randomized controlled trial	Single-level prolapse with exiting and/or traversing nerve root compression and failure of conservative management	$N = 143$/3, 12, and 24 months	MD/TED	VAS, ODI, SF-36	Baseline: VAS in affected leg TED = 6.2 (2.8) vs. MD = 5.8 (2.6) ODI TED = 44 (17) vs. MD = 42 (15) SF-36 PCS TED = 34.1 (6.8) vs. MD = 35.7 (7.1). 2 years: VAS of affected leg significantly lower for TED = 1.9 ± 2.6 vs. MD = 3.5 ± 3.1 ($P < .002$) ODI TED = 18(17) vs. MD 22 (20) SF-36 PCS TED = 47.7 (10.6) vs. MD 47.4 (10.6). There were no major complications reported.	Functional improvements and outcomes were maintained in both groups, with the TED group having a more rapid recovery and less leg pain at 2 years.
Meyer et al[10]	Prospective randomized controlled trial	Symptoms of radiculopathy with corresponding MRI-confirmed LDH and failure of 6 weeks of conservative treatment	$N = 47$/ 12 months	MD /PELD	VAS, ODI	Preoperative: VAS lumbar pain, MD = 6.5 (2.6) vs. ED = 5.4 (2.6) VAS sciatica, MD = 8.7 (1.4) vs. ED = 8.4 (1.7). Postoperative: VAS lumbar pain at 3 months, MD = 3.3 (2.6) vs. ED = 1.6 (2.0) ($P = .009$). VAS sciatica at 12 months, MD = 3 (3.6) vs. ED 2.1 (1.9) ($P < .001$). One dural lesion in the MD group. One postoperative infection in MD group. Three recurrences: 1 in ED group and 2 in MD group.	Endoscopic discectomy is safe, effective, and offers similar results to MD. Less low back pain was reported in the ED group 7 days, 1 month, and 3 months following surgery.

(*continued*)

TABLE 7.1. Continued

Study	Study Type	Inclusion Criteria	Patients (N)/ Follow-up Period	Control/ Active Intervention	Outcome Measures Analyzed	Results	Conclusion
Ruetten et al[11]	Prospective randomized controlled study	Patients with clinically symptomatic disk herniation who underwent discectomies in 2004	$N = 200$/ 24 months	MI/FE	Perioperative complications, recurrences, VAS, ODI	VAS: 79% of MI vs. 85% of FE reported no leg pain after 2 years. No significant differences between groups. Complication rate was significantly elevated in the MI group. Complications included postoperative bleeding, delayed wound healing, transient postoperative dysesthesia, and transient urinary retention. Postoperative pain, work disability, and pain medication use were significantly reduced in the FE group ($P < .01$). No significant differences in the rate of recurrence. Mean operation time was significantly reduced in the FE group (22 vs. 42 minutes). No device- or procedure-related complications were reported.	FE provided safe and clinically comparable outcomes to MI, with significant reduction in postoperative pain and medication use.
Mlaka et al[12]	Prospective observational multicenter two-arm parallel study	Unilateral lumbosacral radicular pain correlated with single-level disk herniation on MRI unresponsive to conservative treatments or transforaminal steroid injections.	$N = 83$ IL and $N = 103$ TF/ 12 months	—/Endoscopic lumbar discectomy via IL and TF	ODI, EQ-VAS	Baseline: IL ODI = 43.36 (SD = 15.98) TF ODI = 39.09 (SD = 14.01). 12 months: IL ODI = 14.75 ($P < .001$) TF ODI = 17.52 ($P < .001$). Statistically significant improvements were observed in both approaches, including reduction in back and leg pain, increase in quality of life, and decrease in ODI.	Endoscopic discectomy via TF or IL provides significant patient relief while decreasing risk of complications and length of hospital stay.

Ahn et al[13]	Observational study	Patients with soft LDH on both MRI and CT, intractable lumbar radiculopathy, and failed nonoperative treatment for a minimum of 6 weeks	$N = 298$/5 years	Open MD/TELD	ODI, VAS	Baseline: VAS TELD = 6.57 ± 2.31 Open = 6.58 ± 1.77. 5 years: VAS TELD = 1.44 ± 1.02 Open = 1.32 ± 1.02. No significant differences between groups in ODI and Macnab criteria. Significantly shorter operative time, hospital stay, and time to return to work in the TELD group.	TELD group had significantly shorter operative time, time to return to work, and hospital stay. Clinical outcomes were comparable in both groups.

Abbreviations: EQ-VAS, ; FE, full endoscopic discectomy; IL, intralaminar approach; LDH, lumbar disk herniation; MD, microdiscectomy; MED, microendoscopic discectomy; MI, conventional microsurgical discectomy; OD, open discectomy; ODI, ; PELD, percutaneous endoscopic lumbar discectomy; PTED, percutaneous transforaminal endoscopic discectomy; QBPDS, ; SF-36, ;TED, transforaminal endoscopic discectomy; TELD, transforaminal endoscopic microdiscectomy; TF, transforaminal approach; VAS, .

Patient Selection and Contraindications

Candidates for the procedure are patients with persistent radicular symptoms or severe pain interfering with activities of daily living caused by structural neural compromise refractory to at least 6 weeks of conservative treatment. The anatomic basis for symptoms should typically correlate with the physical examination and anatomic findings on MRI or CT.

The procedure can be performed under local anesthesia with sedation or with general anesthesia. Due to use of ionizing radiation (fluoroscopy), treatment of parturients is not recommended. Medical contraindications, including sepsis, coagulopathy, and local infection, remain valid.

In combination with posterior interspinous fusion devices or anterior expandable interbody cages and percutaneous instrumentation, segmental stabilization can be performed where translational or angular stability is a relevant concern. The reader is directed to conventional texts of spine surgery for discussion relevant to incorporation or choice of surgical stabilization techniques that are beyond the scope of this chapter.

Relative contraindications to the procedure are a major neurologic deficit, including spinal cord compression, and migration of the herniated disk more than one-third of the vertebral body height. Consideration may be given to the presence of tall iliac crests impeding entry to the L5–S1 level, deformity (anterolisthesis), partial disk space collapse, or listhesis at the planned operative level.

Absolute contraindications to the procedure include unstable spinal fracture, epidural hematoma, Grade II or worse anterolisthesis at the operated level, gross instability, infection, or abscess of the epidural space. Due to the irrigation fluid pressure and that engendered by manual retraction of the dural sac, which would be expected to increase intraneural pressure, patients with myelopathy or cauda equina syndrome should be avoided until evidence demonstrates the safety of endoscopic techniques in these circumstances.

Contraindications must be carefully considered based on clinical context and the medical stability of the patient; however, endoscopic approaches may still provide significant advantages in complicated patient presentations due to a reduction in tissue damage, shortened operative time, avoidance of general anesthesia, reduced infection rate, and more rapid return to function than with conventional spine surgeries.

Pathology addressable with the endoscopic technique is limited by the endoscopist's diagnostic expertise, the mastery of the techniques required, and a full understanding of the complex anatomic features to be encountered. To paraphrase Dr. Stefan Hellinger, "A fool with an instrument is still a fool."

The learning curve for mastery of endoscopic spine surgery techniques is considerably protracted in comparison to that for open surgical procedures, in large measure due to challenges encountered in correlating the limited field of operative view provided by the endoscope with the anatomic orientation of the endoscope, the angulated view provided by the typical 20° to 30° endoscopic lens, and the variability of the field of view and size of spinal structures with depth of scope placement, as well as the need to learn to modify working sleeve placement for both exposure and retraction. Studies have shown that reduced operating times and reduced complications occur with the surgeon's progressive experience with endoscopic techniques; experience with 25 to 50 cases is typically required to achieve facility.

In selecting patients, it may be wise to limit the pathology to be addressed to one or no more than two levels or one level bilaterally, as extended duration of surgery using a prolonged duration of epidural irrigation or prolonged episodes of high irrigant pressure may be deleterious and a potential cause of seizures and/or blindness.

Perioperative Management

Recent imaging studies, usually MRI or CT, are required for endoscopic procedures. CT is especially helpful in planning access to the L5–S1 foramen. As for any surgical procedure, documentation of failure of nonoperative care is customary. Typical laboratory work is limited, with routine CBC, and, where medically merited, electrolytes, glucose, and PT/PTT may be obtained. A history of relevant allergies is scrutinized for concerns related to latex, injected contrast agents, and antibiotics. Due to the reduced tissue damage and physical stress associated with endoscopic techniques as compared to open spine surgeries, a broader patient population may be considered for endoscopic procedures, and medical or cardiology consultation may be appropriate to confirm the patient's candidacy for an endoscopic operative procedure.

Antiplatelet and anticoagulant medications are handled as for any open surgical procedure; these medications are withheld to minimize operative bleeding risk in conjunction with the cardiologist or surgeon who has prescribed them. Unlike knee or shoulder arthroscopy, continuous injection of irrigant under pressure is required to dilate the perineural or epidural spaces to provide adequate visualization and this can be accomplished with pressurized bladders compressing bags of irrigant solution or with an electric pump. Preoperative antibiotics are administered intravenously, as for any spinal surgery, and antibiotics are typically used in the irrigation solution. Aseptic preparation of the surgical site and maintenance of sterile technique, including full surgical dress, is mandatory. Special drapes include pockets to collect endoscopic irrigation fluids and use of water-resistant disposable shoe covers extending to the knee is advisable.

Lumbar and lumbosacral endoscopic spine procedures may be performed under ample local anesthesia with sedation or with general anesthesia. Local anesthesia is placed in the skin, in the subcutaneous tissue, and in the muscular tract extending to the superior articular process or laminar entry target, and typically local anesthetic with epinephrine is injected upon the bony structures to provide comfort and enhance hemostasis. Cervical and thoracic endoscopic techniques typically require general anesthesia.

With use of local anesthesia and sedation, the patient can be instructed to notify the surgeon if pain is experienced; if it is, the patient is asked whether the pain is in the back or in the extremity, with the answer providing information to recommend modification of technique to avoid neural compression, traction, or inadvertent use of an RF probe close to the nerve. Reassuringly, there is experimental evidence finding no long-term damage to spinal nerves when focal thermal lesions were made with bipolar cautery on the circumference of a spinal nerve; however, intraneural and nerve stump injection or thermal injuries are of far greater consequence. Under general anesthesia, consideration is given to use of SSEP neuromonitoring. Especially where substantial distraction or traction of neural structures may be required for interbody fusion, use of neuromonitoring is preferred by some surgeons.

Where upper lumbar levels are being addressed or if there is a pelvic kidney, placement of the initial needle entry for a transforaminal approach may be done using combined fluoroscopic and ultrasound guidance to limit the lateral entry margin and to reduce the risk of renal injury.

Technique

Full-video spinal endoscopic technique can address a broad spectrum of spinal pathologies, including disk herniations in paramedian, lateral recess, foraminal, or far lateral regions. There is considerably reduced trauma to skin and muscle in accessing either the vertebral canal or extraforaminal disk using endoscopic approaches compared with open surgical approaches or even with use of tubular dilator systems, which are often, but incorrectly, referred to as "endoscopic." Preservation of the facet joint is generally achieved, with limited resection of the superior articular process, lamina, or pedicle only as required to provide access to neural elements so that the mechanical stability of the ring structure contributed by the intact posterior elements is minimally disturbed and the mobility enabled by the zygapophysial (facet) joints is not compromised. Endoscopic approaches produce far less bleeding than is encountered in open surgical approaches, and use of flexible RF bipolar probes for coagulation via digitally magnified images results in reduced peridural and perineural fibrosis, which is a frequent cause of postlaminectomy syndrome. Furthermore, focal or extensive ligamentum flavum or facet hypertrophy can be constructively addressed in a more comprehensive fashion via direct endoscopic visualization than can be accomplished with minimally invasive techniques, such as minimally invasive lumbar decompression (MILD), where the imaged thickness of injected epidural contrast is used to indirectly indicate the extent and adequacy of the decompression.

For patients with isolated foraminal pathology, such as a foraminal disk herniation or a hypertrophic facet creating foraminal stenosis, endoscopic technique is efficient. Often a hypertrophic facet joint capsule is accompanied by hypertrophy of the transforaminal ligament extending from the cephalad aspect of the superior articular process to the inferoposterior border of the vertebral body, tethering or compressing the exiting nerve. This ligament may be calcified in whole or in part, meriting dissection of the adherent joint capsule or ligament from the nerve, with resection of the offending ligament or the osseous spur remnant to accomplish a decompressive neuroplasty.

When addressing a far-lateral disk herniation, use of a transforaminal approach to enter the neural foramen and decompress the disk sequentially from medial to lateral will often produce a sudden appearance of the exiting nerve root in the margin of the field of endoscopic view, as the disk will often tether the nerve at the cephalad disk margin. After disk resection, the nerve resumes its usual (and painless) anatomic course. If this happens, inspection of the anatomy for hemostasis is required, and if the nerve demonstrates transmitted cardiac pulsations, the procedure can be terminated with expectation of a salutary outcome.

In circumstances where there is significant translational or angular instability, endoscopic decompression can be paired with interbody fusion using expandable interbody cages and percutaneous pedicle screw instrumentation or with interspinous process fusion using percutaneously placed devices. Endoscopic interbody fusion is likely to be highly successful, because meticulous preparation of the vertebral endplates can be performed using special cutting blades and magnified full-video endoscopy allows visualization of the quality and thoroughness of endplate preparation unachievable by open technique, prior to placement of an expandable interbody fusion cage and bone graft.

Typical contraindications to surgical procedures, including sepsis, local infection at the skin entry site, coagulopathy, and pregnancy, pertain to endoscopic procedures as well. For acute disk space infection, endoscopic irrigation and debridement may provide rapid clinical improvement and superior outcomes compared to extended parenteral antibiotic treatment alone.

With endoscopic technique, the most common limitation to transforaminal approaches is tall iliac crests, which are especially notable in young males and prevent use of a rigid endoscope to access the neural foramen at the L5–S1 level. Interlaminar techniques at L5–S1 pose a higher risk of dural tears than transforaminal approaches at the same level, but literature suggests that the rate of dural tears with interlaminar approaches is no more than 2% to 3%, well below the 10% rate cited for microdiscectomy with hemilaminectomy. Patients with scoliotic angulation of the L4 or L5 lumbar vertebra may also pose access issues, and evaluation with coronal and sagittal plane imaging using MRI or CT may be helpful in surgical planning. Patients with severely narrowed L5–S1 intertransverse spaces pose similar technical challenges. To a degree, lateral decubitus positioning with use of a support or "bump" placed just cephalad to the iliac crest can open access to the lower lumbar levels that might not otherwise be accessible for transforaminal approaches in the supine position.

While most endoscopists prefer prone positioning for its ease and familiarity, the lateral approach offers several advantages, including improved access to lower lumbar and lumbosacral levels, but when the lateral decubitus position is used for operative endoscopic entry into the now "upward" foramen or interspace, the dural sac falls away from the instrumentation, also reducing the risks of dural tear. Furthermore, obese patients or those with compromised airway are easily managed because the anesthesiologist has full access to the airway with the patient in the lateral position, compared to the considerably restricted access available when the patient is prone.

There are several methods for placement of an endoscopic cannula for transforaminal access, and all rely upon anatomic knowledge of Kambin's triangle, the anatomic location of the DRG, vascular structures, and the course of the exiting and transiting spinal nerve roots. Anthony Yeung has written extensively regarding a system of skin markings to guide endoscope placement, but this author finds a fluoroscopically guided approach to be facile. Imaging studies are reviewed preoperatively to determine the approximate angles for access to the targeted neural foramen.

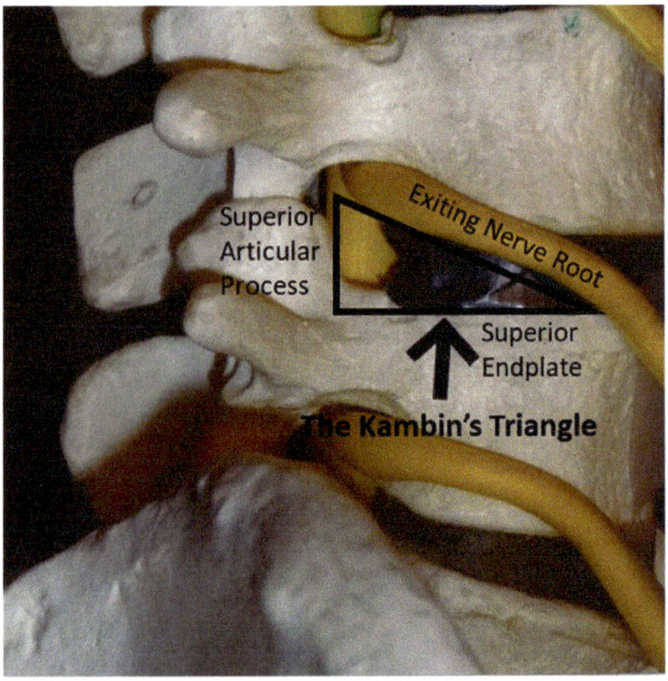

FIGURE 7.2. The anatomic relationships of Kambin's triangle.[14]

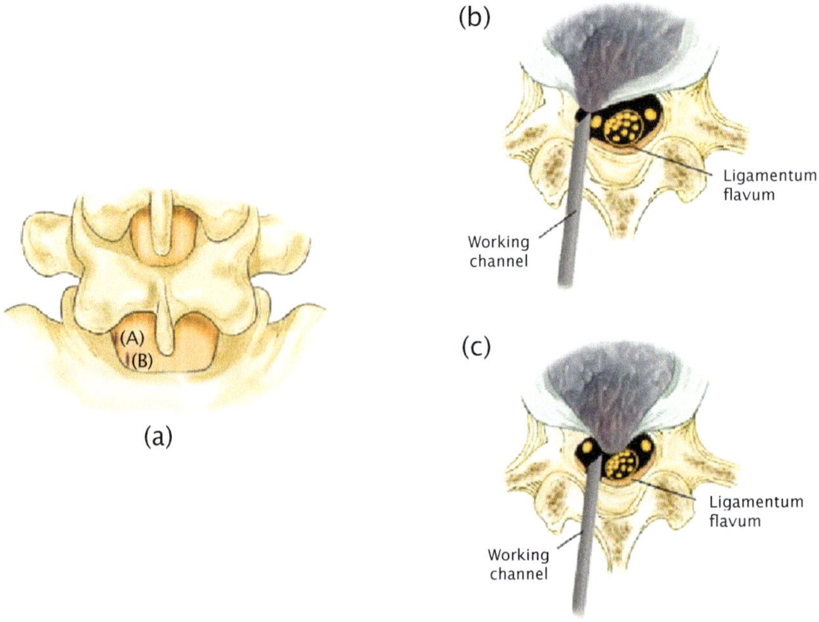

FIGURE 7.3. L5–S1 ligamentum flavum vertical splitting and introduction of the working channel. A & b, A more lateral approach for shoulder-type herniations. B & c, A more caudal approach in axillary-type herniations.[15]

The vertebral levels are enumerated in AP view with identification of the targeted level. The initial target is the tip of the superior articular process (SAP) at the target level. The superior aspect of the inferior vertebral body is squared off by adjustment of the cephalocaudad angle. The C-arm is rotated obliquely to place the SAP over the posterior vertebral body margin but medial to the iliac crest. Additional adjustment of the cephalocaudad angle is used to overlay the disk space with the SAP target, such that the inferior aspect of the foramen will be entered; this angle may be exaggerated with incremental alteration of oblique rotation and additional cephalad angulation so that a straight path can be plotted to target the superior aspect of the SAP. Local anesthetic infiltration of the iliac crest for L5–S1 access is helpful, but not usually necessary with other levels. An 18-gauge needle of suitable length is placed through the local anesthetic skin wheal. The stylet is removed, additional lidocaine with epinephrine is injected, and the needle is then advanced off the SAP and directed to enter the disk nucleus. At this time, injection of a mixture of low osmolality radiocontrast and a basic vital stain will allow endoscopic visualization of the acidic degenerated disk nuclear tissue. Indigo carmine was formerly used to stain nuclear tissue blue, but it is presently unavailable for clinical use; substitutes must be explored.

A semirigid guidewire is passed through the needle inserted into the disk nucleus. It is important to avoid advancing the wire excessively to enter neural, vascular, or peritoneal structures. At this time, with the guidewire in the disk nucleus, additional anesthetic is injected and a stab incision is made through anesthetized skin and into deep fascia along the guidewire. A series of dilators and close-fitting crown reamers of increasing size are sequentially advanced to resect the anterior aspect of the SAP to prepare the foramen for device placement. In AP view, transforaminal reamers must never pass medial to the medial pedicle border, to avoid dural injury. Slightly more lateral placement is used to access the upper lumbar foramina, because the DRGs are slightly more lateral at these levels, whereas in most lumbar levels the DRG is centered within the bony foramen, except that at S1, the DRG is found within the vertebral canal 80% of the time.

For transforaminal approaches, the dilators and crown reamers are removed with maintenance of the guidewire position, and a "bullet" dilator is advanced into the neural foramen, again never passing medial to the medial pedicular line. Additional local anesthetic is sprayed onto the lateral aspect of the SAP, and the bullet dilator remains in place while the guidewire is removed. A working sleeve with a curved distal end is placed over the bullet dilator and is rotated so that the open area faces anteriorly; most working sleeves have an index pin or stub opposite the side of the opening.

If during preparation of the foramen for endoscope placement, radicular pain or pain in an extremity is encountered, rechecking needle or device placement with fluoroscopy is required. If after alteration of approach, radicular pain continues, insertion of the endoscope to visualize the area of concern distal to the foramen may be considered. The possibility of furcal nerves or a tethered cord with caudad location of the exiting nerve may require alteration of approach or discontinuation of the procedure. Transient back pain, especially during tract dilation or reaming of the SAP, is not uncommon.

For endoscopic procedures to be conducted within the intervertebral disk, the bullet dilator is advanced into the disk under fluoroscopic guidance and the working sleeve is

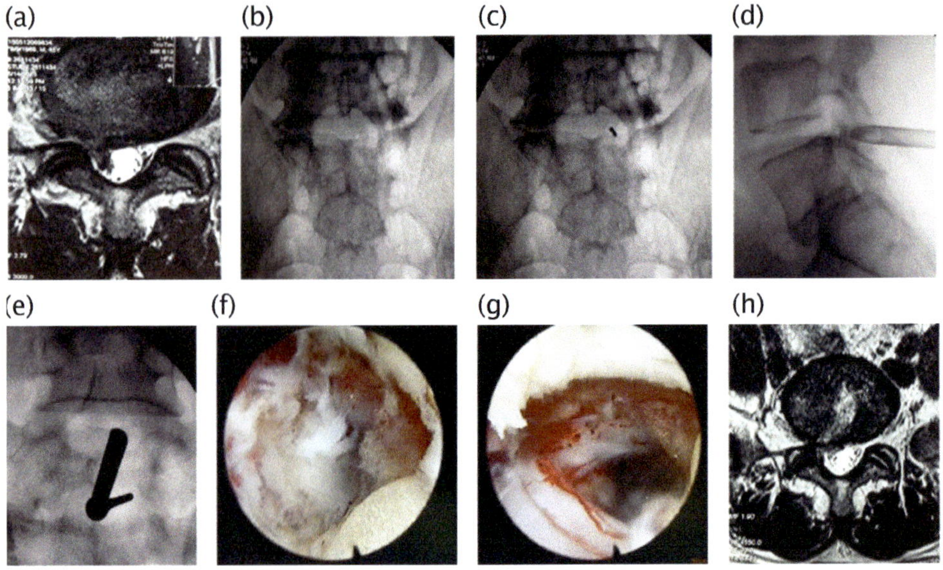

FIGURE 7.4. MRI, CT, and intraoperative endoscopic images of a patient with right-sided L5–S1 lumbar disk herniation.[16]

placed into the disk with the opening oriented posteriorly. The dilator is removed and the endoscope is placed in the working channel.

For endoscopic work within the neural foramen, the bullet dilator is removed, and the endoscope, primed with irrigation fluid, is inserted into the working sleeve with lens and opening facing anteriorly.

The endoscopist must be familiar with the normal and varied appearances of structures within the lumbar spine. Verification of endoscope placement and the location of any instruments or probes can be obtained by AP or lateral fluoroscopic images throughout the case.

Fragments of disk can be removed with pituitaries or forceps, and bipolar RF cautery can be used to shrink soft tissue, including the facet joint capsule and annular fibers. If working within the intervertebral disk, one usually works medially from about the midline, moving sequentially laterally to the medial pedicular line. The endpoint of adequate decompression for intradiscal approaches is noted when the posterior longitudinal ligament flaps freely with variation in the irrigation pressure.

For transforaminal approaches, the annulus is usually resected first with use of pituitaries, forceps, and bipolar cautery. When this has been accomplished, the endoscope and working sleeve are rotated to face posteriorly and the anterior facet capsule is resected sequentially to the tip of the SAP. The location of the exiting nerve relative to the foramen and endoscope should be kept in mind and the nerve identified when seen. Often the anterior aspect of the SAP is heavily calcified, and resection may be performed with endo reamers, with a small chisel, or with a motorized burr. The exiting nerve root should be free and evidencing transmitted cardiac pulsations. Hypertrophic transforaminal ligament should be explored if this is not the case, and it should be resected as necessary.

(a)

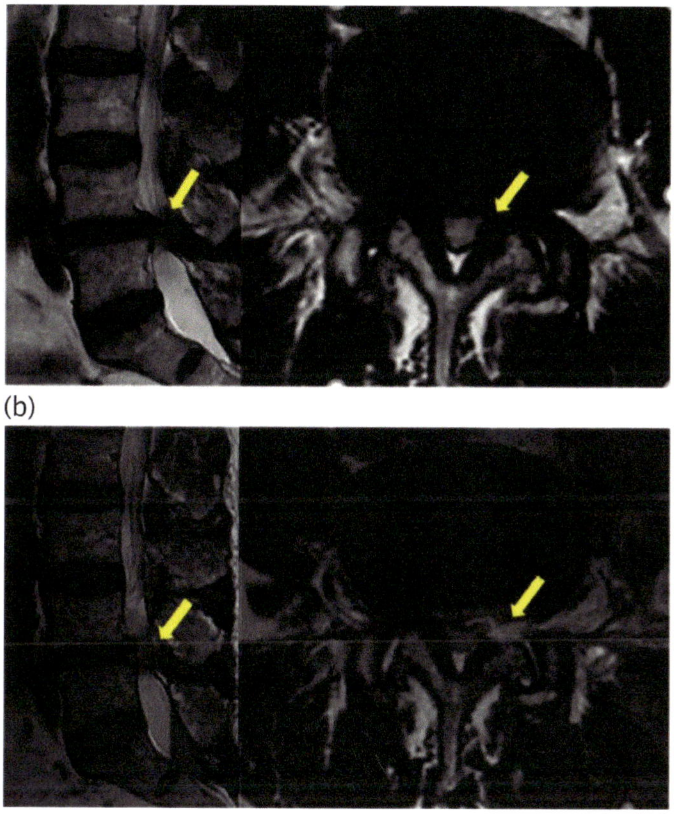

FIGURE 7.5. A, Preoperative and, B, postoperative MRI images of a female patient with left-sided lumbar lateral recess stenosis who underwent percutaneous endoscopic lumbar discectomy.[17]

Where lateral recess pathology is expected, the endoscope is then advanced into the lateral recess, with the appearance of epidural fat and the ligamentum flavum to be resected as needed. The transiting nerve root and dural sac are often seen as this point, and, again, transmitted cardiac pulsations affirm adequate decompression. If necessary, the endoscope is slowly withdrawn and foraminal disk and extraforaminal disk are inspected with additional resection of disk as necessary.

Meticulous hemostasis is obtained by use of bipolar RF cautery, and all instrumentation is removed from the space. The skin incision is usually closed with 4-0 Monocryl and is ressed with a Band-Aid.

When using transforaminal approaches, some physicians will inject the exiting nerve root with a local anesthetic/nonparticulate steroid to reduce post-operative radiculitis.

Postoperative antibiotics are not typically necessary.

The patient's neurologic status should be assessed in the PACU, and most patients are able to ambulate with little or no assistance within 30 minutes of completion of the procedure.

While the spine is not likely unstable from a mechanical standpoint, some physicians prefer use of a compact lumbosacral orthosis (LSO) to reduce risk of postoperative reinjury.

Postoperative analgesics may range from OTC NSAIDs to small doses of hydrocodone or oxycodone for 5 to 7 days.

Restrictions on postoperative showering and bathing, lifting, and twisting are given. The LSO need not be worn while in bed or in the bath and can be weaned after 3 to 4 weeks of use. Many physicians recommend avoidance of driving for 2 weeks postoperatively. Written postoperative instructions are recommended, along with surgeon contact information.

Office follow-up is usually scheduled in 1 week, and if the patient is doing well, a routine postoperative visit is scheduled at 6 weeks.

A more detailed discussion of access techniques for cervical endoscopy as well as interlaminar approaches is beyond the scope of this chapter, and several standard texts, including Daniel Kim's *Endoscopic Spine Procedures*, are recommended for additional detail.

Complications

The complications of endoscopic spine procedures are generally the same as those for any spinal surgery:

- Damage to neural structures, with new motor or sensory deficits
- Bleeding within the vertebral canal, hematoma in deep muscle
- Dural tears or CSF leak: Rates are lower for endoscopic procedures than for open procedures.
- Infection: The infection rate for endoscopic procedures is 40% lower than for microdiscectomy.
- Allergy, hypersensitivity, or drug side effects
- Recurrent disk herniation
- Postoperative radiculitis, which may involve the exiting nerve root or the transiting nerve root
- Unrelieved pain
- Seizures
- Blindness
- Late complications include instability or partial collapse of the disk space, as for any open spinal surgery.

The skills needed to address intraoperative bleeding and for recognition of anatomic features vary significantly from those needed for open procedures, due in part to the use of the digitally magnified images with variable orientation. The long-necked instrumentation, as well as the drills and burrs that are passed through the endoscope working channel, are similar in function to conventional surgical instrumentation, but they are modified for endoscopic use and require different deployment and use from the conventional instrumentation with which an experienced surgeon may be familiar. Bipolar flexible RF probes are used to provide hemostasis. A diamond burr can also provide hemostasis as it removes bone and can be used for resection of the posterior aspect of a vertebral body, undercutting an extruded herniated disk to facilitate disk fragment grasping and subsequent fragment removal. For interventional pain management and radiology physicians, surgical access and imaging may be far less challenging than gaining experience with instrumentation and mastering the sequential task of spinal surgery. Fluoroscopic imaging is vital for initial placement of the working sleeve, and intermittent fluoroscopic visualization is used judiciously throughout the procedure when reorientation or verification of anatomic placement of devices may be useful. No particular specialty of residency training ensures superior outcomes. The often-touted requirement that the individual spinal endoscopist be fully capable of addressing any potential complications, such as the < 1% incidence of dural tears, most of which are asymptomatic, is reminiscent of the requirement for a cardiothoracic surgeon to be immediately available in the early days of coronary angioplasty and stenting, with experience teaching us that with diligence and experience, such precautions are unneeded impediments to qualified endoscopists. Most symptomatic dural tears resolve with a simple epidural blood patch applied using anterior transforaminal or posterior epidural placement as dictated by the mechanism of dural sac injury. Furthermore, anesthesiologists tend to have the most experience addressing symptomatic dural tears or low-CSF-pressure headache. Several techniques are now available for direct endoscopic repair of dural tears using either staples, patches, or glue, and open surgical repair of dural tears may be unneeded in the future.

Conclusions

In addition to treating disk herniations, endoscopic technique is highly valuable for treating foraminal and lateral recess stenosis by providing a minimally invasive alternative to conventional open surgery. Furthermore, avoiding resection of the lamina and the spinal extensor musculature helps preserve normal biomechanical relationships and avoids the requirement for stabilization using instrumented fusion, leading to reduced costs, less postoperative pain, and fewer postoperative mobilization limitations. A study involving German worker's compensation patients showed that time to return to work among endoscopically treated patients was half that among those treated by microdiscectomy. In treatment of lateral disk herniation, endoscopic technique has been shown to have superior patient outcomes, along with reduced blood loss and reduced operating time.

This chapter does not present or elaborate on interlaminar endoscopic technique due in part to concern about a higher rate of dural tears. However, the tears tend to occur early in a physician's experience with the interlaminar technique. The interlaminar approach is quite useful for an experienced endoscopic surgeon, is an extremely efficient use of operating resources, and has a surprisingly rapid postoperative recovery trajectory compared with open microdiscectomy.

Unfortunately, as many readers are aware, the greatest impediment to the widespread use of endoscopic surgical technique is the lack of adequate reimbursement by third-party payers, including Medicare, which for 5 years has failed to establish an economic evaluation benchmark for CPT code 62380 for use with endoscopic surgery.

References

1. Sivakanthan S, Hasan S, Hofstetter C. Full-endoscopic lumbar discectomy. *Neurosurg Clin N Am.* 2020;31(1):1–7. doi:10.1016/j.nec.2019.08.016.
2. Ahn Y. A historical review of endoscopic spinal discectomy. *World Neurosurg.* 2021;145:591–596. doi:10.1016/j.wneu.2020.08.008.
3. Pan M, Li Q, Li S, et al. Percutaneous endoscopic lumbar discectomy: indications and complications. *Pain Physician.* 2020;23(1):49–56.
4. Gore S, Yeung A. The "inside out" transforaminal technique to treat lumbar spinal pain in an awake and aware patient under local anesthesia: results and a review of the literature. *Int J Spine Surg.* 2014;8:28. doi:10.14444/1028.
5. Chen Z, Zhang L, Dong J, et al. Percutaneous transforaminal endoscopic discectomy compared with microendoscopic discectomy for lumbar disc herniation: 1-year results of an ongoing randomized controlled trial. *J Neurosurg Spine.* 2018;28(3):300–310. doi:10.3171/2017.7.SPINE161434.
6. Gadjradj PS, van Tulder MW, Dirven CM, Peul WC, Harhangi BS. Clinical outcomes after percutaneous transforaminal endoscopic discectomy for lumbar disc herniation: a prospective case series. *Neurosurg Focus.* 2016;40(2):E3. doi:10.3171/2015.10.FOCUS15484.
7. Liu X, Yuan S, Tian Y, et al. Comparison of percutaneous endoscopic transforaminal discectomy, microendoscopic discectomy, and microdiscectomy for symptomatic lumbar disc herniation: minimum 2-year follow-up results. *J Neurosurg Spine.* 2018;28(3):317–325. doi:10.3171/2017.6.SPINE172.
8. Ohya J, Oshima Y, Chikuda H, et al. Does the microendoscopic technique reduce mortality and major complications in patients undergoing lumbar discectomy? A propensity score-matched analysis using a nationwide administrative database. *Neurosurg Focus.* 2016;40(2):E5. doi:10.3171/2015.10.FOCUS15479.
9. Gibson JNA, Subramanian AS, Scott CEH. A randomised controlled trial of transforaminal endoscopic discectomy vs microdiscectomy. *Eur Spine J.* 2017;26(3):847–856. doi:10.1007/s00586-016-4885-6. Correction published in *Eur Spine J.* 2017;12.
10. Meyer G, Da Rocha ID, Cristante AF, et al. Percutaneous endoscopic lumbar discectomy versus microdiscectomy for the treatment of lumbar disc herniation: pain, disability, and complication rate—a randomized clinical trial. *Int J Spine Surg.* 2020;14(1):72–78. doi:10.14444/7010.
11. Ruetten S, Komp M, Merk H, Godolias G. Full-endoscopic interlaminar and transforaminal lumbar discectomy versus conventional microsurgical technique. *Spine.* 2008;33(9):931–939. doi:10.1097/BRS.0b013e31816c8af7.
12. Mlaka J, Rapcan R, Burianek M, et al. Endoscopic discectomy as an effective treatment of a herniated intervertebral disc. *Bratisl Lek Listy.* 2020;121(3):199–205. doi:10.4149/BLL_2020_030.
13. Ahn Y, Lee SG, Son S, Keum HJ. Transforaminal endoscopic lumbar discectomy versus open lumbar microdiscectomy: a comparative cohort study with a 5-year follow-up. *Pain Physician.* 2019;22(3):295–304.
14. Zhang B, Zhou F, Wang L, et al. A new decompression technique for upper lumbar fracture with neurologic deficit—comparison with traditional open posterior surgery. *BMC Musculoskelet Disord.* 2019;20:580. https://doi.org/10.1186/s12891-019-2897-1.
15. Lee JS, Kim HS, Jang JS, Jang IT. Structural preservation percutaneous endoscopic lumbar interlaminar discectomy for L5-S1 herniated nucleus pulposus. *Biomed Res Int.* 2016;2016:6250247. doi:10.1155/2016/6250247.
16. Kong W, Liao W, Ao J, Cao G, Qin J, Cai Y. The strategy and early clinical outcome of percutaneous full-endoscopic interlaminar or extraforaminal approach for treatment of lumbar disc herniation. *Biomed Res Int.* 2016;2016:4702946. doi:10.1155/2016/4702946.
17. Lv Z, Jin L, Wang K, et al. Comparison of effects of PELD and fenestration in the treatment of geriatric lumbar lateral recess stenosis. *Clin Interv Aging.* 2019;14:2187–2194. doi:10.2147/CIA.S226295.

8

Uniportal, Percutaneous Microdiscectomy with Annulo-nucleoplasty

Erica R. Eldon and Corey W. Hunter

Introduction

Back pain is the leading cause of disability in the world and is one of the most common reasons a person will go to the doctor. Approximately 80% of people will experience back pain at some point in their lives, and it is the most common cause of missed work in the United States. A variety of etiologies can cause low back pain (LBP): the most common is ligament or muscle strain. Fortunately, this particular cause of LBP tends to be self-limiting in most cases and is easily treated for the most part with rest, anti-inflammatories, and potentially a short course of physical therapy. Conversely, LBP due to discogenic pain resulting from to degenerative disk disease or contained lumbar disk herniation (CLDH) is much less forgiving and may require surgical intervention to resolve.

Over the past 3 decades, opioid use in chronic, nonmalignant pain has increased exponentially, with reported rates of misuse and abuse as high as 40% and drug overdose rates increasing 500%.[1,2] And while open surgical procedures in the lumbar spine are effective for treating certain types of disk-related LBP, they carry failure rates as high as 40% and reoperation rates as high as 80%.[3] Therefore, there is an obvious need for a minimally invasive treatment that could provide an alternative to both chronic opioid therapy and invasive surgeries, with a lower probability of failed back surgery syndrome, shorter recovery time, and most importantly, a favorable risk profile that would not preclude patients with significant comorbidities.[4] This chapter presents such a minimally invasive treatment: the uniportal, percutaneous microdiscectomy with annulo-nucleoplasty using the Disc-FX® System (Elliquence®, Baldwin, New York).

Background and Historical Perspective

Treatment of discogenic back pain spans a broad range from conservative physiotherapy to invasive procedures, such as spinal fusion or interbody fixation. For patients with a small CLDH or lumbar radiculopathy who fail conservative management, minimally invasive discectomy and annuloplasty may provide symptomatic relief by removing tissue from the nucleus pulposus to reduce intradiscal pressure and decompress the disk, subsequently relieving pressure off the neural tissue, such as nerve roots.[5] Radical surgery and open discectomy methods damage the back muscles, require longer recovery time, have greater infection risk, and decrease mobility of the lumbar spine. As the benefits of minimally invasive surgical procedures have become prominent in the literature, new technologies and techniques have been introduced to the market. Percutaneous microdiscectomy with or without annulo-nucleoplasty is a minimally invasive method to reduce CLDH that has been shown to reduce postoperative complications, to reduce hospital stays, and to lead to shorter rehabilitation and early return to work, therefore reducing the cost of treatment.[5]

Anatomy

The intervertebral disk consists of a collagenous nucleus pulposus within a fibrous annulus fibrosus and functions to absorb axial compression from the spinal column while allowing for flexion and extension. The nucleus pulposus is positioned slightly posteriorly and consists of crisscrossing type II collagen and elastin within a gelatinous proteoglycan matrix. The surrounding annulus fibrosus is formed by three concentric lamina. The inner two lamina consist of organized type II fibrocartilage, and the outermost lamina consists of dense type I cartilage fibers that contribute to its tensile strength and attaches to the vertebral end plates at the epiphyseal rings. The intervertebral disk decreases in height from the cervical to the lumbar spine.

The intervertebral disk becomes avascular by the third decade of life and gains nutrition through diffusion. The outer annulus is innervated by sinuvertebral nerves posteriorly,[6] the adjacent ventral primary rami and gray rami communicantes posterolaterally, and the rami communicantes laterally.[6,7] In healthy disks, the outer annulus has nociceptors to a depth of a few millimeters and the nucleus pulposus has no nociceptive innervation. Damaged disk releases substance P, which stimulates neoinnervation, an ingrowth of nerve endings, and sensitization. Sensory nerves have been found penetrating deep into disrupted nucleus pulposus in degenerated disks, contributing to disk degeneration as a pain generator.[6]

Pathology

Disk herniation is defined as general or focal displacement of disk material beyond the intervertebral disk space and may consist of nucleus pulposus, cartilage, fragmented apophyseal bone, or annular tissue.[8] Disk herniations are classified as incomplete or contained—when the outer annulus fibrosis remains intact—and complete or uncontained—when the nucleus pulposus protrudes through non-intact outer annulus fibrosis or posterior longitudinal ligament (PLL). Disk herniation occurs most commonly in the posterior aspect, where the PLL is thin and the annular fibers are less dense. The anterior longitudinal ligament (ALL) is broad, and the annular fibers are most abundant anteriorly and laterally, protecting against annular fissures and anterior disk herniation. Posterior disk herniations are most common at the L4–L5 disk level and compress the traversing nerve root exiting at the next spinal level. Far posterolateral disk herniations may compress the exiting nerve root ganglion at the level of the disk herniation[9] and cause radicular symptoms. Furcal nerve, also known as a link nerve, is an independent nerve with ventral and dorsal rootlets, most commonly arises at the L4 level, is located superior and ventral to the L4 nerve root, and gives branches to the femoral nerve, lumbosacral trunk, and obturator nerve. Furcal nerves are a known cause of atypical presentation of radicular symptoms, with an incidence of 15% in patients with low back pain.[10,11]

The dorsal wall of the spinal canal is formed by ligamentum flavum between the lamina of each vertebra. Nerve roots exit via the transverse foramen, which is formed by superior and inferior pedicles, the vertebral body and disk, and the facet joint. Kambin's triangle (Figure 8.1) is a transforaminal access corridor that is considered a "safe zone" for interventional spine procedures because it is largely free of vasculature. It is bordered by inferiorly

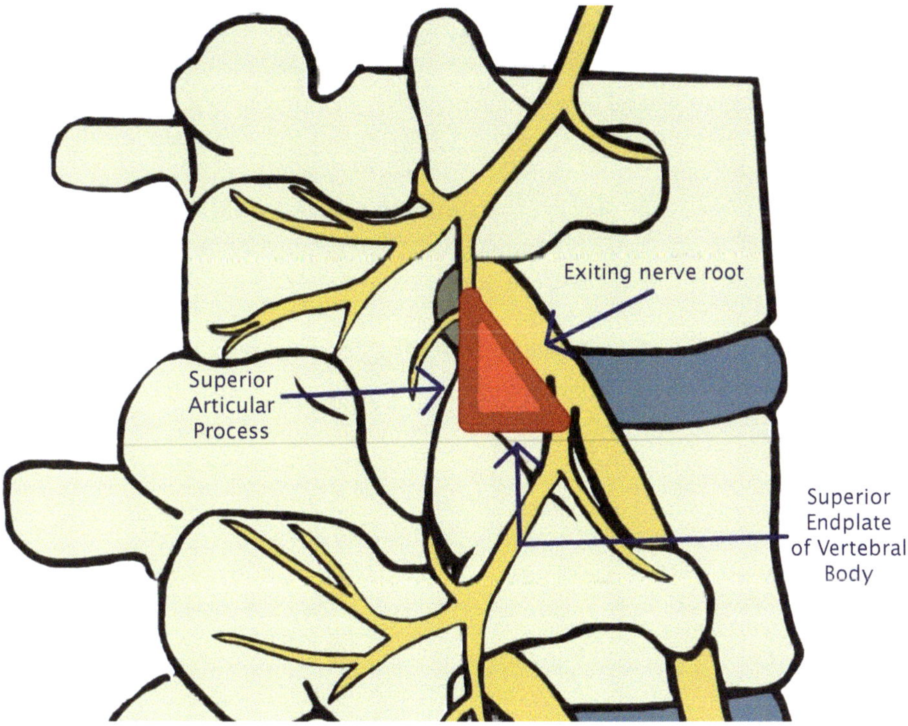

FIGURE 8.1. Kambin's triangle identified by red triangle. Figure redrawn by Erica Eldon based on: Yeung A, Gore S. Endoscopic foraminal decompression for failed back surgery syndrome under local anesthesia. *Int J Spine Surg.* 2014;8:22. doi:10.14444/1022.

(at the base) by the superior plate of the inferior vertebral body, posteriorly (height) by the superior articular process (SAP) of the inferior vertebra, and anteriorly (hypotenuse) by the exiting nerve root. The medial (deep) border is the thecal sac and traversing nerve root, and thus it has been suggested that the name be changed to Kambin's prism to account for all four borders[12]; however, the space is largely referred to as a triangle in the existing literature. Anatomic variants and degeneration may distort Kambin's triangle. Apical disk herniations displace the nerve root inferiorly, which reduces the size of the triangle. Osteophytes, facet joint hypertrophy, vertebral body osteochondrosis, and calcified annulus fibrosus can make accessing the disk difficult and lead to complications.[7]

Uses and Indications

The Disk-FX® system combines percutaneous manual discectomy, nucleus ablation, and annular modification in one procedure.[13,14] The indicated target for Disk-FX® is a CLDH, which is defined as a focal disk prolapse with thinning of the annulus fibrosus and protrusion of the nucleus pulposus or as diffuse annular bulge without thinning or protrusion. Patient selection and exclusion criteria are shown in Table 8.1.

Evidence for Efficacy

Patients who underwent this procedure for discogenic back pain refractory to conservative management experienced good outcomes, with 65.2% reporting successful pain reduction and 62.9% reporting successful reduction in disability.[16] Comparatively, Disc-FX® has been shown to have favorable outcomes at 2 and 4 years in patients with symptomatic degenerative disk disease, with 78% of patients reporting excellent or good outcomes 2 years after the procedure[5] and 83% of patients reporting they were "satisfied" or "very satisfied" with quality of life 4 years after the procedure.[14] However, outcomes were negatively affected by high body mass index and smoking status at 6 months and 12 months after the

TABLE 8.1. Inclusion and Exclusion Criteria for Percutaneous Microdiscectomy

Inclusion Criteria	Exclusion Criteria
Age between 18 and 60 years old	Back pain due to causes other than degenerate disk or radiculopathy due to CLDH
Axial back pain due to degenerate disk or back pain with radicular symptoms due to CLDH confirmed on MRI	MRI revealing acute disk prolapse/ sequestrated disk
Symptoms unresponsive to at least 6 months of conservative management	Presence of spondylolisthesis/instability
Visual Analog Scale (VAS) score ≥5	Presence of infection
MRI revealing degenerate/symptomatic disks at not more than 3 levels	Presence of malignant spinal conditions
Disk level falls within Pfirrmann Grade II to IV	Cauda equina syndrome
Greater than one-half disk height preserved	

[5,7,15]

procedure.[5] Of patients with loss of function due to lumbar radiculopathy who underwent microdiscectomy, 85% showed significant improvements in function and clinical outcomes at 3 and 12 months.[17] The 2007 evidence-based best practice guideline for interventional techniques reported moderate evidence for percutaneous disk decompression, and limited evidence for nucleoplasty.[18] The MIST guidelines (2018) reported Level 1 evidence that percutaneous image-guided lumbar decompression was superior to lumbar epidural steroid injection in the treatment of lumbar spinal stenosis.[19]

Preparation for the Procedure

Standard preoperative precautions and testing before the procedure include:

- Basic metabolic panel
- CBC
- PT, PTT, and INR
- Medical clearance where indicated
- Anticoagulation withheld in accordance with the most recent ASRA Guidelines

Equipment and Supplies

Equipment and supplies needed are:

- Chlorhexidine
- Utility drapes
- Laparotomy drape
- 1% Lidocaine with epinephrine (1:100,000)
- 0.25% Bupivacaine
- Iohexal contrast
- Spinal needle (16-gauge × 8-inch)
- Guidewire
- Soft tissue dilator
- Microtubular system
- Trephine
- Depth stopper
- Pituitary grasping forceps
- Trigger-Flex bipolar system
- Dissolvable suture

Technique

The following technique is adapted from the microtubular decompression and nucleotomy as described by Hellinger[14] and percutaneous microdiscectomy with annulo-nucleoplasty as described by Kumar.[7,20] The Disc-FX system is used with a posterolateral approach. The patient is positioned prone with a bolster or cushion under the pelvis to decrease lumbar lordosis. Patients unable to tolerate the prone position may be placed in the lateral decubitus position with the symptomatic side up. Fluoroscopic imaging is used to identify key structures, and an entry point is marked on the skin:

- Tilt should be adjusted to "square off" the endplates of the index level.
- Oblique should be rotated ipsilaterally to the intended entry side until the SAP is approximately one-third of the way across the disk.

The skin entry point should allow a transforaminal trajectory for access to the posterolateral annulus fibrosis, at the posterior third of the index disk. Under fluoroscopic imaging, the skin overlying the middle aspect of the disk, immediately anterior to the SAP, is marked as the skin entry point.

Prepare and drape the skin in typical sterile fashion. Inject local anesthetic subcutaneously at the entry site and along the intended needle tract aiming toward Kambin's triangle. With a 16/18-gauge × 8-inch spinal needle under intermittent fluoroscopic guidance and using a "gun barrel approach," enter the posterolateral corner of the annulus fibrosis. There are two technique variations at this point:

- Hellinger technique: target is the inner pedicle line in AP view and the posterior third of the disk in lateral view.[13,14]
- Kumar technique: target is lateral to the SAP and medial to the exiting nerve root.[20]

Once the needle is felt to have entered the disk, adjust the C-arm and take an AP image to visualize the lateral-to-medial location of the needle tip. Then adjust the C-arm and take a lateral image to visualize the anterior-to-posterior position of the needle tip.

Once needle tip placement is confirmed in AP and lateral fluoroscopic imaging, a discogram is performed to confirm and document the disk morphology.[5] Injection of a contrast mixture containing Omnipaque™ (iohexol) and indigo carmine dye will allow for fluoroscopic visualization as well as direct visualization of light blue staining of the disk tissue and annular defects.[7]

Remove the stylet and pass a flexible blunt guidewire until it is viewed just beyond the needle tip in the nucleus pulposus. Carefully advance the guidewire tip until the tip is located within the middle of the disk as visualized on AP and lateral views. Guidewire advancement should be performed under lateral imaging because the guidewire is rigid enough to pierce the disk and enter the peritoneum if advanced too far.

Remove the needle while maintaining the guidewire in place inside the nucleus pulposus. At this point, inject additional local anesthetic into the skin around the guidewire, making a skin wheal with a radius of approximately 5 mm. Using a scalpel, make a 2- to 3-m incision on either side of the guidewire to allow for the access cannula to be placed over the guidewire. Secure a depth stop over the access cannula and then advance the access cannula over the guidewire into the disk. Careful attention should be paid to ensure that

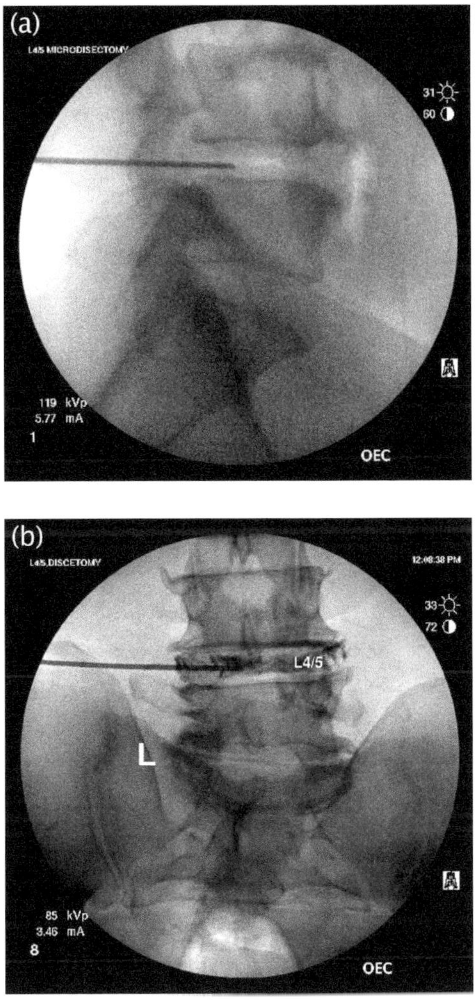

FIGURE 8.2. (a) Fluoroscopic lateral view of needle placement. Note the needle tip is at the posterior 1/3 line. (b) Fluoroscopic AP view of discogram. Original images by Cory Hunter, HPI redacted by Erica Eldon.

the guidewire is not inadvertently advanced in the process of advancing the access cannula. A "pop" will be felt once the annulus has been breached. At this point, the guidewire is removed. Once the tip of the access cannula is in proper position, pituitary rongeurs are inserted through the access cannula, into the disk.

Under direct visualization, decompress the disk by performing a nucleotomy of approximately 1 cm^3 of nucleus material.[14] Each bite should be done under live imaging to ensure proper placement of the rongeurs. If indigo carmine is utilized, will be seen on the pathologic portions of disk being removed.

After the manual debulking is completed, the next step is to perform the ablation of the nucleus. Insert the Trigger-Flex® steerable probe through the cannula to ablate the nucleus. Careful attention should be paid to the location of the tip of the Trigger-Flex® when recoiled and when fully deployed to ensure it is not extended too far. Six passes will be

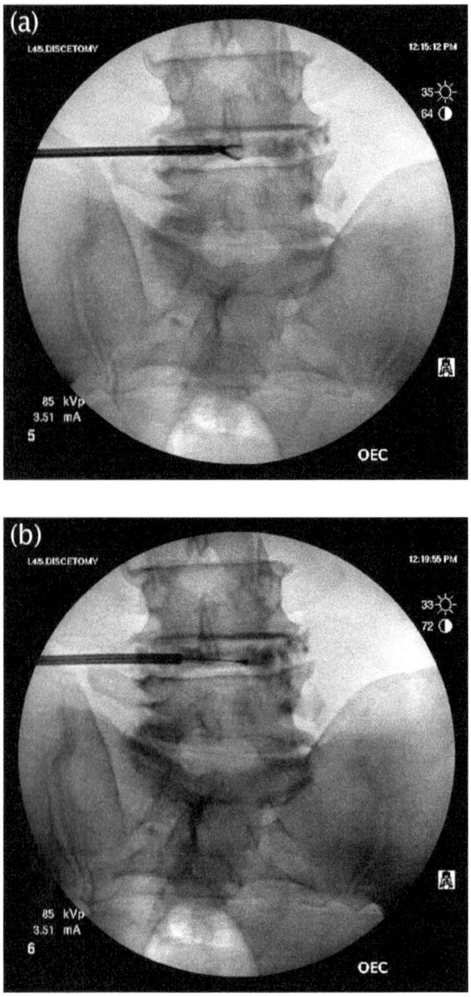

FIGURE 8.3. (a) Fluoroscopic view of debulking forceps in the intradiscal space during nucleotomy. (b) Fluoroscopic view of intradiscal radiofrequency probe during modulation annulotomy. Original images by Cory Hunter, HPI redacted by Erica Eldon.

made, with the handle positioned, respectively, at 12 o'clock, 2:30, 4:30, 6, 8:30, and 10:30. With the Trigger-Flex® apparatus remaining stationary, squeeze the handle to deploy the probe for each pass—an ablation is performed for a total of 6 seconds (3 seconds with then probe moving outward and 3 seconds with the prove returning inward).

Hellinger described using the Bipolar-Hemo Waveform with a limit of 6 applications of 6 seconds each, power setting 25 on both Bipolar-Turbo and Bipolar-Hemo. Kumar described performing nucleus ablation with a Surgi-Max generator set at Bipolar-Turbo mode. He used 6 strokes at 6 locations around the nucleus, followed by irrigation of the disk using antibiotic-laced saline.

The access cannula is then retracted until the tip is located at the midpedicular line. Ablation is performed once again, this time along the posterior-inner aspect of the annulus.

The Trigger-Flex® probe is then placed under the pathological annulus in Bipolar-Hemo mode. With slight downward force onto the cannula, the Trigger-Flex® probe is deployed and activated to modulate the posterior annulus. Four passes are made, with the handle positioned at 4, 5:30, 6:30, and 8 o'clock.[20] In contrast to the first use of the Trigger-Flex®, this time the probe is fully deployed first by squeezing the handle and then manually by advancing the whole Trigger-Flex® apparatus in a sawlike motion—3 seconds forward and 3 seconds back. With the probe fully deployed and a downward force being applied, one should have a tactile feel of the probe rubbing against the posterior aspect of the inner annulus. Modulation shrinks and thickens the herniation site, and the RF probe can be used to cauterize small bleeding vessels. Once this aspect is completed, one may elect to irrigate the disk an additional time. At this point, the access cannula is retracted from within the disk to just outside the disk, and a small amount of dexamethasone suspended in bupivacaine can be injected to provide postprocedure analgesia and decrease any irritation to the exiting nerve root. After removal of the access cannula, imaging is repeated to ensure no hardware remains. Depending on the size of the wound, a small suture may be placed on the skin. The entry site is then covered with a sterile adhesive dressing.

Postprocedural Care

An advantage of minimally invasive procedures in comparison to more invasive, open approaches is same-day discharge as well as the short recovery time. Patients should be observed for 45 to 60 minutes after completion of the procedure for any neurological deficits.[20] Standard postoperative instructions and precautions apply. Follow-up should be in 10 to 14 days, when sutures are removed and the wound is assessed to ensure it is healing appropriately.

The patient should be educated about avoiding positions and activities that increase intradiscal pressure, such as lumbar flexion or lifting. A lumbar orthosis can be worn to provide stability and support during the 1- to 2-week recovery period. If symptoms improve, the patient may participate in strengthening and training program with a physical therapist.[7]

References

1. Warner M, Anderson RN. Drug poisoning deaths in the United States, 1980–2008. 2011;81:8.
2. Cheatle MD. Prescription opioid misuse, abuse, morbidity, and mortality: balancing effective pain management and safety. *Pain Med.* 2015;16(suppl 1):S3–S8. doi:10.1111/pme.12904.
3. Hunter CW, Carlson J, Yang A, Deer T. Spinal cord stimulation for the treatment of failed neck surgery syndrome: outcome of a prospective case series. *Neuromodulation Technol Neural Interface.* 2018;21(5):495–503. doi:10.1111/ner.12769.
4. Manabe H, Yamashita K, Tezuka F, et al. Thermal annuloplasty using percutaneous endoscopic discectomy for elite athletes with discogenic low back pain. *Neurol Med Chir (Tokyo).* 2019;59(2):48–53. doi:10.2176/nmc.oa.2018-0256.
5. Kumar N, Zaw AS, Kumar N, Sonawane D, Hey HWD, Kumar A. Annulo-nucleoplasty using Disc-FX in the management of degenerative lumbar disc pathology: how long can the effect last? *Glob Spine J.* 2018;8(4):365–373. doi:10.1177/2192568217726525.

6. Devereaux MW. Anatomy and examination of the spine. *Neurol Clin.* 2007;25(2):331–351. doi:10.1016/j.ncl.2007.02.003.
7. Yang A, Diwan S. Minimally invasive percutaneous endoscopic discectomy: transdiscal approach. In: Diwan S, Deer TR, eds. *Advanced Procedures for Pain Management: A Step-by-Step Atlas.* Springer International Publishing; 2018:53–65. doi:10.1007/978-3-319-68841-1_5.
8. Fardon DF, Williams AL, Dohring EJ, Murtagh FR, Gabriel Rothman SL, Sze GK. Lumbar disc nomenclature: version 2.0—Recommendations of the combined task forces of the North American Spine Society, the American Society of Spine Radiology and the American Society of Neuroradiology. *Spine J.* 2014;14(11):2525–2545. doi:10.1016/j.spinee.2014.04.022.
9. Thompson J. *Netter's Concise Orthopaedic Anatomy Updated Edition.* 2nd ed. Elsevier; 2002.
10. Haijiao W, Koti M, Smith FW, Wardlaw D. Diagnosis of lumbosacral nerve root anomalies by magnetic resonance imaging. *J Spinal Disord.* 2001;14(2):143–149. doi:10.1097/00002517-200104000-00009.
11. Harshavardhana NS, Dabke HV. The furcal nerve revisited. *Orthop Rev.* 2014;6(3). doi:10.4081/or.2014.5428.
12. Fanous AA, Tumialán LM, Wang MY. Kambin's triangle: definition and new classification schema. *J Neurosurg Spine.* 2019;32(3):390–398. doi:10.3171/2019.8.SPINE181475.
13. Hellinger S. Disc-FX—a new combination procedure for minimal invasive disc surgery. *Spinal News.* 2007;(4):14.
14. Hellinger S. Treatment of contained lumbar disc herniations using radiofrequency assisted microtubular decompression and nucleotomy: four-year prospective study results. *Int J Spine Surg.* 2014;8:24. doi:10.14444/1024.
15. Mallick S. Radiofrequency-assisted minimally invasive manual lumbar discectomy using Disc-FX system: outcome of nine cases. *J Recent Adv Pain.* 2017;3(1):7–13. doi:10.5005/jp-journals-10046-0059.
16. Lee JH, Lee S-H. Clinical efficacy and its prognostic factor of percutaneous endoscopic lumbar annuloplasty and nucleoplasty for the treatment of patients with discogenic low back pain. *World Neurosurg.* 2017;105:832–840. doi:10.1016/j.wneu.2017.06.112.
17. Tampin B, Slater H, Jacques A, Lind CRP. Association of quantitative sensory testing parameters with clinical outcome in patients with lumbar radiculopathy undergoing microdiscectomy. *Eur J Pain.* 2020;24(7):1377–1392. doi:10.1002/ejp.1586.
18. Boswell MV, Trescot AM, Datta S, et al. Interventional techniques: evidence-based practice guidelines in the management of chronic spinal pain. *Pain Physician.* 2007;10(1):7–111.
19. Deer TR, Grider JS, Pope JE, et al. The MIST guidelines: the Lumbar Spinal Stenosis Consensus Group guidelines for minimally invasive spine treatment. *Pain Pract.* 2019;19(3):250–274. doi.org/10.1111/papr.12744.
20. Kumar N, Kumar A, Siddharth MS, Sambhav PS, Tan J. Annulo-nucleoplasty using Disc-FX in the management of lumbar disc pathology: early results. *Int J Spine Surg.* 2014;8. doi:10.14444/1018.

PART 3

Spinal Implants

9

Indirect Lumbar Decompression

Jessica Jameson, Sean Li, Steven Bhutra,
Lynn Kohan, and Arti Ori

Indirect Lumbar Decompression

Lumbar spinal stenosis (LSS) is a degenerative process that occurs as a result of normal aging, which results in narrowing, or stenosis, of the spaces around the neural elements of the spine, leading to compression.[1] This stenosis occurs in three different locations—the central, foraminal, or lateral recess—leading to characteristic symptoms, including pain that radiates to the buttocks, thighs, or lower extremities, with or without low back pain.[2] The pain may be unilateral when stenosis involves the nerve foramen or lateral recess and can then follow a specific dermatomal pattern. Patients may also report numbness, weakness, and muscle cramps in the lower extremities. The symptoms of neurogenic claudication worsen with standing and walking, and improve with sitting or leaning forward ("shopping cart" sign), since flexion of the spine creates more space in the spinal canal and neural foramina, thus relieving compression.

Diagnosis of LSS is established by the presence of the above symptoms and is correlated with specific radiographic findings. The first line of treatment is conservative therapy, comprised of physical therapy, chiropractic treatment, acupuncture, and use of anti-inflammatory drugs and opioid analgesics, as well as epidural and facet injection therapies. When conservative management fails to provide relief of symptoms, surgery is then offered, including decompressive laminectomy or laminectomy with pedicle fixation at one or more levels. However, in patients who are unable to tolerate invasive surgery due to comorbid conditions, including advanced age, high body mass index (BMI), and cardiopulmonary disease, or in patients with LSS that is not severe enough to warrant surgical intervention, the use of interspinous spacers to provide indirect lumbar decompression makes additional options available that restore function and quality of life.[3] These outpatient procedures have a shorter surgical time and require only small incisions, which allow the use of local anesthesia with mild sedation, avoiding the risks of general anesthesia.[3]

Invasive surgery relieves stenosis by increasing the space via removal of the posterior spinal elements, including the lamina, facet joints, osteophytes, and ligament. However, the removal of structural elements leads to an alteration in spinal anatomy that can cause instability. Additional surgery, often fusion, is then required. Indirect lumbar decompression using interspinous process spacers alters spinal alignment and increases space in the spinal canal while preserving spinal anatomy. Studies have shown that the spinal canal lengthens with flexion and shortens with extension. Dimensions of cadaver lumbar spines were measured using MRI during flexion and extension before and after placement of an interspinous spacer, and it was demonstrated that the use of interspinous spacers prevents narrowing of the spinal canal and foramina in extension.[4] Interspinous spacers block extension, creating a relative flexion, without altering anatomy and while maintaining spinal alignment. Use of an interspinous process implant still allows for flexion, rotation, and lateral bending, thus preserving mobility. In addition, interspinous process spacers have been shown to reduce facet loading at the implanted level without altering facet loading at the adjacent levels.[5] Studies have also demonstrated that interspinous process decompression relieves disk pressure at the implanted level without altering disk pressure at the adjacent levels.[6]

In summary, interspinous lumbar decompression has been shown to be a minimally invasive, low-risk procedure for the treatment of LSS that maintains spinal alignment and preserves mobility.[7]

Types of Devices

Currently, there are two interspinous/interlaminar process spacers that are FDA approved—the Coflex® device and the Superion® Interspinous Spacer (Figure 9.1; previously VertiFlex®). The differences between the two are that Coflex is implanted after surgical decompression of the canal has been performed, while Superion is a "stand-alone" device not requiring prior decompression surgery.[8] With the Superion device, a dilator is used to open up the interspinous space, and the device, made of titanium, is deployed percutaneously through

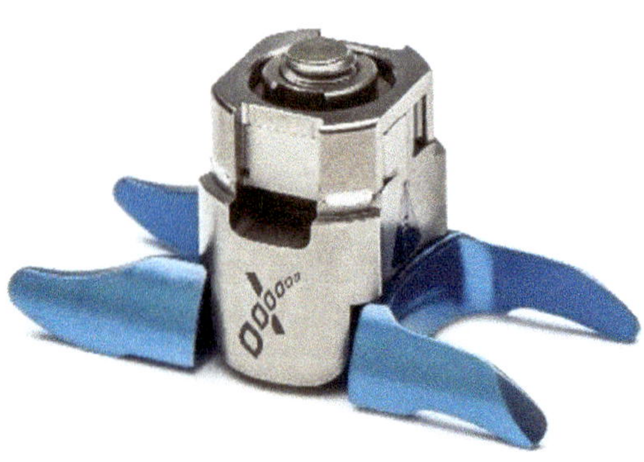

FIGURE 9.1. Size 10 Superion implant deployed. Image provided courtesy of Boston Scientific. ©2020 Boston Scientific Corporation or its affiliates. All rights reserved.

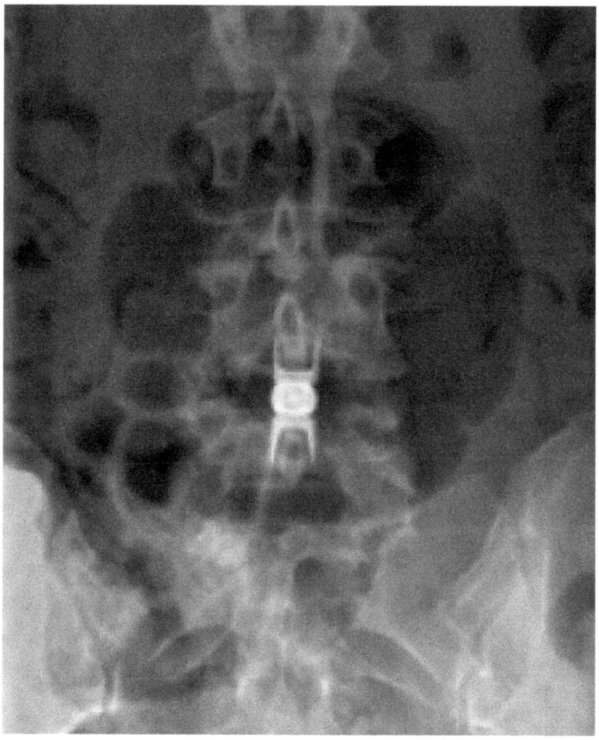

FIGURE 9.2. AP view of Superion implant at L4–L5. Image provided courtesy of Boston Scientific.

a cannula (Figures 9.2 and 9.3). The Coflex Interlaminar Technology provides interlaminar stabilization by being implanted at the midline between adjacent lamina after decompression of stenosis at the affected level.[8] It is a single-piece, U-shaped implant made of titanium alloy, with two pairs of serrated wings. One pair of wings extends from the upper long arm and the other pair extends from the lower long arm of the U. After the U portion is positioned between two adjacent spinous processes, the device is pressed into place. Both of the interspinous process spacer devices may be implanted at one or two adjacent lumbar levels. The X-STOP® Interspinous Process Decompression (IPD) System (Figure 9.4) received FDA premarket approval in 2005; however, research with longer-term follow-up demonstrated minimal benefit. There was also a relatively high rate of complications, which included spinous process fracture.[9] Premarket approval was withdrawn in 2015, and Medtronic discontinued use of the device.

Indications

The Superion Indirect Decompression System (IDS) is used to treat skeletally mature patients suffering from pain, numbness, and/or cramping in the legs (neurogenic intermittent claudication) secondary to a diagnosis of moderate degenerative LSS, with or without Grade 1 spondylolisthesis. Spinal stenosis is confirmed by x-ray, MRI, and/or CT evidence of thickened ligamentum flavum, narrowed lateral recess, and/or central canal or foraminal

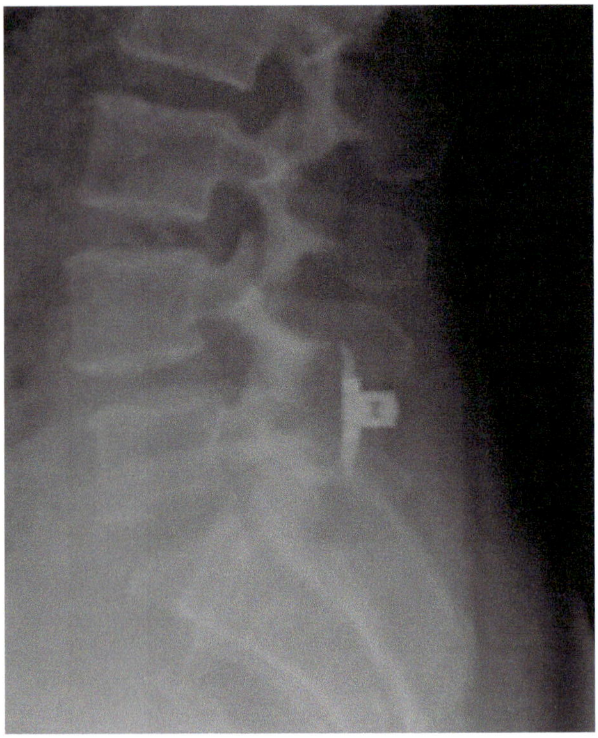

FIGURE 9.3. Lateral view of Superion implant at L4–L5. Image provided courtesy of Boston Scientific.

narrowing. The device is indicated for patients with impaired physical function who experience relief in flexion from symptoms of leg/buttock/groin pain, numbness, and/or cramping, including patients with or without back pain. The patients must have undergone at least 6 months of nonoperative treatment.[10] The Superion may be implanted at one or two adjacent lumbar levels from L1 to L5.[11]

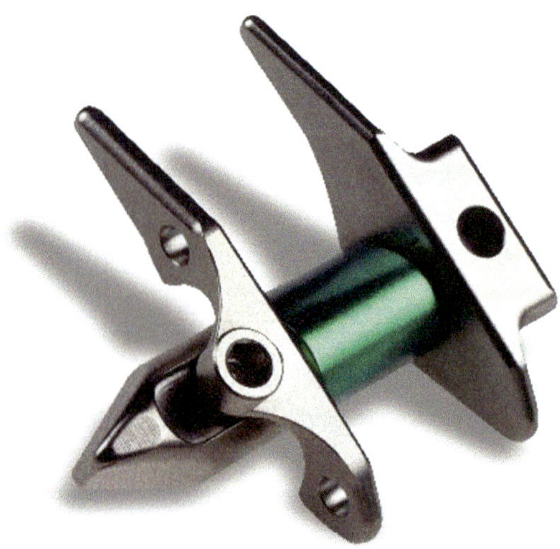

FIGURE 9.4. X-stop device.
Reproduced with permission from Boston Scientific

Moderate degenerative LSS was defined as 25% to 50% reduction in central canal and/or nerve root canal (subarticular, neuroforaminal) compared to the adjacent levels on radiographic studies, with radiographic confirmation of any one of the following:

- Evidence of thecal sac and/or cauda equina compression
- Evidence of nerve root impingement (displacement or compression) by either osseous or nonosseous elements
- Evidence of hypertrophic facets with canal encroachment

and association with the following clinical signs:

- Moderately impaired physical function (PF), defined as a score of ≥ 2.0 on the Zurich Claudication Questionnaire (ZCQ)
- Ability to sit for 50 minutes without pain and to walk 50 feet or more

Evidence

In a study comparing the Superion Interspinous Spacer to decompressive laminectomy, Lauryssen et al showed that both treatments provide effective and durable relief of claudicatory symptoms.[12] However, patients treated with the interspinous spacer had greater improvements in back pain (65% vs. 52%) and leg pain (70% vs. 62%). When outcomes for disability were evaluated for Superion compared to decompressive laminectomy, the Superion showed a slightly higher improvement in outcomes on the Oswestry Disability Index (ODI; 51% vs. 47%), ZCQ symptom severity (ZCQss; 37% vs. 29%), and PF (36% vs. 32%).

Patel et al demonstrated durable clinical improvement consistently across all clinical outcomes for the Superion in the treatment of moderate spinal stenosis.[13] In their study, Superion was evaluated in the treatment of patients 45 years old or older suffering from symptoms of intermittent neurogenic claudication secondary to a confirmed diagnosis of moderate degenerative LSS at one or two contiguous levels from L1 to L5. The study included 391 patients randomized to groups consisting of 190 Superion devices and 201 X-STOP controls. The four components to the primary endpoint were improvement in physical function measured with the ZCQ, no reoperations at the index level, no major procedure-related complications, and no clinically significant confounding treatments. At 3 years, the proportion of patients achieving the primary endpoint was greater for Superion (63/120, 52.5%) than for X-STOP (49/129, 38.0%). In addition, the success rates for each of the four individual components of the primary endpoint exceeded 80% in the Superion group.[14]

The same study was followed up at 4 years, and 75 of 89 patients with Superion (84.3%) demonstrated clinical success on at least two of three ZCQ domains.[15] The responder rates for the four individual components were 83% (74/89), 79% (70/89), and 87% (77/89) for ZCQss, ZCQpf, and ZCQpatient satisfaction (ZCQps); 78% (67/86) and 66% (57/86) for leg and back pain on the Visual Analog Scale (VAS); and 62% (55/89) for the ODI. Patients with Superion also demonstrated percentage improvements over baseline of 41%, 40%, 73%, 69%, and 61% for ZCQss, ZCQpf, leg pain VAS, back pain VAS, and ODI.

During a 5-year follow-up of the same study, 84% of patients (74 of 88) demonstrated clinical success on at least two of three ZCQ domains. Individual ZCQ domain success rates were 75%, 81%, and 90% for ZCQss, ZCQpf, and ZCQps, respectively.16 Leg and back pain success rates were 80% and 65%, respectively. The success rate for ODI was 65%.

At 5 years, 75% of interspinous process device patients were free from reoperation, revision, or supplemental fixation at their index level.

Merkow et al performed a literature review to separately evaluate the effectiveness and safety of minimally invasive lumbar decompression (MILD) and interspinous process device with Superion. Thirteen studies were reviewed, and based on the available evidence, MILD and Superion were found to be safe and modestly effective minimally invasive procedures for patients with symptomatic LSS.[17]

Deer et al looked at emerging evidence showing that percutaneous interspinous process decompression systems can be used as a salvage treatment for persistent structural neurogenic claudication in postlaminectomy syndrome or after spinal cord stimulator implantation.[18] In a pragmatic trial of patients who underwent interspinous process decompression for lumbar stenosis with intermittent neurogenic claudication, 63% of patients maintained improvement in VAS leg pain, 61% in VAS back pain, and 78% in function, and 88% reported satisfaction with treatment at 12-month follow-up. In a small case series of seven individuals with postlaminectomy adjacent-segment disease, postoperative satisfaction scores were 3 or 4 on a 0 to 4 scale. These patients were also able to decrease or wean completely off pain medications. In another study, there was a significant decrease in average leg pain (60% improvement) and axial low back pain (58% improvement) in patients who underwent one- or two-level percutaneous interspinous process decompression as a rescue treatment for reemerging neurogenic claudication after spinal cord stimulator implantation.

A postmarket registry (PRESS) and patient phone survey were used to determine real-world data on clinical outcomes with use of the Superion device.[19] At 12 months, it was found that patient satisfaction was 80%, while responder rates were 75% for leg pain and 67% for back pain. The rate of revision rate was 3.6%.

Using data from the 5-year IDE (Investigation Device Exemption) trial, Nunley et al examined the type, dosage, and duration of opioid medications through 5 years of follow-up after Superion implant.[20] The patient data demonstrated a marked decrease in the need for opioid medications to manage symptoms related to LSS. At 5 years there was an 85% decrease in the percentage of subjects using opioids.

All in all, the evidence shows that indirect interspinous decompression is an effective minimally invasive low-risk procedure for treatment of spinal stenosis.

Patient Selection and Contraindications

The most important factor for implant success is patient selection. Candidates for implant are patients with symptomatic central canal stenosis who have not responded to conservative therapies but are not candidates for surgery or who choose not to have invasive surgery. Symptomatic spinal stenosis is regarded as inability to walk unsupported for more than 300 feet, lower back pain, and bilateral leg pains and/or numbness that is relieved by sitting or bending forward.

There should be no structural abnormality of the spine at the level of interest that would prevent implantation of the device or cause the device to be unstable. A prior fusion or decompression procedure at the level of interest is a contraindication.

Anything more than Grade 1 spondylolisthesis at the level of interest (≤ 3 mm of anterolisthesis on lateral flexion-extension radiograph views) is not acceptable due to risk of posterior migration of the implant. Other contraindications are an ankylosed segment at the affected level; fracture of the spinous process, pars interarticularis, or laminae (unilateral or bilateral); and scoliosis (Cobb angle >10°).

An absolute indication for surgery (rapidly progressive neurologic decline, motor deficits, or cauda equina syndrome) is a contraindication to implant.

Exclusion criteria include the presence of significant mechanical back pain (in addition to those symptoms associated with neural compression) that is judged unlikely to improve with decompression alone. This type of back pain is present at rest, with movement, or while standing and does not have characteristics consistent with neurogenic claudication.

Further, the Superion® IDS is contraindicated in patients with an allergy to titanium or titanium alloy. Also, severe osteoporosis, defined as bone mineral density (from DEXA scan) in the spine or hip that is more than 2.5 SD below the mean of adult normal is is a contraindication due to the risk of spinous process fracture. Finally, active systemic infection or infection localized to the site of implantation is a contraindication, as is morbid obesity, defined as a BMI greater than 40.

Perioperative Management

The perioperative management of patients undergoing indirect lumbar decompression procedures aims to improve safety and to decrease potential complications. The implanting physician must know, understand, and subsequently implement guideline recommendations from established organizations, such as the Centers for Disease Control and Prevention, Surgical Care Improvement Project (SCIP), and others. There are no specific recommendations that apply to indirect lumbar decompression outside of those that apply to any surgical procedure. While indirect lumbar decompression is not a neuromodulatory procedure, many physicians have adopted the Neuromodulatory Appropriateness Consensus Committee's (NACC) recommendations for infection control.[21] The recommendations below are based partially on the NACC recommendations as adapted for indirect lumbar decompression. The various perioperative and intraoperative considerations are discussed here with the associated evidence where applicable.

Medical History

The medical history is the first step in determining perioperative management of a patient undergoing indirect lumbar decompression. The history should focus on the patient's previous surgeries and the occurrence of previous infection or poor wound healing, in addition to underlying comorbidities that may affect or interfere with the procedure. Optimizing hemoglobin A_{1c} and glucose control prior to considering an implantable device is suggested based on the literature that shows that uncontrolled glucose affects wound healing. In addition, smoking cessation is an important factor to consider in the perioperative period. Four weeks of smoking cessation is suggested. If this is not possible, transdermal nicotine patches as a replacement for smoking for 4 weeks is an alternative that has been found to lower incision infection rates among smokers to a level similar to that of nonsmokers.[22] A discussion should also be had with patients about BMI. Body weight is of course important for the patient's overall health and pain control, and it affects the ability to perform the procedure. A BMI over 40 is a relative contraindication, because it not only affects the technical aspects of the procedure but also may increase complication rates in the postoperative period.

Management of Anticoagulation Therapy

The presence of hematoma following the procedure can lead to complications that include wound dehiscence and secondary infection. The NACC as well as American Society of Regional Anesthesia have made recommendations on reduction of bleeding risks that are important to consider when performing this procedure.[23,24] A thorough discussion of the bleeding risks secondary to the procedure should be had with the patient. The patient should be asked about not only prescription medications but also over-the-counter medications. Discontinuing anticoagulation therapy does have some intrinsic risk for the patient, and it is important to discuss this with the patient and the prescribing physician. The final decision should be left to the prescribing physician, who can assess the risk and then determine the safest perioperative plan for use of the medications.

Preoperative Screening for Methicillin-sensitive *Staphylococcus aureus* (MSSA) and Methicillin-resistant *Staphylococcus aureus* (MRSA)

Approximately 30% of all surgical site infections (SSIs) are caused by *S. aureus*.[25] In orthopedic and neurosurgical cases, the percentage increases to 50% to 60%.[26] Carriers of *S. aureus* often harbor it in multiple areas, including the nares and perianal and groin regions. A high level of nasal carriage of *S. aureus* was found to be the most important risk factor for SSIs.[27] Decolonization protocols are effective in reducing the risk of SSI and involve mupirocin nasal ointment applied twice daily and bathing with chlorhexidine daily. Decolonization typically is performed daily for 5 days before surgery.[28] Bode et al,[29] in a randomized, double-blind placebo-controlled, multicenter trial, showed a significant reduction in SSIs through the use of rapid screening for *S. aureus* and subsequent decolonization for nasal carriers of *S. aureus*. The protocol resulted in a nearly 60% reduction in SSIs; the rate of SSI was 3.4% in the decolonization group and 7.7% in the placebo group. In addition, the effect of decolonization was most pronounced in preventing deep SSIs: the rate of a deep surgical infection was 4.4% in the placebo group and 0.9% in the mupirocin + chlorhexidine group. While specific studies relating to decolonization and indirect decompression do not exist, the literature indicates that this infection control process should be considered.

Preoperative Laboratory Testing

The bulk of preoperative laboratory testing should be based on the individual patient's comorbidities. The testing addresses not only the concerns of the surgeon, but also the concerns of the anesthetist about providing safe anesthesia care. Many surgeons will order a CBC to assess for anemia and/or infection at baseline. If the patient has a cardiac history, an electrocardiogram can be useful for assessing intraoperative changes compared to baseline and for detecting any unidentified rhythm abnormalities. A retrospective study assessed whether preoperative labs correlated with any adverse outcomes in a posterior fusion population. The study determined that INR, platelets, sodium, and creatinine correlated with adverse events, with sodium and platelets being associated with minor events and INR and creatinine being associated with major events.[30] There has been a recent trend for surgeons to order baseline C-reactive protein (CRP) and erythrocyte sedimentation rate (ESR), which have long been used as markers of infection.[31] It is important to note that other factors, such as advanced age, anemia, pregnancy, drugs, and obesity, can cause elevations in ESR and CRP as well. Obtaining ESR and CRP values preoperatively can allow the surgeon to compare them to postoperative levels in the case of a questionable infection. Overall, perioperative lab work should be based on both the risks associated with the surgery and the patient's underlying medical comorbidities.

Preoperative Antibiotics

Preoperative antibiotics have been shown in both preclinical and clinical studies to significantly reduce the risk of SSIs.[32] Failure to optimize antimicrobial therapy has been proven to increase the risk of infection from two to six times.[33] The agent selected for preoperative antibiotics must be effective against *S. aureus* and *S. epidermidis,* because they are commonly expected pathogens. Community and local hospital organism and resistance patterns are also important considerations. In the majority of patients, a single dose of cephalosporin is recommended. For patients with true beta-lactam allergy, clindamycin or vancomycin may be utilized. The serum and tissue levels of the agent must exceed the minimum inhibitory concentration (MIC) prior to incision and throughout the procedure. Customized weight-based dosing is needed for each individual to achieve this. Forse and colleagues noted that the rate of SSIs in morbidly obese patients who underwent gastroplasty was significantly higher than that in normal weight individuals, despite the fact that both groups had received 1 g of cefazolin prior to incision. The hypothesis was that 1 g may not lead to adequate antibiotic tissue and serum levels in morbidly obese individuals. When patients were randomized to receive either 1 g or 2 g of cefazolin, serum and tissue levels exceeded bacterial MIC only with the 2-g dose. When weight-based dosing was implemented, SSI rates decreased from 16.5% to 5.6% for morbidly obese patients.[34] Cefazolin and clindamycin should be administered within 30 to 60 minutes of incision, while vancomycin should be given within 120 minutes.

Technique

Certain anatomic considerations have been associated with an increased risk of spinous process fractures, while others may increase the difficulty of the procedure itself. Thin or "gracile" spinous processes usually measure less than 20 mm in superior–inferior dimension and increase the likelihood of a postoperative spinous process fracture. When spinous processes are in very close approximation or are in direct contact ("kissing"), there is increased difficulty with the procedure. When spinous processes do not "open up" in the flexed position, fracture and difficulty may both be increased. To reduce the potential for postoperative fracture, it is important to locate the implant body sufficiently anterior and to confirm the final position fluoroscopically.

The procedure includes a set of single-use instruments that are necessary to deliver the implant (Figure 9.1).

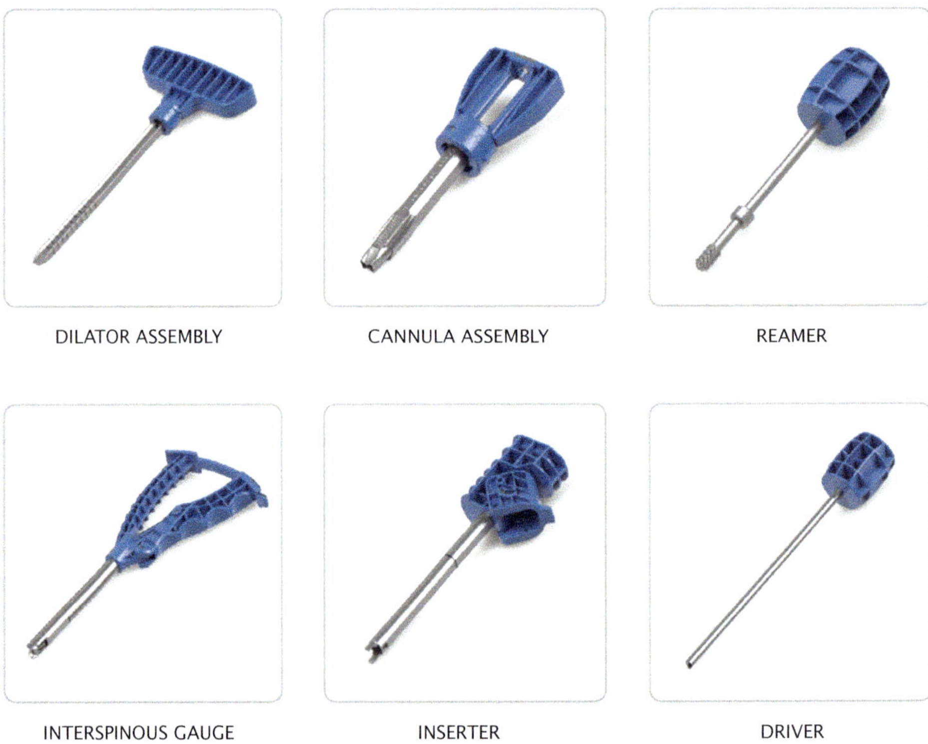

The procedure itself is divided into ten steps. The first step involves positioning the patient. The patient should be positioned in the prone position on a radiolucent table. Flexion of the lumbar spine is imperative at this stage, either with a Wilson frame or with towels or blankets. The surgical field should be prepared and draped in sterile fashion. The second step involves identifying the level to be treated. It is suggested that a radiopaque marker be used to identify the correct level as well as the midline position. The next step involves the surgical approach. This can be done through the fluoroscopically guided technique or direct visualization (mini-open). In the fluoroscopic technique, a scalpel is used to make a

12- to 15-mm midline incision at the operable level. Dissection is carried out to the depth of the supraspinous ligament (SSL). With AP and lateral fluoroscopy for guidance, the blade is advanced to produce a longitudinal split of the SSL at midline. In the direct visualization approach, the same initial approach is used as in the fluoroscopically guided technique. After dissection, a retractor is inserted to allow visualization of the SSL. Next, a longitudinal split of the SSL at midline is produced with a blade. The next step of the procedure is dilation. The cannula assembly is advanced manually or using a mallet, taking care to ensure the dilator does not advance further than the assembly. The assembly is advanced until the distal tip reaches the dorsal aspect of the facet shadow, as evidenced by lateral fluoroscopy. The dilator is then removed, and the cannula assembly handle is unlocked and removed. This leaves only the outer cannula (hereinafter referred to as the cannula). The distal end of the cannula at this point will be positioned about 10 mm dorsal to the spinolaminar junction and beyond the apexes of the spinous process. The position should be confirmed with AP and lateral fluoroscopy. It is important to note that dural injury may result if the cannula assembly is advanced too deeply. The next step utilizes the interspinous reamer to prepare the interspinous space for the implant. The reamer is inserted through the cannula into the interspinous space, with care that it does not go further than the facet shadow or the spinolaminar junction. Again, it is important to realize that dural injury may result from advancing the reamer too far. Next is the implant gauging step. Insert the interspinous gauge through the cannula to determine proper implant size selection. Confirm the depth under lateral fluoroscopy. The distal tips of the gauge should contact the spinous process dorsal to the spinolaminar junction of the superior lamina. Measurement is obtained by firmly actuating the trigger until resistance is detected and is read on the interspinous gauge scale. Utilizing an AP fluoroscopic view, confirm the midline positioning and that the distal tips of the gauge contain the spinous processes, then the gauge may be removed. Next, the implant is loaded. First, the arrow on the body of the implant is aligned with the arrow on the distal end of the inserter. Flip the lever so the bottom of the lever aligns with the bottom of the handle and pulls the proximal third of the implant into the shaft of the inserter. Next, the driver is inserted through the proximal entry point on the insterter and is gently rotated until the distal end of the driver has engaged the implant. Under lateral fluoroscopic guidance, the inserter is introduced into the cannula to minimum insertion depth. Turn the driver clockwise to partially deploy it in the lateral view. When the implant has been deployed approximately 30%, utilize the AP view to ensure bilateral containment of the superior and inferior spinous process. At this point, continue rotating the driver clockwise until the implant's superior and inferior cam lobes have been completely deployed. Do not force deployment or implant breakage or damage to bony structures may result. Potential causes for resistance include:

- The implant and driver are not completely inserted through the cannula.
- There is soft tissue obstruction of the implant.
- The cam lobes are breaching or are obstructed by a spinous process.
- The cam lobes are deploying outside (lateral to) the spinous processes.
- The implant is too far ventral and is engaging the lamina.

Under these circumstances, it is not advisable to manipulate the position. After implant deployment, the implant should be driven ventrally by removing the driver and gently tapping on the inserter. Once the proper implant depth is achieved and has been confirmed in AP and lateral views, rotate the lever upward to disengage and withdraw the inserter and the cannula. Irrigate and suture the incision in routine fashion. Final imaging may be taken at this time.[35]

Postoperative Management and Follow-up

Prevention is always the best approach to managing postoperative complications, and preventive measures often begin before the patient leaves the operating room. The practice of meticulous surgical technique, with proper irrigation of the surgical bed and efficient skin closure, will help decrease postoperative infection. The use of bio-occlusive dressing will limit the entry of bacteria and allow for effective wound healing.

Postoperative Analgesia

The degree of postoperative pain varies among patients; however, most will require 3 to 5 days of analgesic medications. The postoperative analgesia regimen for elderly patients with symptomatic spinal stenosis requires additional care and restraint. In Food and Drug Administration approved IV acetaminophen in 2010. The use of preoperative acetaminophen as preemptive analgesia remains controversial, but the practice has been shown to improve patient satisfaction.[36] In addition to its added cost, IV acetaminophen has not shown significant benefit over oral acetaminophen in patients with functional gastrointestinal tracts.[37] Infiltration of local anesthetics in the surgical bed can also decrease the need for opioid. The introduction of extended-release liposomal bupivacaine has provided another option for patients who are unable to tolerate oral opioids. Despite its causing noticeable pain relief compared to placebo, liposomal bupivacaine has not shown clear benefit over bupivacaine hydrochloride.[38]

Postoperative Antibiotics

The use of postoperative antibiotics remains controversial. Current CDC guidelines for preventing SSIs do not advocate the use of postoperative antibiotics for clean incisions once they are closed.[39] In the literature on spinal cord stimulator implantation, the use of postoperative antibiotics (for an average 7.6 days) has been shown to significantly decrease the postoperative infection rate.[40] In the same multicenter retrospective review of 2,737 permanent spinal cord stimulator implants,[40] the use of bio-occlusive dressing was also shown to decrease postoperative infection.

Bracing

The routine use of a lumbar brace after indirect interspinous decompression is not recommended and has not been shown to add any clinical benefit. The interspinous decompression procedure does not weaken the existing lumbar architecture and thus does not require postoperative stabilization. The use of lightweight abdominal binders has been reported by experienced implanters to add temporary compression to help decrease postoperative bleeding and fluid collections.

Follow-up

Despite the minimally invasive nature of the procedure, patients benefit from a postoperative wound check at 1 to 2 weeks. Any patient-reported signs and symptoms of wound issues, such as bleeding or infection, should never be ignored and must be attended to immediately. Most patients will return to normal function by 3 months and can resume their usual activities, although their exact schedule is at the discretion of the physician.

Physical Therapy

Physical therapy after indirect interspinous decompression is not mandatory. Many patients with chronic symptomatic neurogenic claudication are physically deconditioned due to inactivity. With the insertion of a spacer device, neurogenic claudication symptoms may improve but patients may lack the physical stamina for expected activities. Postoperative physical therapy may complement the recovery process by restoring atrophied muscle groups and thereby help prevent injuries.

Complications and Management

Bleeding

The midline interspinous space tends to have limited vasculature, and the minimally invasive serial dilation process of this procedure has an inherently low risk for bleeding. Meticulous surgical technique and hemostasis also help minimize the incidence of postoperative bleeding. Most postprocedure bleeding will stop with applied pressure and conservative care. If conservative options fail, one may need to reexplore the incision and apply surgical hemostasis.

Infection

Overall, SSI after interspinous spacer implantation is rare. The rate of infection reported in the Superion Investigational Device Exemption (IDE) trial was 1.1% in 190 patients.[41]

Revision and Explantation

The interspinous spacer device implantation is reversible. In the rare circumstance when the device must be removed, the device is surgically exposed via a small incision and the removal steps are performed in the reverse sequence of the steps for implantation. There may be osteophytic growth around the implant over time requiring debridement. Removal of the device(s) can also be achieved during open laminectomy. In the Superion IDE trial, the revision/reoperation rate was 20% at 24 months.[42] The postmarket registry for the device showed only a 3.6% revision/reoperation rate during the 6 to 12 months after implantation.

Specifically with the interspinous spacer device, spinous process fracture can occur during implantation or in the postoperative period. The fracture rate was reported to be 16.3% during the Superion IDE study. If the spacer remains in adequate position, conservative therapy is recommended, allowing the fractured spinous process to heal without intervention. *Pend PRESS data on fractures.

Device migration or dislodgement has also been reported. Radiographic evidence of device migration should be correlated with clinical presentation. Revision or removal should be considered only if there are clinically significant findings.

Conclusion

Indirect lumbar decompression and the associated evidence for the procedure's efficacy and safety have significantly added to patient treatment options for LSS. The devices provide a safe and minimally invasive treatment strategy and should be considered in the algorithmic approach to treating LSS with neurogenic claudication.

References

1. Jackson RP, McManus AC, Moore J. Lumbar spinal stenosis: Treatment options for an aging population. *Mo Med.* 2012;109(6):466–469.
2. Diwan S, Sayed D, Deer TR, Salomons A, Liang K. An algorithmic approach to treating lumbar spinal stenosis: an evidenced-based approach. *Pain Med.* 2019;20(suppl 2):S23–S31. doi:10.1093/pm/pnz133.
3. Hartman J, Granville M, Jacobson RE. The use of Vertiflex® Interspinous Spacer device in patients with lumbar spinal stenosis and concurrent medical comorbidities. *Cureus.* 2019 Aug; 11(8):e5374.
4. Richards JC, Majumdar S, Lindsey DP, et al. The treatment mechanism of an interspinous process implant for lumbar neurogenic intermittent claudication. *Spine.* 2005;30(7):744–749.
5. Wiseman CM, Lindsey DP, Fredrick AD, et al. The effect of an interspinous process implant on facet loading during extension. *Spine.* 2005;30(8):903–907.
6. Wilke H-J, Drumm J, H€aussler K, et al. Biomechanical effect of different lumbar interspinous implants on flexibility and intradiscal pressure. *Eur Spine J.* 2008;17(8):1049–1056.
7. Falowski SM, Sayed D, Deer TR, Brescacin D, Liang K. Biomechanics and mechanism of action of indirect lumbar decompression and the evolution of a stand-alone spinous process spacer. *Pain Med.* 2019;20(suppl 2):S14–S22.
8. Gala R, Russo GS, Whang PG. Interspinous implants to treat spinal stenosis. *Curr Rev Musculoskelet Med.* 2017;10(2):182–188.
9. Gazzeri R, Galarza M, Neroni M, et al. Failure rates and complications of interspinous process decompression devices: a European multicenter study. *Neurosurg Focus.* 2015;39(4):E14.
10. Guyer R, Musacchio M, Cammisa FP Jr, Lorio MP. ISASS recommendations/coverage criteria for decompression with interlaminar stabilization—coverage indications, limitations, and/or medical necessity. *Int J Spine Surg.* 2016;10:41.
11. *Decision Memo for Percutaneous Image-guided Lumbar Decompression for Lumbar Spinal Stenosis* (CAG-00433N) American Society of Anesthesiologists. https://www.asahq.org.
12. Lauryssen C, Jackson RJ, Baron JM, et al. Stand-alone interspinous spacer versus decompressive laminectomy for treatment of lumbar spinal stenosis. *Expert Rev Med Devices.* 2015;12(6):763–769.
13. Patel VV, Whang PG, Haley TR, et al. Two-year clinical outcomes of a multicenter randomized controlled trial comparing two interspinous spacers for treatment of moderate lumbar spinal stenosis. *BMC Musculoskelet Disord.* 2014;15:221.

14. Patel VV, Nunley PD, Whang PG, et al. Superion® Interspinous Spacer for treatment of moderate degenerative lumbar spinal stenosis: durable three-year results of a randomized controlled trial. *J Pain Res.* 2015;8:657–662.
15. Nunley PD, Patel VV, Orndorff DG, Lavelle WF, Block JE, Geisler FH. Superion Interspinous Spacer treatment of moderate spinal stenosis: 4-year results. *World Neurosurg.* 2017;104:279–283.
16. Nunley PD, Patel VV, Orndorff DG, Lavelle WF, Block JE, Geisler FH. Five-year durability of stand-alone interspinous process decompression for lumbar spinal stenosis. *Clin Interv Aging.* 2017;12:1409–1417.
17. Merkow J, Varhabhatla N, Manchikanti L, Kaye AD, Urman RD, Yong RJ. Minimally invasive lumbar decompression and interspinous process device for the management of symptomatic lumbar spinal stenosis: a literature review. *Curr Pain Headache Rep.* 2020;24(4):13.
18. Deer TR, Sayed D, Malinowski MN, et al. A review of emerging evidence for utilization of a percutaneous interspinous process decompression device to treat symptomatic lumbar adjacent-segment degeneration. *Pain Med.* 2019;20(suppl 2):S9–S13.
19. Tekmyster G, Sayed D, Cairns KD, Raso LJ, Kim C, Block JE. Interspinous process decompression with the Superion Spacer for lumbar spinal stenosis: real-world experience from a device registry. *Med Devices.* 2019;12:423–427.
20. Nunley PD, Deer TR, Benyamin RM, Staats PS, Block JE. Interspinous process decompression is associated with a reduction in opioid analgesia in patients with lumbar spinal stenosis. *J Pain Res.* 2018;11:2943–2948.
21. Deer TR, Provenzano DA, Hanes M, et al. The Neurostimulation Appropriateness Consensus Committee (NACC) recommendations for infection prevention and management. *Neuromodulation.* 2017;20(1):31–50. doi:10.1111/ner.12565. Erratum in *Neuromodulation.* 2017;20(5):516. PMID: 28042909.
22. Sorensen LT, Karlsmack T, Gottrup F. Abstinence from smoking reduces incisional wound infection: a randomized controlled trial. *Ann Surg.* 2003;238:1–5.
23. Deer TR, Narouze S, Provenzano D, et al. The Neuromodulation Appropriate Consensus Committee (NACC) recommendations on bleeding and coagulation management in neuromodulation devices. *Neuromodulation.* 2017;20:51–62.
24. Narouze S, Benzon HT, Provenzano D, et al. Interventional spine and pain procedures in patients on antiplatelet and anticoagulant medications (second edition). *Reg Anesth Pain Med.* 2018;43:225–262.
25. Perl TM, Cullen JJ, Wenzel RP, et al. Intranasal mupirocin to prevent postoperative *Staphylococcus aureus* infections. *N Engl J Med.* 2002;346:1871–1877.
26. Parvizi J, Matar WY, Saleh KJ, Schmalzried TP, Mihalko WM. Decolonization of drug-resistant organisms before total joint arthroplasty. *Instr Course Lect.* 2010;59:131–137.
27. Kalmeijer MD, van Nieuwland-Bollen E, Bogaers-Hofman D, de Baere GA. Nasal carriage of *Staphylococcus aureus* is a major risk factor for surgical-site infections in orthopedic surgery. *Infect Control Hosp Epidemiol.* 2000;21:319–323.
28. Chen AF, Wessel CB, Rao N. *Staphylococcus aureus* screening and decolonization in orthopaedic surgery and reduction of surgical site infections. *Clin Orthop Rel Res.* 2013;471:2383–2399.
29. Bode LG, Kluytmans JA, Wertheim HF, et al. Preventing surgical-site infections in nasal carriers of *Staphylococcus aureus. N Engl J Med.* 2010;362:9–17.
30. Lakomkin N, Goz V, Cheng JS, Brodke DS, Spiker WR. The utility of preoperative laboratories in predicting postoperative complications following posterolateral lumbar fusion. *Spine J.* 2018;18(6):993–997. https://doi.org/10.1016/j.spinee.2017.10.010.
31. Markanday A. Acute Phase Reactants in Infections: Evidence Based Review and a Guide for Clinicians. *Open Forum Infect Dis.* 2015;2(3):ofv098.
32. Fletcher N, Sofianos D, Berkes MB, Obremskey WT. Prevention of perioperative infection. *J Bone Joint Surg Am.* 2007;89:1605–1618.
33. Burke JP. Maximizing appropriate antibiotic prophylaxis for surgical patients: an update from LDS Hospital, Salt Lake City. *Clin Infect Dis.* 2001;33(suppl. 2):S78–S83.
34. Forse RA, Karam B, MacLean LD, Christou NV. Antibiotic prophylaxis for surgery in morbidly obese patients. *Surgery.* 1989;106:750–757.
35. *Superion IDS Surgical Technique Manual.* Boston Scientific; 2017.

36. Apfel CC, Souza K, Portillo J, Dalal P, Bergese SD. Patient satisfaction with intravenous acetaminophen. *J Healthcare Quality.* 2015;37(3):155–162.
37. Jibril F, Sharaby S, Mohamed A, Wilby K. Intravenous versus oral acetaminophen for pain: systemic review of current evidence to support clinical decision-making. *Can J Hosp Pharm.* 2015;68:238–247.
38. Hamilton TW, Athanassoglou V, Mellon S, et al. Liposomal bupivacaine infiltration at the surgical site for the management of postoperative pain. *Cochrane Database Syst Rev.* 2017;2(2):CD011419.
39. Berríos-Torres SI, Umscheid CA, Bratzler DW, et al. Centers for Disease Control and Prevention guideline for the prevention of surgical site infection, 2017. *JAMA Surg.* 2017;152(8):784–791
40. Hoelzer BC, Bendel MA, Deer TR, et al. Spinal cord stimulator implant infection rates and risk factors: a multicenter retrospective study. *Neuromodulation.* 2017;20(6):558–562.
41. *FDA: Summary of Safety and Effectiveness Data.* 2017. https://www.accessdata.fda.gov/cdrh_docs/pdf14/p140004b.pdf.
42. Nunley PD, Shamie AN, Blumenthal SL, Orndorff D, Block JE, Geisler FH. Interspinous process decompression: expanding treatment options for lumbar spinal stenosis. *Biomed Res Int.* 2016;2016:1–5.

10

Minimally Invasive Posterior Lumbar Fusion—A New Approach to a Standard Procedure

Behnam Myers and Alaa Abd-Elsayed

Introduction

Background

Posterior lumbar/intertransverse fusion dates to the earliest forms of fusion. In 1911, a crude version of a posterolateral fusion (PLF) was developed by Albee. Bone was taken from the patient's tibia (autologous bone), was chopped up (morselized), and was packed between adjacent spinous processes. The goal was to fuse the two spinous processes into one segment. [1,2] In 1953, Watkins and Campbell pioneered the modern version of PLF, which involved fusion of the facet joints, pars interarticularis, and bases of the transverse processes.[2] This was achieved by making a large midline incision and exposing outward through soft tissue to the transverse processes. Wiltse later described the final modification of the procedure, which simply included fusion of the lamina in addition to the previously mentioned posterior elements.

Until recently, physicians would dissect all the tissue (including fascia, ligaments, and muscle) from the posterior elements of the vertebrae involved in the fusion, which included the transverse processes of both vertebrae, the lateral facet joints, and perhaps the lateral lamina. Once the extensive dissection was complete, decortication (removal of the bony cortex) was accomplished by grinding the outer covering (the cortex) off the bones to prepare the area for fusion. The oozing bone was needed to supply the bone graft with the blood, mesenchymal stem cells (MSC), and growth factors necessary for fusion to take place. All three of these components are essential to provide the osteoinduction, osteoconduction, and osteogenesis needed for healing to occur.[3] Today, however, there is a new technique that allows for the same bony decortication but without the extensive tissue dissection. With advances in medical devices, physicians now have the ability to perform this procedure using a minimally invasive approach that can significantly decrease blood loss, scarring, and healing time.

Facet-Mediated Low Back Pain

Facet-mediated low back pain is estimated to cause approximately 25% to 40% of low back pain.[4] The percentage is even higher with adjacent-level disease from prior fusions or spinal intervention. Modalities that can cause facet pain include kyphoplasty and vertebral augmentation procedures. Other conditions that can contribute to facet-mediated low back pain include disk degeneration, spondylolisthesis, inflammatory arthritis, instability, and traumatic injuries.[5] On MRI or CT, findings can be facet cyst or facet arthritic changes. A smaller subset of facet-mediated pain can be a result of prior surgical intervention at the same level. This often requires MRI of the facet joints, because after surgery, the joint can become compromised by arthritic changes or aberrant movement, resulting in facet-mediated pain.

Facet-mediated low back pain is a common cause of disability. In addition to the causes just described, some common causes are:

- Repetitively lifting heavy objects
- Sudden flexion-extension injuries from a motor vehicle accident
- Excessive muscle strain due to prolonged sitting or wrong positioning
- Prolonged use of high-heeled shoes
- Poor posture
- Obesity
- Sports injuries

To understand the natural history of facet-mediated back pain, one needs to understand the anatomy of the lumbar spine. Although generally people have five lumbar vertebrae, it's estimated that around 5% of adults have a sixth lumbar vertebra.[6] This is often called a transitional vertebra and should not cause any particular issues in a healthy person. Between the lumbar vertebrae are the lumbar disks. Over time, when subjected to one of the above causes of injury, patients may begin to experience low back pain. Most often, but not always, the pain is the result of disk degeneration and loss of integrity in the anterior column. Because the disk is unable to withstand the stress across the lower back, the facet joints can begin to become a source of pain.[7] The facet joints located in the lumbar spine (Figure 10.1) are most susceptible to facet damage because as the lumbar spine bears the most weight and endures the greatest amount of stress/strain. The intervertebral disks and facet joints can wear down with years of strain and activity. Intervertebral disks are composed primarily of water, and age-related degenerative changes affect disk hydration—the net effect being a loss of disk height and changes to the alignment of the facet joints. This deterioration and malalignment can lead to facet joint pain. That is why facet joint syndrome often coexists with other spinal degenerative disorders, including degenerative disk disease, spondylolisthesis, and

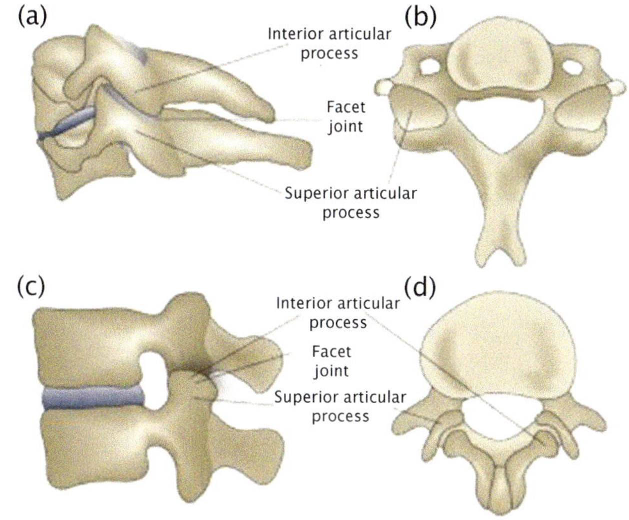

FIGURE 10.1. Cervical and lumbar facet joint anatomy.

a. Lateral view of adjacent cervical vertebrae demonstrating the facet joint and articulating processes.

b. Axial view of a cervical vertebra showing the vertebral foramen and facet joint orientation.

c. Lateral view of adjacent lumbar vertebrae with an intervertebral disc, demonstrating the facet joint and articulating processes.

d. Axial view of a lumbar vertebra showing the vertebral foramen and facet joint orientation.

spondylosis (spinal osteoarthritis). Low back pain is commonly caused by facet joint syndrome. Pain may be felt in the lower back and sometimes in the buttocks and/or thighs.[5] Inflammation of the joints can cause stiffness and difficulty standing up straight or sleeping on a flat surface. The symptoms are often relieved by leaning forward and often are aggravated by extension.

Indications

The main objective of posterolateral intertransverse/facet arthrodesis is fusion of the identified pain generators, with the goal of alleviating symptoms and allowing the patient to return to activities of daily living. Patients who are candidates for the procedure have undergone a workup that has determined that a pain generator is located at the facet joint or joints (Figure 10.2). In either scenario, fusion is always accomplished bilaterally because it stabilizes the joint and prevents global movements. Before a posterolateral intertransverse/facet arthrodesis is decided upon, the patient should try conservative therapies, such as physical therapy and oral anti-inflammatory medication. In physical therapy, it's important to focus on core stabilization and body mass index (BMI) optimization. Patients who fail the conservative regimen are often given diagnostic and therapeutic facet blocks. Well-established procedures, such as facet joint blocks, medial branch blocks, and rhizotomies, are used to diagnose and treat chronic facet pain.[5] Gender, age, and weight significantly influence the probability that the facet joint is the origin of the patient's low back pain. Older age correlates with an increased incidence of facet joint disease from the accumulated degeneration of the joint. Higher BMI is associated with higher probability of facet-mediated

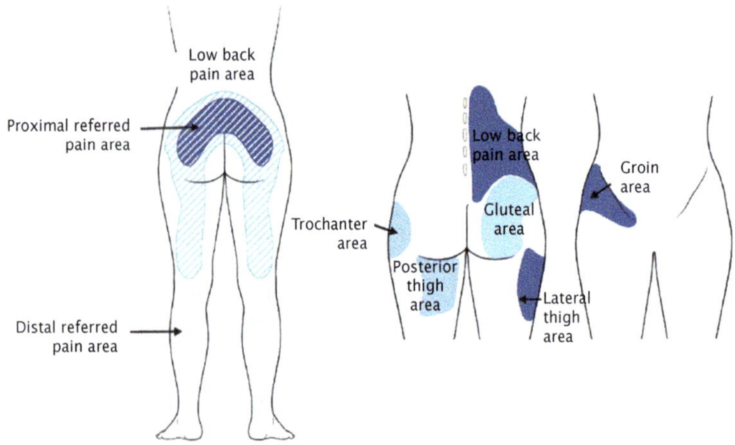

FIGURE 10.2. Diagram of areas of facet-mediated pain.

pain if a patient presents with low back pain, due to the increased weight distributed on the facet joints. Furthermore, previous lumbosacral spine surgery predisposes a patient to the development of facet joint pain at adjacent levels. The adjacent disk and facet joints act as shock absorbers and allow for global range of motion, but they experience increased stress and load that might expedite degeneration across the articular surfaces.

Patient Selection

Almost always, procedural success is related to appropriate patient selection. Often, the source of back pain is multifactorial, but if the source of pain has been determined to be facet-mediated, facet-mediated low back pain is treatable. To avoid selecting patients who may not obtain good results, the following contraindications should be taken into account. Patients with spondylitic spondylolisthesis or patients with a mobile listhesis on flexion or extension views are not ideal candidates. Additionally, patients with morbid obesity should be carefully evaluated, as this condition can complicate the surgical procedure and postoperative recovery. Rheumatoid arthritis itself is not a contraindication. Patients are also encouraged to maintain a normal blood glucose level. A hemoglobin A_{1c} of 8.5 or greater incurs an increased risk of infection. It is commonly recommended that HIV-positive patients have a negative viral titer prior to surgery. Assessment of contraindications and other risk factors, such as smoking, obesity, and infections, is also very important (Boxes 10.1 and 10.2).

Preoperative Workup

Patients under the age of 40 who are relatively healthy and who have no associated medical comorbidities generally require minimal workup. Preoperative surgical blood work is often requested. For females, a pregnancy test and urinalysis will be requested. For individuals over the age of 40, in addition to getting blood work, physicians may request

BOX 10.1. Contraindications to the FacetCore Fusion System

The device is intended to be used by a physician familiar with the possible side effects, typical findings, limitations, indications, and contraindications of facet fusion procedures.

Overall, the contraindications can be applied to other allograft facet implants.[9] Contraindications are:

- Morbid obesity
- Pregnancy
- Grossly distorted anatomy due to congenital abnormalities
- Any medical or surgical condition that would preclude the potential benefit of spinal implant surgery, such as the presence of tumors, congenital abnormalities, elevated white blood cell count (WBC), or a left shift in the WBC differential count
- Rapid progressive joint disease, bone absorption, osteopenia, osteomalacia, or osteoporosis (although osteopenia and osteoporosis are relative contraindications)
- High-grade instability
- Grade 2 or higher spondylolisthesis
- Inability to lie prone throughout the procedure
- Allergy to procedural drugs (e.g., iodinated contrast)
- Trauma

medical clearance from a qualified perioperative physician. Patients are provided with preoperative instructions that they have nothing orally after midnight before the procedure. It is also requested that all patients stop any anti-inflammatory medication, herbal supplements, and anticoagulants (with permission of the prescribing physician) according to published guidelines. Smoking cessation is recommended before surgery. Finally, lumbar flexion and extension x-rays are often requested prior to surgery if mobile listhesis is suspected.

Once the patient has been evaluated and worked up, the patient is seen in the office for a final preoperative consultation. The physician should review the procedure and the medical clearance and answer any final questions prior to surgery.

Technique

There are several different methods for accomplishing posterolateral fusion; however, this chapter focuses on the procedure for the 3D GraftRasp System[9] used in combination with the FacetCore Fusion System[10] by SurGenTec.

Box 10.2. Contraindications to the 3D GraftRasp System

The component is intended to be used by a physician familiar with the possible side effects, typical findings, limitations, indications, and contraindications of bone graft delivery. The component should be used only on patients who are suitable for such procedures, and only for the delivery of hydrated allograft, autograft, or synthetic bone graft materials as directed by a licensed physician. The component is not to be used for filling closed voids/bond defects where undesired pressurization may occur. The contraindications include:

- Active infectious process, particularly in or adjacent to the spine or spinal structures
- Gross joint instability or dislocation
- Morbid obesity
- Pregnancy
- Grossly distorted anatomy due to congenital abnormalities
- Any medical or surgical condition that would preclude the potential benefit of spinal implant surgery
- Osteopenia, osteomalacia, or osteoporosis
- Any patient in whom implant utilization would interfere with anatomic structures or expected physiological performance
- Trauma
- High-grade instability
- Tumors
- Spondylolysis (pars fracture)
- Grade 2 or complicated anatomy
- Distorted or complicated anatomy
- Progressive neurologic deficit
- Chronic smoker
- Acute disk herniation
- Allergy to procedural drugs (e.g., iodinated contrast)
- Open wound or skin ulceration
- Poorly controlled diabetes
- Inability to lie prone for the duration of the procedure
- Intraoperative recognition of foraminal trespass or epidural placement
- Severe nerve root pain during procedure

The patient is placed on a radiolucent table in the prone position. The patient's lumbar spine should be optimally flexed in the neutral position, so that the facet joints are visible on imaging. The use of gel rolls (optional) is recommended to position the patient properly and to achieve optimal fluoroscopic imaging (Figure 10.3).

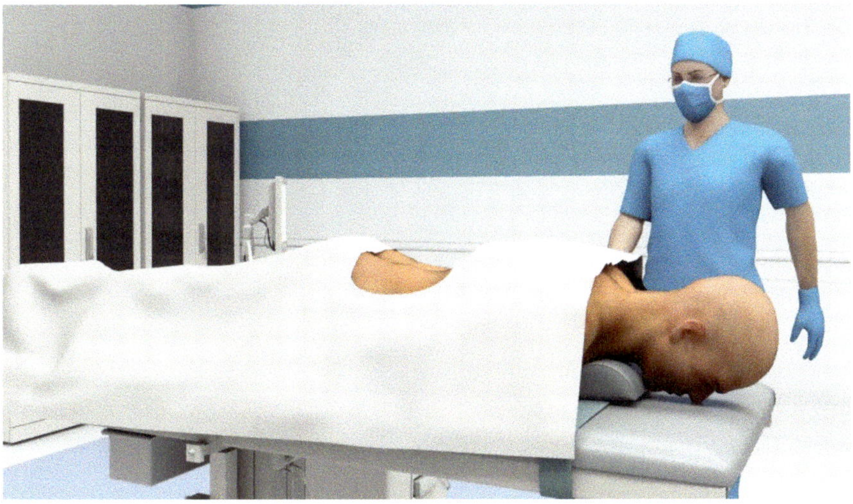

FIGURE 10.3. Patient on table in prone position.

Anesthesia is accomplished by use of local anesthesia with sedation or general anesthesia. The anticipated duration of the procedure is 30 to 60 minutes.

Surgery Steps

Cortical Allograft Implant Placement with FacetCore Fusion System

1. Approximately a 1-inch incision is made approximately one fingerbreadth lateral to the facet (Figure 10.4).
2. The facet joint is located with a guidewire and imaging (Figure 10.5).
3. The facet locator is inserted over the guidewire into the facet joint (Figure 10.6).
4. The drill guide is docked on the facet joint (Figure 10.7).
5. An orthopedic drill is used to prep the insertion site (Figure 10.8).
6. Cortical allograft implant is inserted into the facet joint (Figure 10.9).
7. The procedure is repeated on the contralateral side

Decortication of Transverse Process and Application of Bone Graft with the GraftRasp

1. Palpation with blunt dissection or dilators are used to retract the muscle and to locate the facet joint and transverse process (Figure 10.10).
2. Cobb is inserted through the same 1-inch incision and is used to remove the soft tissues from the transverse processes.
3. The GraftRasp is used to decorticate both transverse processes and facet joints (Figure 10.11).
4. The GraftGun is inserted down the cannula of the GraftRasp and is actuated to dispense graft across the adjacent transverse processes and over the facet joints (Figures 10.12 to 10.14).

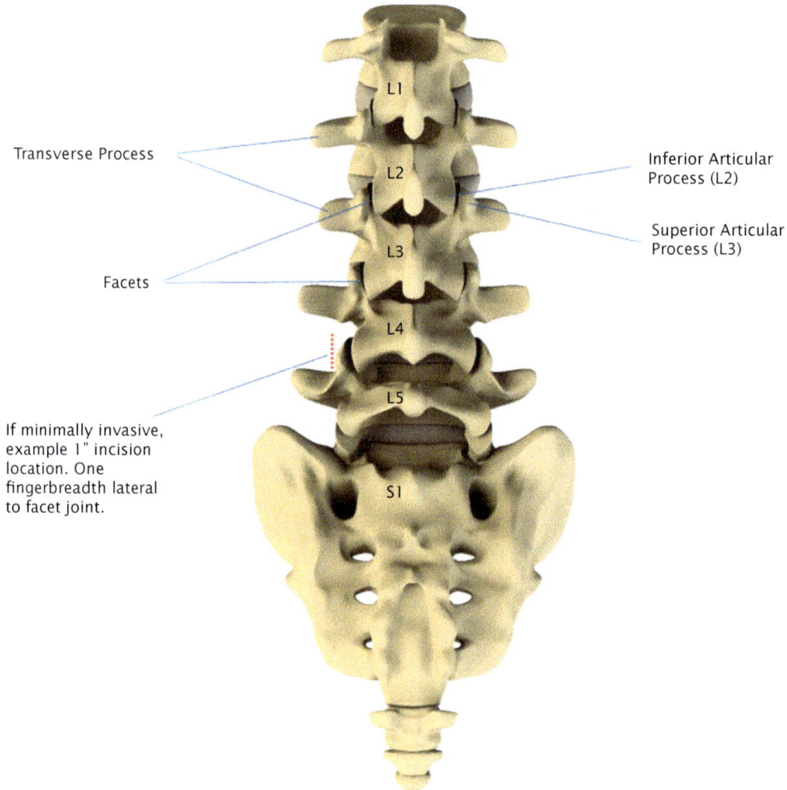

FIGURE 10.4. Incision and lumbar anatomy.[10]

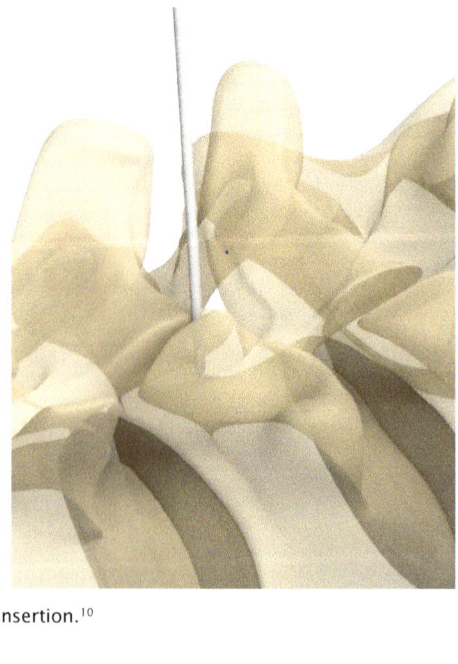

FIGURE 10.5. Guidewire insertion.[10]

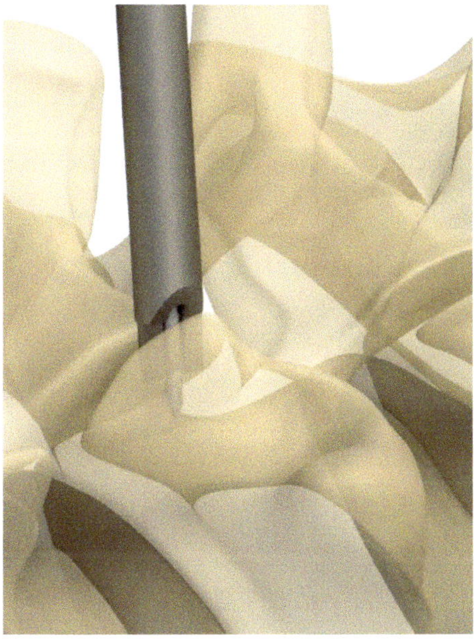

FIGURE 10.6. Facet locator placed in the facet joint.[10]

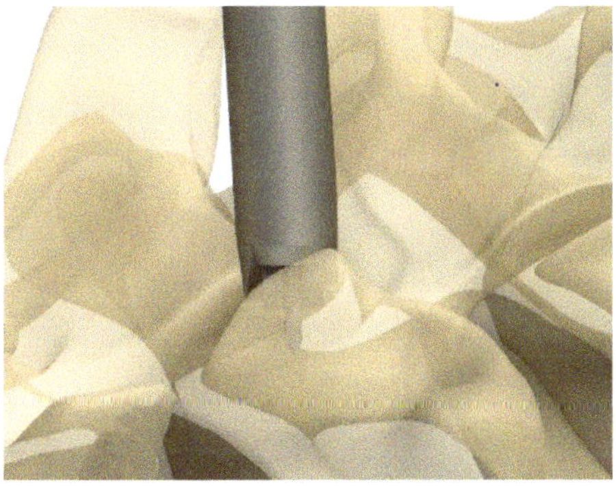

FIGURE 10.7. Drill guide placement.[10]

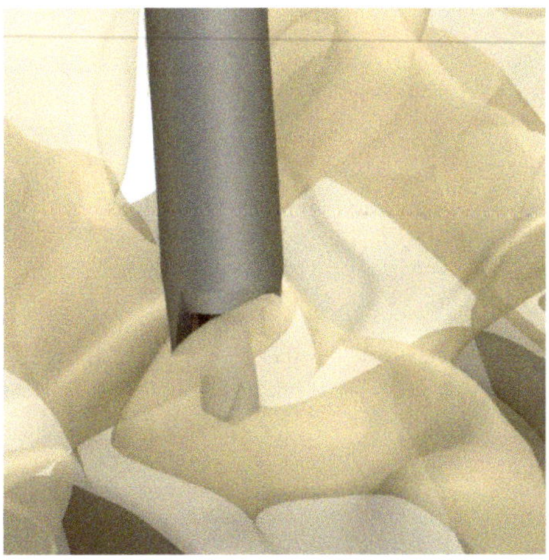

FIGURE 10.8. Drill bit fully inserted into drill guide.[10]

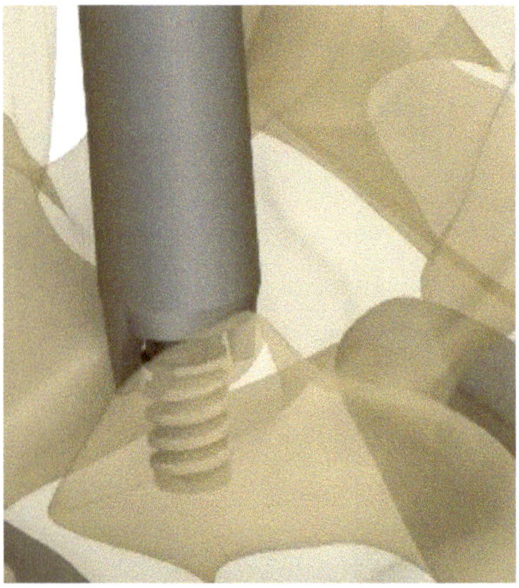

FIGURE 10.9. Cortical allograft insertion.[10]

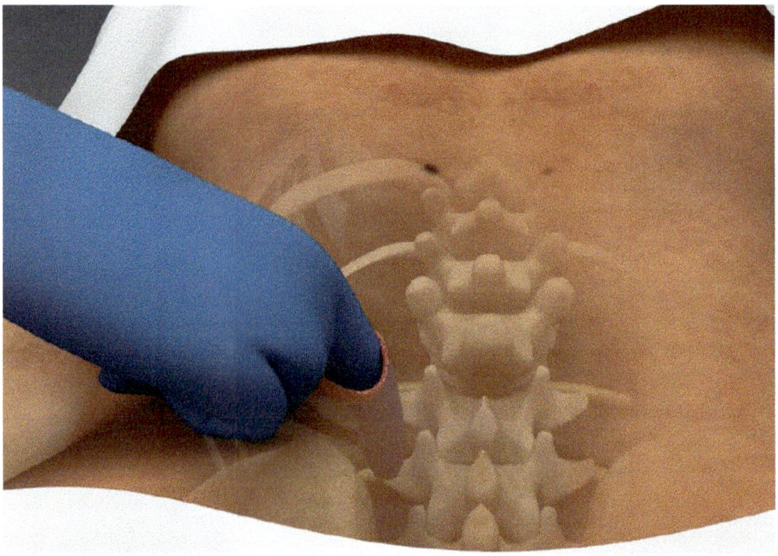

FIGURE 10.10. Blunt tissue dissection.[9]

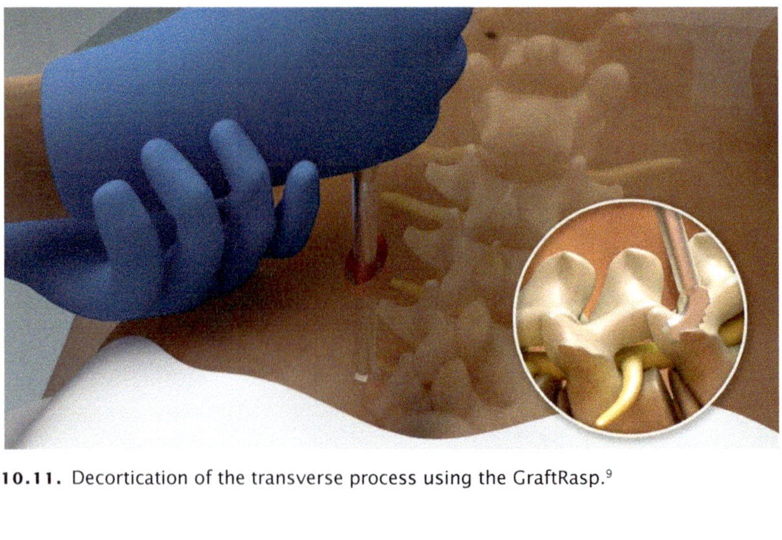

FIGURE 10.11. Decortication of the transverse process using the GraftRasp.[9]

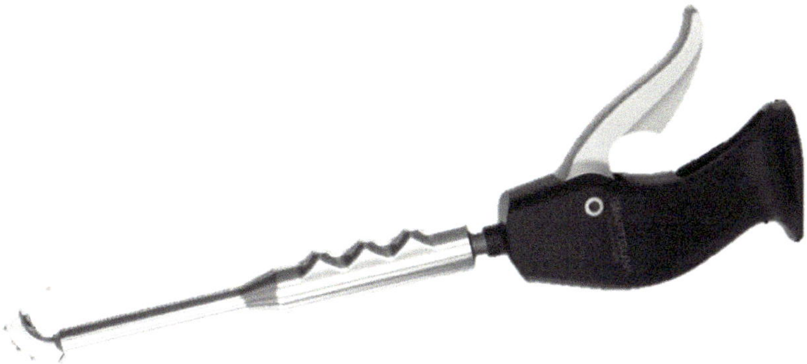

FIGURE 10.12. Graftgun inserted into GraftRasp.[9]

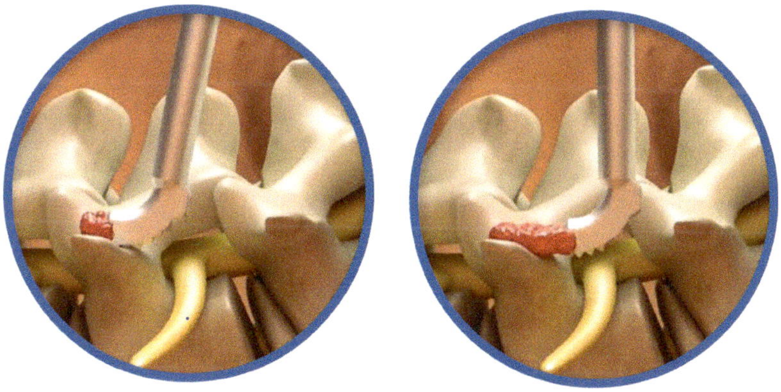

FIGURE 10.13. Delivery of bone graft onto the transverse process using the GraftRasp.[9]

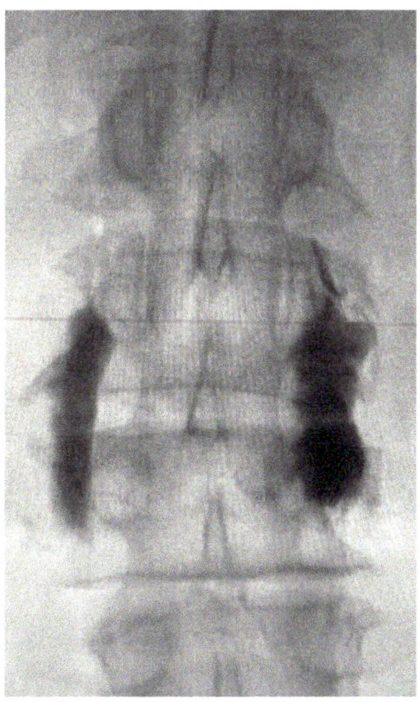

FIGURE 10.14. Minimally invasive posterior lumbar fusion: Radiographic image demonstrating ideal placement of bone graft across the transverse process.

Postoperative Management

The first follow-up visit should occur no later than 1 week after surgery. Postoperatively, patients are instructed to wear a lumbar sacral orthosis brace for a minimum of 6 weeks, but no longer than 8 weeks because this can lead to a deconditioned back. Patients are instructed not to lift anything more than 5 pounds for the first 6 weeks. Patients are allowed to shower 72 hours after surgery, and they can allow water to run over the incision if it is covered by Steri-Strips. Patients are checked for allergies and are given postoperative antibiotic, usually Keflex 500 mg 4 times a day for 3 days. Patients also are given postoperative pain medications as needed.[11]

At the 6-week visit, the brace is discontinued. The patient is now allowed to lift up to 15 pounds, but nothing more.

At the 3-month postoperative follow-up, AP/lateral x-rays may be taken at the physician's discretion. At this time, bony callus formation may be seen. A bone growth stimulator is often used at this time to help augment the fusion.

At the 6-month follow-up, the patient undergoes a repeat set of x-rays of the lumbar spine.

At 1 year postoperatively, if the patient is doing well and has no complaints, they may be discharged. If pain is lingering, x-rays and a CT scan are taken to assess fusion.

Potential Complications

Infection

It is important that the patient's temperature be taken and the incision be assessed at every visit. Should the patient complain of fever, or should the incision appear to be reddened or inflamed, further workup is required to rule out an infection. Soft tissue infection or septic arthritis is uncommon with this procedure given its minimal access and sterile technique.[12] In addition, prior to the incision the patient receives prophylactic antibiotics, typically 1 to 2 g of Ancef depending on the patient's weight and allergies.

Facet Fracture

There is a risk of facet fracture, but it is very rare. Should a unilateral facet fracture occur, then the facet should continue to be stabilized with the allograft implant and bone graft. The intertransverse fusion between the transverse processes should also be performed. The patient should be maintained in a brace and should be given a bone growth stimulator.

Transverse Process Fracture

Transverse process fractures are rare, but they are more likely than a facet fracture. Bone graft is to be maintained over the transverse process and the intertransverse fusion should be completed. The patient is maintained in a brace and should be given a bone growth stimulator.

CSF Leak

CSF leak is uncommon, but it can occur if the guidewire is placed in the dural canal. Patients complaining of postoperative headache should be worked up for potential CSF leak, especially if the patient has a postural headache after the procedure. Treatment may include observation, blood patch, or a formal surgical closure.

Hematoma

Hematoma usually occurs in the subfascial layer; however, without any physical decompression of neural elements, the hematoma will be benign, and it will usually resolve on its own over time.

Damage to the Nerve Root

Nerve root damage is highly unlikely. It is best avoided by staying within the facet joint and out of the neural foramen.

Nonunion

Nonunion can occur in both instrumented and noninstrumented fusions. Nonunion of a posterolateral intertransverse and facet fusion does not preclude the patient from getting any further procedures. The patient can expect to undergo an exploration of fusion and revision without disruption from the prior surgery.

Conclusion

Posterolateral intertransverse arthrodesis is a procedure that has been performed for over 100 years. Until recently, the technique required extensive dissection with significant soft tissue debridement. Today, there is an alternative method of access that uses enhanced medical devices to obtain the same goals. The modified procedure and technique allow for stabilization and fusion of the lumbar spine without hardware. Through advanced bone preparation and graft placement, the system allows physicians to create multiple contact surfaces between bleeding bone and bone graft, thus giving patients the best possible chance at successful fusion. The key advantages of the technique are minimal soft tissue disruption and decreased bleeding, which yield faster recovery and less scarring.

References

1. Virk S, Qureshi S, Sandhu H. History of spinal fusion: where we came from and where we are going. *HSS J*. 2020;16(2):137–142.
2. Peek RD, Wiltse LL. History of spinal fusion. In: Cotler JM, Cotler HB, eds. *Spinal Fusion*. New York, NY: Springer; 1990: 3–4. https://doi.org/10.1007/978-1-4612-3272-8_1.
3. Canto FR, Garcia SB, Issa JP, Marin A, Del Bel EA, Defino HL. Influence of decortication of the recipient graft bed on graft integration and tissue neoformation in the graft-recipient bed interface. *Eur Spine J*. 2008;17(5):706–714.

4. Manchikanti L, Pampati V, Rivera J, Fellows B, Beyer C, Damron K. Role of facet joints in chronic low back pain in the elderly: a controlled comparative prevalence study. Pain Pract. 2001;1(4):332–337. doi.10.1046/j.1533-2500.2001.01034.x.
5. Perolat R, Kastler A, Nicot B, et al. Facet joint syndrome: from diagnosis to interventional management. *Insights Imaging*. 2018;9(5):773–789. doi:10.1007/s13244-018-0638-x
6. Yan Y, Li Q, Wu C, et al. Rate of presence of 11 thoracic vertebrae and 6 lumbar vertebrae in asymptomatic Chinese adult volunteers. *J Orthop Surg Res*. 2018;13(124). https://doi.org/10.1186/s13018-018-0835-9.
7. Dunlop R, Adams M, Hutton W. Disc space narrowing and the lumbar facet joints. *J Bone Joint Surg Br.* 1984;66-B(5):706–710.
8. Mooney V, Robertson J. The facet syndrome. *Clin Orthop Relat Res*. 1976;(115):149–156. PMID: 130216.
9. The 3D GraftRasp System. *Surgical Technique Guide*. Boca Raton, FL: SurGenTec 2021.
10. FacetCore™ Fusion System. *Surgical Technique Guide*. Boca Raton, FL: SurGenTec 2021.
11. Bajwa SJ, Haldar R. Pain management following spinal surgeries: An appraisal of the available options. *J Craniovert Junction Spine*. 2015;6(3):105–110.
12. Mueller K, Zhao D, Johnson O, Sandhu FA, Voyadzis J-M. The difference in surgical site infection rates between open and minimally invasive spine surgery for degenerative lumbar pathology: a retrospective single center experience of 1442 cases. *Operative Neurosurg*. 2019;16(6):750–755. https://doi.org/10.1093/ons/opy221.

PART 4

Vertebral Augmentation Procedures

11

Vertebroplasty

Johnathan Goree and Mark Malinowski

Conflicts of Interest
Dr. Goree is a consultant for Abbott Laboratories and Stratus Medical. Dr. Goree also has research support from SPR Therapeutics. Dr. Malinowski is a consultant for Abbott Laboratories, Nalu Medical, LLC, and SI-Bone, Inc., and has research with Abbott.

Introduction

Osteoporosis is a common degenerative bone disease that makes patients susceptible to fractures, including femoral neck fractures and vertebral compression fracture (VCF). Approximately 10 million Americans over 50 years old have osteoporosis, and another 33 million Americans are predisposed to fractures due to low bone mass.[1] While osteoporosis can occur at any stage of life, the incidence increases with each additional decade of life, and the disease most frequently affects non-Hispanic White women.[1,2]

The most common type of osteoporotic fracture is the VCF.[3] The incidence is more than 700,000 annually, accounting for thousands of office visits and over 50,000 hospitalizations every year.[4] While VCFs are associated with pain, morbidity, and decreased quality of life, they are also associated with increased mortality risk. Women with one or more VCF have a 1.2-fold increased age-related mortality risk.[5] The total healthcare cost of osteoporotic fractures, including VCFs, is over 10 billion dollars a year.[6–7]

Vertebral augmentation is a class of minimally invasive procedures that have been proven to improve function, mortality risk, and quality of life after a VCF. A percutaneous cannula is used to inject cement into the compressed vertebral body to stabilize the fracture, restore height, and relieve pain. There are two types of vertebral augmentation, vertebroplasty (VP) and kyphoplasty. VP involves accessing the compressed vertebral body through the posterior elements and injecting cement, whereas kyphoplasty also includes using a balloon or other device to restore physiologic height prior to cement injection. This chapter details the indications, risks, benefits, patient selection, technique, and postprocedural management of VP.

Indications

Percutaneous VP is most commonly performed for patients with painful acute or subacute VCF, especially those who have failed conservative treatment, including bracing, ibuprofen, other oral analgesics, and rest (4–6 weeks).[8,9] While direct VP treatment without a trial of bracing and medication is indicated for patients with intractable pain, concern for increased mortality risk in elderly patients with conservative care has made this more common in recent years.[10] Other indications include treatment of pathologic fractures and palliative treatment for spinal instability in which surgical intervention is not indicated.

Evidence

Evidence for VP is often mixed due to multiple underpowered studies, poorly designed clinical trials, and poorly chosen outcomes. Despite those challenges, there are many well-designed clinical trials that prove both acute and durable benefit after VP for VCF.

In a 2020 systematic review by Sanli and colleagues, 18 studies were evaluated to determine both short- and long-term benefit from VP in comparison to conservative management. Pooled results showed significant pain relief at day 1, day 180, and day 360.[11] For measures of functional outcomes, VP showed a significant improvement in Oswestry Disability Index and Roland Morris Disability Questionnaire at 6 months.[11] In a single-center, sham-controlled trial, similar findings were demonstrated. A significant percentage of patients who underwent VP had pain scores less than 4 at 14 days, 1 month, 3 months, and 6 months, better results than for sham VP with subcutaneous lidocaine.[12]

Hinde et al evaluated all-cause mortality outcomes after VP. In a meta-analysis of over 2 million patients with osteoporotic compression fractures, VP decreased 10-year mortality by 22%.[13] Some studies have compared kyphoplasty to VP, and results are mixed. A meta-analysis from 2018 by Wang and colleagues demonstrated no significant difference between the two procedures, except for a reduction in cement extravasation and improvement in vertebral body height with kyphoplasty.[14]

Contraindications

Absolute Contraindications

VP should not be performed on patients who have radiographic findings without symptoms or are improving with conservative management.[8] Uncorrectable coagulopathy or current anticoagulant therapy is a contraindication. Also, to prevent potential systemic infection, local infections over the site of cannula entry are also contraindications. Last, previous allergic reaction to any materials needed to complete the procedure is an absolute contraindication.[8]

Relative Contraindications

Patients with fracture disruption of the posterior wall of the vertebral body of interest or tumor invasion of the spinal canal are at risk of cement extravasation during the procedure.[8] This could lead to neural compromise. Severe compression, called vertebra plana, is a contraindication because of the inability to safely perform the procedure.[8] Table 11.1 lists all contraindications, absolute and relative.

Perioperative Management

The typical patient who presents with pathological compression fractures will have comorbidity. The preoperative evaluation of these patients requires standardized pretesting and optimization of the comorbid conditions. While the VP procedure may be done in the office setting, it may also be done in the ambulatory surgical setting or commonly as a traditional inpatient operative case under monitored anesthesia care or general endotracheal anesthesia. Proper preoperative cardiopulmonary evaluation is needed, including, but not limited to, electrocardiogram, echocardiography, or stress testing. Laboratory tests typical for surgical cases include complete blood count and coagulation studies (PT, aPTT, INR). Presurgical infection risk assessment includes urinalysis with culture and methicillin-resistant *Staphylococcus aureus* (MRSA) screening. Diabetic patients will often be tested for hemoglobin A_{1c}, although this value is more pertinent to risk stratification rather than an absolute contraindication in the inpatient setting. Nonetheless, perioperative glucose control is the standard of care and is known to directly correlate with the postoperative course. Preoperative antibiosis is the standard of presurgical care. Extended-spectrum antibiotics directed at gram positive cocci are typical, and the choice of agent may vary from region to region based on known local sensitivities. For MRSA, weight-based vancomycin dosing is the standard of care. For active infections without absolute contraindication, antibiotic sensitivities will drive the decision. However, antibiotics with good spinal penetration are the preferred choice when the case is to proceed to the operating room.[15] Perioperative coagulation is critical to address when the patient presents on antiplatelet or other anticoagulants. The American Society of Regional Anesthesia and Pain Medicine has published

TABLE 11.1. Contraindications to Vertebroplasty

Absolute Contraindications	Relative Contraindications
Asymptomatic compression fracture	Disruption of the posterior wall
Uncorrectable coagulopathy	Tumor invasion into the spinal canal
Local or systemic infection	Severely compressed fracture
Allergy to polymethylmethacrylate (PMMA) or alternative bone cement	

widely accepted guidelines for regional anesthesia in the presence of antithrombotic or thrombolytic therapy.[16]

Preoperative imaging is a critical for diagnosing and evaluating fracture location, morphology, and etiology. Radiographs of the affected spine are commonly the initial step. Subsequent imaging includes magnetic resonance imaging (MRI) and/or computed tomography (CT) with or without contrast enhancement. CT is well known to visualize osseous structures more prominently than MRI, but MRI is best when soft tissue involvement in the pathological process is of concern. In addition, MRI will best detect the nature and extent of neurologic injury, such as spinal cord compression, nerve root impingement, or other localized compressive pathology, when it is suspected. Location of the level of the fracture is critical and determines whether VP can be done under fluoroscopic guidance or CT guidance, if at all. The morphology of the fracture is very important to understand, as not all fractures may be repaired using VP. Burst fractures are common after axial load injury. They result in multidirectional fragmentation of the vertebral body and will often lead to breach of the posterior cortex of the vertebral body, retropulsion, and spinal canal compromise. Last, other pathology related to the fracture that requires strong consideration includes, but is not limited to, hematoma, infection/abscess, hemangiomas, advanced disk disease, unstable spondylolisthesis with canal compromise, and local or widespread malignancy.

Neuromonitoring, if not the standard of care, has become a widely accepted method for anticipating and mitigating neural injury in neurosurgery. Similarly, neuromonitoring is increasingly used in minimally invasive surgery, but it remains an option rather than a rule. The use of neuromonitoring for VP has not been a clear practice in the past, although it has gained some acceptance. However, the use neuromonitoring should not supplant the standard of proper technique and direct visualization, nor the mitigation of potential injury by the device or by PMMA cement extravasation.

Technique

VP is performed using sterile technique with the patient in the prone position and with image guidance. Most commonly, fluoroscopy is biplanar, using serial anterior-posterior (AP) and lateral visualization with one or two fluoroscopes. The *en face* approach is another technique: it uses an oblique angle, with direction visualization and trajectory of the pedicle shadow in a dorsolateral to ventromedial fashion. Also, because VP may be performed in a variety of settings from the office to the operating room, the choice of anesthesia and analgesia may vary, but the selection should be tailored to safety and the medical profile of the patient.

After preparation of the patient in the prone, padded position using sterile technique, the images are optimized. Classically, when using fluoroscopy for an interventional procedure, the superior endplate of the level is aligned. However, this is often not possible in the presence of VCF with superior endplate deformity. Therefore, when using the transpedicular technique, the physician should angle the imaging so as to identify the oval pedicle shadow and to maximize visualization of the medial and lateral borders of the pedicle. With the extrapedicular technique, the trajectory of the instrument should maintain the instrument lateral to the costovertebral angle and lateral to the medial aspect of the pedicle shadow; therefore, positioning for AP imaging for this technique will vary slightly from that for the transpedicular technique. The lateral view of the vertebral body should maximize the view of the inferior neuroforamen as well as the anterior borders of the vertebral body. As a rule of thumb, the AP view designates direction, and the lateral view designates depth, to maximize the safety of the procedure.

Once direct visualization is optimized, the patient's skin is anesthetized with an amide local anesthetic (e.g., lidocaine, bupivacaine) with or without epinephrine. The author includes epinephrine when it is not contraindicated to minimize local soft tissue bleeding and to maximize the duration of local anesthetic effect. An 11- or 15-blade scalpel is used to make an incision of 1 to 2 cm in the skin lateral to the pedicle shadow at the 1 to 3 o'clock position on the right or the 9 to 11 o'clock position on the left. The position of the incision is directly influenced by the trajectory needed to safely obtain access to the vertebral body inferior to a fractured superior endplate (or superior to a fractured inferior endplate). A 9 or 3 o'clock position affords a shallow approach to the endplate, while a 1 or 11 o'clock position facilitates a steeper approach.

The different trocar gauges vary by manufacturer. The size of the trocar and overlying cannula needed depends on the size of the vertebra and associated pedicle. A 10-gauge trocar is typical of most companies and most procedures. The tip of the trocar may have either one beveled surface to facilitate directionality of the tip or three or four bevels to facilitate access.

The tip of the trocar is inserted into the incision and is advanced until bony contact is made with the pedicle shadow. The tip is then "docked" into the bone to create stability. Guided by serial AP and lateral imaging views, the tip of the needle is advanced either by direct pressure or by mallet through the pedicle. As a rule, when the tip of the trocar is placed at the lateral edge of the pedicle shadow, then in the lateral view, the tip of the needle should be seen posteriorly (Figure 11.1). When the trocar is in the middle of the pedicle shadow in the AP view,

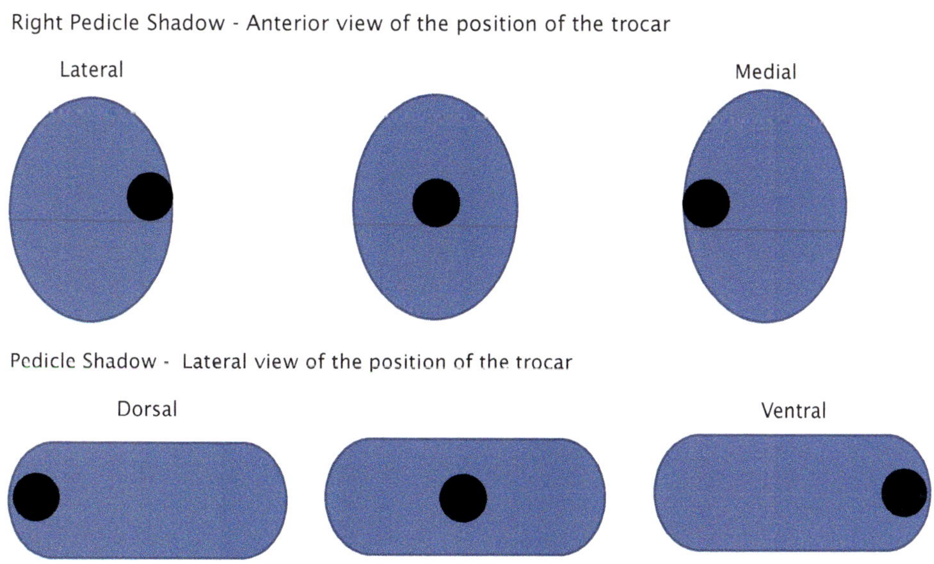

FIGURE 11.1. Position of the trocar needle in anterior and lateral views, transpedicular technique.

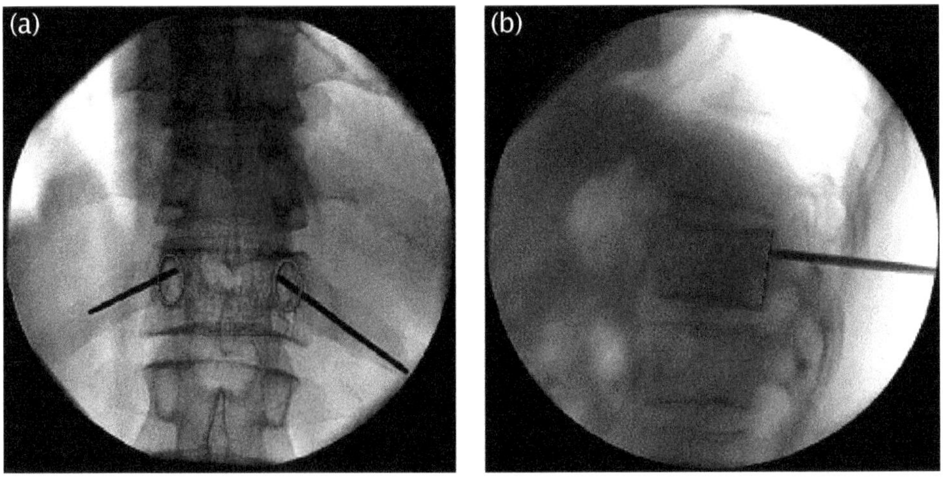

FIGURE 11.2. Position of trocar in the lateral view when trocar tip is most medial on the pedicle shadow. Adapted from Park J, Baek SJ, Baek SH, and Kim ED. Response to Transforaminal Epidural Block as a Useful Predictive Factor of Postherpetic Neuralgia. *Journal of Clinical Medicine.* 2019; 8(3):323.

then in the lateral view, the tip of the needle should be at the midpoint of the pedicle shadow. Subsequently, when the tip of the needle is at the most medial edge of the purple shadow in the AP view, then the tip of the trocar should be near the breach of the posterior wall of the vertebral body shadow. If the extrapedicular approach is taken, then the trocar tip will be seen first laterally at the midpoint of the pedicle shadow, culminating in tip placement most medially under AP view at the medial border of the pedicle shadow, with corresponding position at the posterior aspect of the vertebral body under lateral view (Figures 11.2).

Typically, the trocar is advanced slightly into the posterior aspect to the vertebral body enough that the corresponding cannula enters the posterior aspect of the vertebral body as well. The trocar is then removed, leaving the cannula in place. If a bone biopsy is required or chosen, then a bone biopsy needle is advanced through the cannula into the vertebral body proper, with core biopsy taken and sent to pathology for further evaluation. After biopsy, another device, such as a drill, is used to tunnel further into the midpoint or anterior third of the vertebral body shadow as seen on lateral view. Typically, it is at this point in the procedure that the polymethylmethacrylate (PMMA) bone cement is prepared. The timing of the chemical reaction needed to create doughy cement is important to understand. The more quickly the cement is used following mixture, the less viscous the substance will be. Conversely, waiting longer will produce a more viscous product as the cement transitions to hardening (Figure 11.3).

The PMMA bone cement can be delivered via a few different systems specific to the company selected. More importantly, during delivery of the cement, it is very important that the surgeon remain diligent in assessing spread of the bone cement so as to prevent extravasation dorsally through the pathway of the cannula, inferiorly toward the neuroforamen, or dorsally through fracture lines into the ventral epidural space or further. The amount of cement applied unilaterally varies and depends on the size of the vertebra as well as the extent of the fracture lines. Anywhere between 1 and 3 mL of cement is typical. Cement delivery

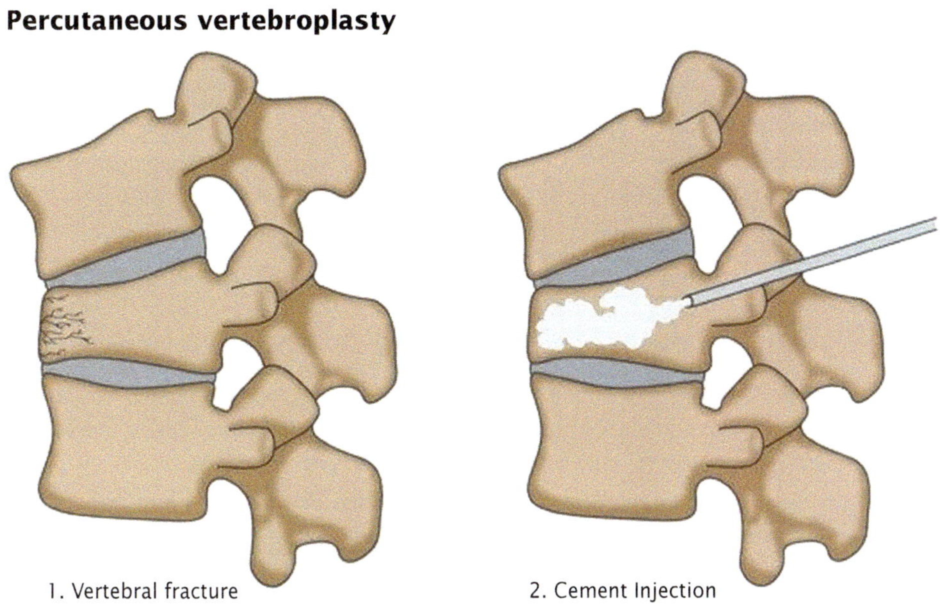

FIGURE 11.3. Transpedicular approach and cement delivery.

may be performed unilaterally or bilaterally, depending on the structure of the fracture as well as the extent of bilateral spread, if needed, upon unilateral delivery. When delivery of the cement is completed and satisfactory, then the delivery device is removed, and a trocar is placed in the cannula to displace any cement remaining in the cannula. Then, the trocar and cannula are withdrawn from the patient. Typically, the incision is then covered with Steri-Strips and a small occlusive bandage. Sometimes, the incision may need an absorbable suture rather than a Steri-Strip.

Postoperative Management and Follow-up

Postoperative care directs attention to wound healing and prevention of further fractures. While some surgeons may prescribe postoperative bracing for a limited time, the practice is specific to the surgeon and is not a standard of care. Postoperative care classically involves the patient's primary care provider or specialist, and the patient should be evaluated for pharmacological optimization, such as improvement of bone density in an osteoporotic patient.

Complications and Management

The complications of VP vary from critical or life-threatening to mild. Mild complications include, but are not limited to, bruising, bleeding, postoperative swelling, and pain. More serious complications include superficial and deep wound infection requiring culture and appropriate antibiotics. Direct trauma will most commonly present with immediate postoperative findings. Severe neurologic injury caused by compressive, noninfectious pathology may present immediately or over days. These severe complications require immediate specialty consultation with neurosurgery or orthopedic spine surgery. Trauma resulting in vascular injury may take time to develop or may be apparent immediately intraoperatively or postoperatively. Vascular injury is a surgical emergency if it involves the aorta, inferior vena cava, and their associated branches. An infectious pathology requiring urgent surgical consultation may develop over days to weeks. If neurologic effects linger, then long-term rehabilitation may be warranted.

Conclusion

VP is a safe, effective way to treat painful VCF. While many interventional providers are shifting to balloon kyphoplasty or other types of vertebral augmentation, VP provides a lower cost, less painful option that can be done quickly with local anesthesia only. With increasing diagnosis of osteoporosis in the aging population, this procedure provides an avenue for decreasing morbidity and mortality from VCF.

References

1. Wright NC, Looker AC, Saag KG, et al. The recent prevalence of osteoporosis and low bone mass in the United States based on bone mineral density at the femoral neck or lumbar spine. *J Bone Miner Res.* 2014;29(11):2520–2526. doi:10.1002/jbmr.2269.
2. Heaney R. Pathophysiology of osteoporosis. *Endocrinol Metab Clin North Am.* 1998;27:255–265.
3. Genant HK, Cooper C, Poor G, et al. Interim report and recommendations of the World Health Organization Task-Force for Osteoporosis. *Osteoporos Int.* 1999;10(4):259–264. doi:10.1007/s001980050224. PMID:10692972.
4. McCarthy J, Davis A. Diagnosis and management of vertebral compression fractures. *Am Fam Physician.* 2016;94(1):44–50. PMID:27386723.
5. Kado DM, Browner WS, Palermo L, Nevitt MC, Genant HK, Cummings SR. Study of Osteoporotic Fractures Research Group. Vertebral fractures and mortality in older women: a prospective study. *Arch Intern Med.* 1999;159(11):1215–1220.
6. Cosman F, de Beur SJ, LeBoff MS, et al. National Osteoporosis Foundation. Clinician's guide to prevention and treatment of osteoporosis. *Osteoporosis Int.* 2014;25(10):2359–2381. Correction in Osteoporosis Int. 2015;26(7):2045–2047.
7. National Osteoporosis Foundation. 2023. www.nof.org.
8. Jay B, Ahn SH. Vertebroplasty. *Semin Intervent Radiol.* 2013;30(3):297–306. doi:10.1055/s-0033-1353483
9. McGraw J, Cardella J, Barr J, et al. Society of Interventional Radiology quality improvement guidelines for percutaneous vertebroplasty. *J Vasc Intervent Radiol.* 2003;14:827–831.
10. Hirsch JA, Chandra RV, Carter NS, Beall D, Frohbergh M, Ong K. Number needed to treat with vertebral augmentation to save a life. *AJNR Am J Neuroradiol.* 2020;41(1):178–182. doi:10.3174/ajnr.A6367. PMID:31857326; PMCID:PMC6975314.
11. Sanli I, van Kuijk SMJ, de Bie RA, van Rhijn LW, Willems PC. Percutaneous cement augmentation in the treatment of osteoporotic vertebral fractures (OVFs) in the elderly: a systematic review. *Eur Spine J.* 2020;29(7):1553–1572. doi:10.1007/s00586-020-06391-x. PMID: 32240375.
12. Clark W, Bird P, Gonski P, et al. Safety and efficacy of vertebroplasty for acute painful osteoporotic fractures (VAPOUR): a multicentre, randomised, double-blind, placebo-controlled trial. *Lancet.* 2016;388(10052):1408–1416. doi:10.1016/S0140-6736(16)31341-1. Erratum in *Lancet.* 2017;389(10069):602. PMID:27544377.
13. Hinde K, Maingard J, Hirsch JA, Phan K, Asadi H, Chandra RV. Mortality outcomes of vertebral augmentation (vertebroplasty and/or balloon kyphoplasty) for osteoporotic vertebral compression fractures: a

systematic review and meta-analysis. *Radiology*. 2020;295(1):96–103. doi:10.1148/radiol.2020191294. PMID:32068503.

14. Wang B, Zhao CP, Song LX, Zhu L. Balloon kyphoplasty versus percutaneous vertebroplasty for osteoporotic vertebral compression fracture: a meta-analysis and systematic review. *J Orthop Surg Res*. 2018;13 (1):264. doi:10.1186/s13018-018-0952-5. PMID:30348192; PMCID:PMC6196425.
15. Mangram AJ, Horan TC, Pearson ML, Silver LC, Jarvis WR. Guideline for prevention of surgical site infection, 1999. Centers for Disease Control and Prevention (CDC) Hospital Infection Control Practices Advisory Committee. *Am J Infect Control*. 1999;27(2):97–132. PMID:10196487.
16. Narouze S, Benzon H, Provenzano D, et al. Interventional spine and pain procedures in patients on antiplatelet and anticoagulant medications (second edition): guidelines from the American Society of Regional Anesthesia and Pain Medicine, the European Society of Regional Anaesthesia and Pain Therapy, the American Academy of Pain Medicine, the International Neuromodulation Society, the North American Neuromodulation Society, and the World Institute of Pain. *Reg Anesth Pain Med*. 2018;43(3):225–262. doi:10.1097/AAP.0000000000000700.

12

Vertebral Augmentation

Vinicius Tieppo Francio, Hemant Kalia, and
Alexander Escobar

Introduction

For decades, the treatment of osteoporotic vertebral compression fractures (VCFs) has focused on pain management, without reduction, fixation, and restoration of the treated vertebrae, yet these basic orthopedic principles for the management of fractures aim to optimize healing and to correct the compression deformity. This chapter focuses on two specific vertebral augmentation techniques in the treatment of vertebral fractures (VFs), percutaneous balloon kyphoplasty (BKP) and titanium implantable vertebral augmentation devices (TIVAD).

Vertebral augmentation techniques first became popular in the late 1990s and early 2000s. BKP, which was first introduced in 1998,[1–2] was designed to reduce pain, to improve function, and to decrease the incidence of cement leakage during the injection, which is not usually symptomatic but is a complication of other vertebral augmentation techniques.[2–5] BKP is a minimally invasive fluoroscopy-guided intervention that uses an inflatable balloon to create a cavity within the vertebral body for injection of the bone cement, usually polymethylmethacrylate (PMMA), into a fractured vertebral body, with the goal of restoration of the vertebral body height.[6]

BKP differs from percutaneous vertebroplasty (VP), which does not use a balloon to create a cavity within the vertebral body and involves direct injection of cement percutaneously via a large-bore access needle under fluoroscopy guidance. BKP is the most widely used modification of vertebral augmentation technique and was developed specifically for use in osteoporotic VFs.[2] The general goals are pain relief and improvement of quality of life and musculoskeletal function secondary to VFs, restoration of vertebral stiffness and load sharing toward normal values, and prevention of refractures long term.[7–8] Mechanical vertebral body stabilization is a very important aspect specifically relevant to vertebral augmentation, which has been shown to restore the vertebral stiffness of fractured bodies to prefracture levels, with a resultant reduction in axial mechanical pain and pressure.[6] Recently, the revolutionary new method, TIVAD, which addresses the key principles of fixation and restoration of vertebral body height, has gained approval and clearance from the Federal Drug Administration (FDA). TIVAD is now commercially available in the United States and Europe, and two biomechanical studies discussed the use of TIVAD in VFs.[9–10]

Nowadays, there are multiple treatment options for patients with VFs, particularly osteoporotic fractures. The management options range from conservative nonsurgical treatment (NST), such as oral analgesics, bed rest, physical support, therapy, opioids, gabapentin, and bisphosphonates, all the way to minimally invasive interventions, such as percutaneous VP, BKP, and TIVAD. Although the majority of VFs may be managed with NST, a subset (~ 40%) with significant vertebral height loss, mechanical disruption, and uncontrollable pain warrant vertebral augmentation.[11] Not only do VFs create a heavy burden on those suffering from them, they also create a significant financial burden: in the United States, healthcare costs for VFs are over $1 billion dollars annually.[12] This chapter discusses the most up-to-date indications, evidence, and procedural techniques for BKP and TIVAD in the management of VFs.

Indications

In short, vertebral augmentation using specific FDA-approved devices is considered medically necessary for the treatment of symptomatic thoracolumbar osteoporotic VFs that have failed to respond to at least 6 weeks of conservative NST, and for the treatment of severe pain due to osteolytic lesions of the spine related to multiple myeloma or metastatic malignancy. However, conflicting data from medical subspecialties, medical societies, insurance companies, and governmental agencies regarding the indications for vertebral augmentation and appropriate management of VFs make the approaches not as straightforward as would be ideal.

The Centers for Medicare and Medicaid Services[13] endorses specific patient selection for the use of vertebral augmentation for painful VFs associated with osteoporosis and osteolytic destruction; however, the Official Disability Guidelines[14] advocate that vertebral augmentation is not recommended for osteoporotic VFs, but may be an option for osteolytic VFs. Hirsch et al aimed to bridge this gap: in a unique and important publication, they provided an evidence-based clinical care pathway for VFs developed by a multidisciplinary panel.[15]

More recent reviews on vertebral augmentation have discussed practice parameters and have suggested three main indications for vertebral augmentation:

1. Painful osteoporotic VFs or VFs refractory to medical therapy
2. VFs secondary to neoplasm
3. Symptomatic vertebral body microfractures documented by nuclear imaging but without loss of vertebral height

All the above indications must be associated with symptomatic back pain, vertebral body injury, and failed conservative management.[6,16–17] It is important to understand these indications, but it is most important to understand specific aspects of the indications, such as when the medical therapy and NST failed and the appropriate time to consider vertebral augmentation. Patients experiencing failure of medical therapy/conservative treatment are classified as:

1. Patients experiencing severe VF-related pain that persists and prevents ambulation for more than 24 to 48 hours, despite aggressive analgesic therapy
2. Patients with significant pain from VF persisting at that level, with no response to bed rest, bracing, analgesic therapy, and physical therapy
3. Patients with VF and unacceptable side effects from the analgesic therapy necessary to reduce pain to a tolerable level.[16]

Therefore, although some guidelines suggest NST trial for at least 6 weeks prior to consideration of vertebral augmentation, this is only a recommendation; to make a treatment decision, it is imperative to consider numerous clinical factors, such as the patient's ambulatory status, the patient's ability to tolerate therapy and NST while suffering from a painful VF, the adverse effects of potent analgesics, and the probability of adjacent fracture or worsening refracture.

Documentation requirements for proper insurance coverage include a relevant history, physical examination, and recent radiological evidence of painful osteolytic lesions of the spine related to multiple myeloma or metastasis or acute painful osteoporotic fractures that have failed to respond to at least 6 weeks of conservative treatment.[13–15]

In summary, vertebral augmentation is approved for, and is covered by medical insurance for, patients with the following:

- Inclusion criteria (all are required):
  - Acute (< 6 weeks) painful osteoporotic VFs (from T5 to L5) confirmed by recent (within 30 days) advanced imaging (MRI/CT scan)
  - Symptomatic VFs
    - In hospitalized patients with severe pain (pain scale > 8)
    - In nonhospitalized patients with moderate to severe pain (pain scale > 5) despite optimal NST, with the following:
      - Worsening pain
      - Kyphotic deformity
      - Loss of > 25% vertebral body height
      - Severe impact of VFs on daily musculoskeletal function (measured by disability index)

Evidence

BKP

The evidence regarding the use of vertebral augmentation, such as percutaneous VP and BKP, in VFs has been controversial since the intervention's conception in the late 1990s and early 2000s, yet most anecdotal data and published studies at that time seemed to show positive benefits from the treatments.[18–19] In 2009, two randomized controlled trials (RCT) suggested that vertebral augmentation techniques did not confer any benefit over active sham.[20–21] However, at the same time, data from larger observational studies and open-label RCTs comparing vertebral augmentation with NST were highly positive and supported the use of percutaneous VP and BKP for VFs.[22–23] Since then, multiple societies, insurance companies, governmental agencies, and practice guidelines have gone back and forth on the management of VFs with VP and/or BKP, and the landscape continues to change.

In 2016, the first sham/placebo-controlled RCT of vertebral augmentation for the management of VFs was performed and demonstrated positive results. In this study, the sham intervention was a subcutaneous injection of local anesthetic.[24] In contrast, 2 years later, a RCT with sham versus VP failed to show benefit of vertebral augmentation, due to the high level of pain relief seen in the active sham arm.[25]

Recently, in research assessing mortality risk, survival benefits with vertebral augmentation for VFs have been the focus, and studies point out that the use of BKP conferred a > 50% 1-year mortality benefit and reduced the 10-year mortality by up to 24% compared to NST.[26] On the basis of this information, in 2019 Hirsch et al calculated the number needed to treat (NNT) to save 1 life at 1 and 5 years for VFs treated with vertebral augmentation and found that both vertebral augmentation modalities (VP and BKP) conferred a prominent mortality benefit over NST with a low NNT. The adjusted NNT to save 1 life for NST versus BKP ranged from 14.8 at 1 year to 11.9 at 5 years. The adjusted NNT for NST versus VP ranged from 22.8 at 1 year to 23.8 at 5 years.[27] These claims-based study data demonstrated a relative mortality advantage of BKP over percutaneous VP versus NST and revealed that only 15 patients need to be treated to save 1 life. This is an obvious clinically impactful and statistically significant finding that vertebral augmentation treatment for VFs provides a powerful mortality benefit over NST with a low NNT.[27] These data are especially important when considering the burden on the United States healthcare system caused by VFs, which cost the industry over $1 billion annually.[11] Not only are BKP and VP safe and effective, but also these interventions, when properly used, can lower the healthcare cost of VFs, with a low NNT to save lives.

The evidence on BKP specifically has shown that balloon-augmented vertebral bodies have preserved height more readily, and the preservation of sagittal alignment and vertebral body height has been shown to have contributed to palliation of pain, improvement in function, and perhaps even the mortality advantage of BKP.[24–27] BKP has been shown to significantly decrease the kyphotic wedge angle, to increase the postoperative vertebral body height, and to decrease the risk of cement leakage, in contrast to VP.[28] Furthermore, BKP was found to result in the greatest reduction of refractures at the initial level, while also reducing the risk of subsequent adjacent-level fracture, when compared to VP.[7] Yuan et al performed a meta-analysis to evaluate which intervention (NST, BKP, or VP) yielded better pain relief. It was found that both VP and BKP resulted in more pain relief and better quality of life (QoL) than NST, with perhaps a slightly better acute pain relief with VP than with BKP.[29] Yet, more recent studies have demonstrated that when pain was measured using the Visual Analog Scale (VAS), pain reduction was comparable among all procedures, including VP, BKP, and vertebral body stents.[7,28,30] Studies have shown that VP has the highest probability of being the most effective for acute pain reduction and improvements of function, as measured by the Oswestry Disability Index (ODI) and the Roland Morris Disability Questionnaire (RMDQ).

In contrast, BKP has been consistently shown to have the highest probability of improving function and QoL as measured by the Short-Form 36 (SF-36) and of reducing the risk of subsequent/adjacent VFs and refractures at the treated level.[7] Nevertheless, a Cochrane meta-analysis of high-quality RCTs suggested that there is no role for VP in treating acute or subacute VFs in routine practice, with no demonstrable clinically important benefits compared with placebo (sham procedure).[31] However, the review was current to 2017 data, and since then at least a handful of high-quality meta-analyses have been published that contest these data. In 2018, a meta-analysis of multiple level I and level II studies revealed that BKP resulted in significantly better pain reduction, disability scores, and vertebral body height restoration than percutaneous VP.[30] In 2020, a comprehensive review of the literature discussed the concept of vertebral augmentation in the management of VFs and favored the use of BKP. The summary of the data reviewed showed that analysis of level I and II studies favored BKP and found BKP to be significantly better in pain reduction than VP and nonsurgical management, and BKP tended to yield better height restoration than VP.[32]

Since the 2009 sham trials published in the *New England Journal of Medicine*, more than 250 publications dedicated to vertebral augmentation have been produced annually. The role of vertebral augmentation in the management of VF has been supported by multiple RCTs,[33–37] meta-analyses,[38–39] and registry outcomes; however, the literature regarding vertebral augmentation in the management of VFs does not provide consistent guidance, remains controversial, and exhibits reporting bias. Therefore, formulating clinical care pathways for the optimal management of VFs is essential to establish a recognized pattern of efficacious procedural outcomes in vertebral augmentation, independent of the site, proceduralist bias, and other possible confounders, therefore allowing for heterogeneity in the treatment of VFs with augmentation. The studies of Hirsch et al and Shonnard et al used consistent data collection that allowed a highly sensitive analysis, which revealed that vertebral augmentation for VFs resulted in significant improvements in pain and function scores, demonstrating real-world outcomes and meaningful clinical impact.[15,27,40]

A 2017 study revealed that BKP was associated with greater pain relief, fewer back-related disabilities, and better QoL,[41] and a multicenter, prospective, single-arm study[42] concluded that activities of daily living (ADLs), QoL, and vertebral deformity showed greater improvement with BKP for acute VFs with poor prognostic factors at 6 months after injury, reinforcing the importance of early intervention to improve outcomes. The study suggested a strategy for BKP intervention early on, according to the presence or absence of poor prognostic MRI findings, such as high-intensity or diffuse low-intensity areas in the VFs on T2 images, which are predictive of delayed union.

Overall, the evidence suggests that BKP is a safe and effective procedure, with level I evidence suggesting its use when proper criteria are met. Since VFs have been associated with increased morbidity and mortality, and considering the abundance of high-quality information, multiple medical societies favor and confidently advocate the use of BKP to improve spinal mechanics, pain, function, and QoL in patients with VFs.

TIVAD

TIVAD (commercially known as SpineJack™) has been demonstrated to yield superior sagittal middle vertebral height restoration and preservation in comparison to BKP. Current level I evidence demonstrates TIVAD's non-inferiority to BKP. The 12-month prospective randomized SAKOS study, which directly compared TIVAD and BKP, established the clinical safety and efficacy of TIVAD and, interestingly, found a decreased incidence of adjacent-segment fractures in the TIVAD group compared to the BKP group. The BKP group's rate of adjacent fractures was more than double (27.3% vs. 12.9%) and its rate of nonadjacent fractures nearly three times higher (21.9% vs. 7.4%) than the rates in the TIVAD group. The need for oral pain medications on postoperative day 5 was also greatly reduced in the TIVAD group compared to the BKP group (7.4% and 21.9%, respectively).[9–10]

Presently there is no consensus about which vertebral augmentation approach is best for treating VFs. The decision to choose one vertebral augmentation system over another is physician dependent, with similar outcomes of improved QoL, functionality, and pain relief. However, the SAKOS study made clear that TIVAD not only is a practical option, but also may be the preferred treatment when clinical conditions are met.[10] In our practice, when treating VFs close to thoracolumbar junction, middle vertebral body height loss is > 30%, and or there is evidence of retropulsion, TIVAD is considered first.

Patient Selection

Proper patient selection is perhaps the most important factor in predicting a successful vertebral augmentation procedure, along with correct technique and an individualized therapeutic strategy. Most guidelines[6,13–14] require all the following patient selection criteria for BKP surgery:

1. Presence of severe pain and functional deficits due to the VF
2. Lack of satisfactory improvement with NST
3. Absence of alternative causes for pain, such as discitis or disk herniation
4. At least one-third loss of vertebral height
5. Fracture age not exceeding 3 months

Contraindications

If there is a clear discrepancy between clinical presentation, physical exam findings, and radiological findings (lack of bone marrow edema on MRI that would suggest a subacute or chronic fracture), vertebral augmentation should be reconsidered, and a clear discussion with the patient about expectations should be held.[43] Generally, based on most clinical guidelines, contraindications to BKP can be classified as absolute and relative. (Numerous case reports have appeared in the literature regarding adverse events related to vertebral augmentation, and it is beyond the scope of this section to report each individual adverse event; however, general complications and postoperative management are discussed later in this chapter.) Most subspecialty society guidelines report the absolute contraindications as including, but not being limited to:

- Allergy to bone cement or opacification agent
- Uncontrollable coagulopathy (INR > 1.2, platelets less than 100,000)
- Active vertebral body/spinal infection with or without discitis
- Spinal cord compression
- Complete or significant posterior vertebral body collapse (which could increase the risk of cement leakage into the spinal canal)
- Loss of posterior vertebral wall integrity
- Pregnancy
- Spinal tumor
- Septicemia/systemic infection
- Healed fracture, old fracture, nonpainful lesion

Relative contraindications[6,16–17,44–46] include, but again are not limited to:

- Retropulsion of vertebral body fragments
- Posterior vertebral body cortical breach
- Epidural tumor expansion with significant central canal encroachment
- Active neurologic symptoms unrelated to vertebral body fracture

Perioperative Management

Initial Consultation

Once a patient has been identified as a good candidate for vertebral augmentation, an initial consultation should be arranged, preferably to occur in the presence of interested family members. Involvement of family members in the patient's care is particularly important for elderly and debilitated patients. Alternatively, with patients who are unable to have a face-to-face meeting for any identified reason (COVID19 pandemic, long distance from the facility, etc.), an appropriate telemedicine platform should be utilized for the initial consultation. The initial consultation not only is helpful for evaluating the premorbid status of a patient but also helps to screen for anticoagulant medications, allergies, and history of obstructive sleep apnea or other medical comorbidities that could affect procedural outcomes. Advanced imaging like MRI should be performed prior to the consultation. If MRI is contraindicated, a bone scan can be utilized to distinguish between acute/subacute and chronic compression fracture.

This consultation also provides an opportunity to discuss how the procedure is performed at your institution and to review your specific protocols in preparation for the procedure.

Preoperative Evaluation and Perioperative Optimization

Evaluation should be individualized to the patient. It generally starts with a thorough history and physical examination. Risk stratification tools can be utilized to assess morbidity and mortality risk. Complete blood count, prothrombin time/partial thromboplastin time, INR or activated clotting time, and platelet count should be obtained before vertebral augmentation. If intraosseous venography is considered, blood urea nitrogen and creatinine levels should also be tested.

Vertebral augmentation can be performed under local anesthesia with monitored anesthesia care (MAC). Intraoperative standard monitoring, including electrocardiogram, noninvasive blood pressure, pulse oximetry, and expired carbon dioxide monitoring via nasal cannula, is sufficient in most cases. Blood pressure should be monitored at short intervals (every 2 minutes) during cement injection. Bradycardia, loss of consciousness, and hypertension can be signs of fat or PMMA embolism.

Technique

Transpedicular Approach

Percutaneous access to lumbar and lower thoracic vertebrae can be successfully achieved by the bilateral transpedicular approach, perhaps the most commonly used method.[47–49] The transpedicular approach is a standard and safe approach that protects postganglionic nerve roots and that can be achieved by bilateral needle insertion and deployment of two balloons for adequate cement fill.[47–48]

In the transpedicular approach, the upper thoracic spine can be a bit challenging for perfect midline access and deployment of balloons due to costochondral junctions and the presence of ribs within the trajectory. Lack of medial placement of balloons or instruments may compromise adequate fracture reduction and lead to lateral cortex violation before fracture reduction is achieved.

It is important to visualize the entire path of the working channel from the skin insertion point, through the pedicle within two-thirds of the vertebral body and ending at the midline.

Once appropriate imaging is confirmed, an incision is made 1 cm superior and 2 cm lateral to the entry point on the pedicle. The authors routinely use this approach for access, but some interventionalists may prefer the "bull's eye" approach straight down the barrel through the pedicle; this view can be obtained after about 10° to 30° of ipsilateral oblique angulation from the true AP orientation (Figure 12.1). It is important to reinforce here that the AP view is utilized to guide medial and lateral corrections and the lateral view is used for superior and inferior correction.

The landmarks, including pedicles, spinous process, and endplates, should be clearly visualized in true AP and lateral images (Figure 12.2). A Jamshidi needle is introduced and "docked" at the superolateral border of the pedicle (10 o'clock position on the left and 2 o'clock position on the right). A lateral view can be obtained to visualize the trajectory and to confirm that the needle tip is at the posterior margin of the pedicle. A mallet should

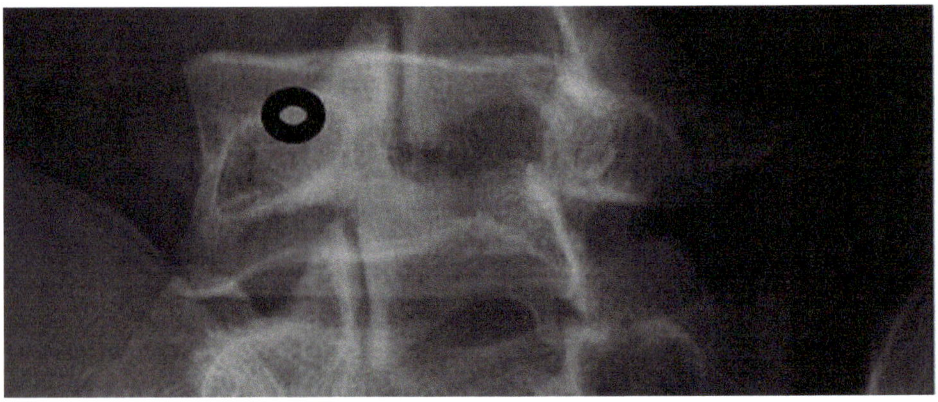

FIGURE 12.1. Transpedicular access: ipsilateral 20° oblique "bull's eye" view of the upper outer quadrant of pedicle.

Image courtesy of Hemant Kalia, MD, MPH.

be used to gently tap in the needle through the pedicle. It is critical to respect the medial border of the pedicle: the medial border of the pedicle should never be breached in the AP view until the tip of the needle is either at or past the posterior border of the vertebral body in the lateral view. Once it is in the posterior vertebral body, the needle is advanced approximately 0.5 to 1.0 cm toward the midline, and then a drill or biopsy needle is passed to reach approximately 0.3 to 0.5 cm from the anterior cortex of the vertebral body. A balloon is inserted through each tract created by the drill bilaterally, and each balloon is inflated while both AP and lateral views are scrutinized, manometric pressures are monitored, and the balloons are inflated to desired pressure in small increments (Figure 12.3).The end point is achieved when any of the following is true: contact of cortical wall, adequate creation of cavity, fracture reduction, or maximum volume of inflation. Height restoration can be

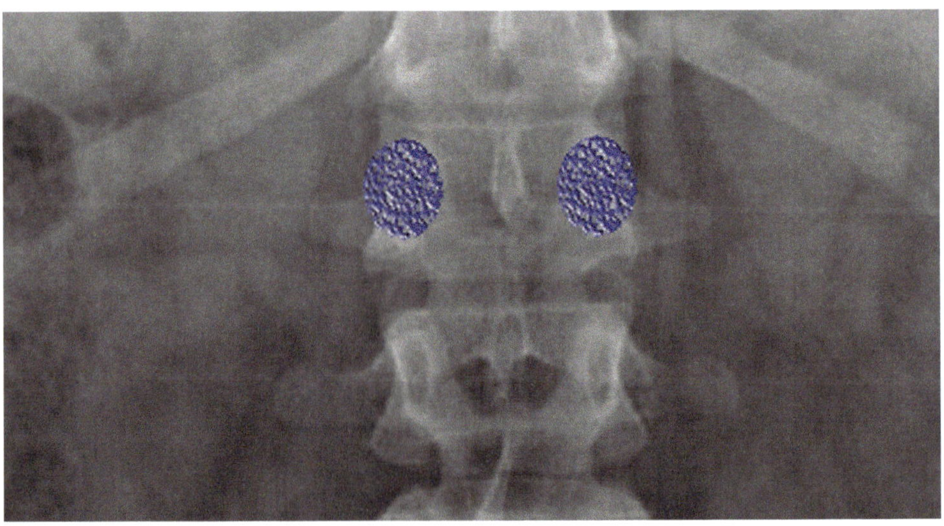

FIGURE 12.2. True AP view: Spinous process bisecting the pedicles (blue) with squared off endplates.

Image courtesy of Hemant Kalia, MD, MPH.

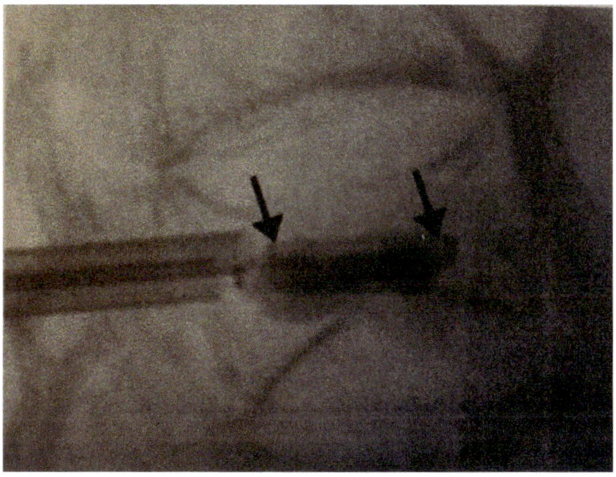

FIGURE 12.3. Balloon kyphoplasty.
Image courtesy of Hemant Kalia, MD, MPH.

attempted safely after the void has been created in the vertebral body. Internal fixation is achieved with injection of cement into the void created by the balloons (Figure 12.4).Once there is adequate interdigitation of cement into the cancellous bone, the working cannulas can be removed safely.[47–49]

The TIVAD third-generation vertebral augmentation system uses percutaneous bipedicular access similar to that just described, followed by a series of cannulated steps and insertion of bilateral expandable titanium implants that come in three sizes—4.2 mm, 5.0 mm, and 5.8 mm—prior to filling of the cavity with bone cement. Implant size pertains to the width of the instrumented pedicle; thus, it requires careful measurements, and it is recommended that 0.8 mm be added to the implant size for appropriate device selection (i.e., a minimum 5.0-mm pedicle width would require a 5.8-mm implant; Figures 12.5 and 12.6).[9–10]

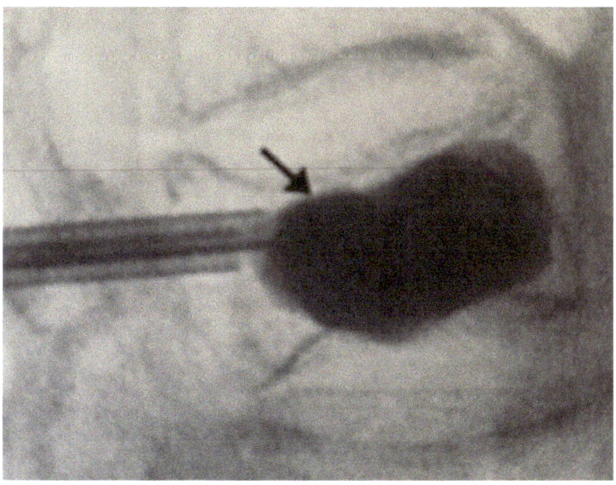

FIGURE 12.4. Balloon kyphoplasty: height restoration.
Image courtesy of Hemant Kalia, MD, MPH.

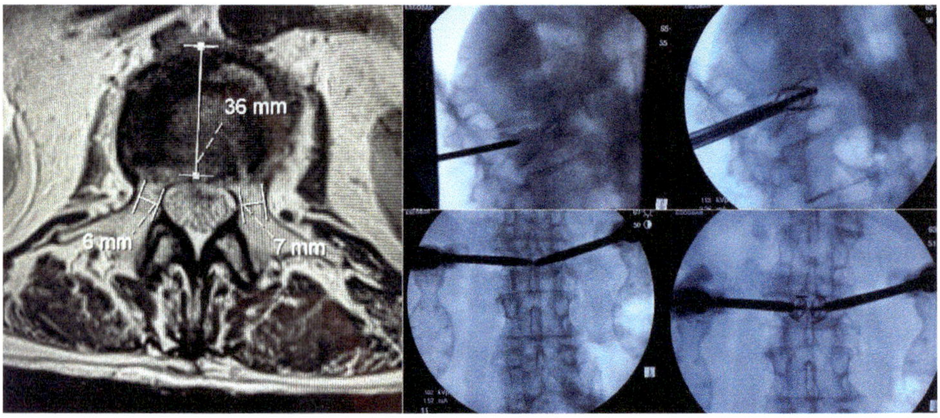

FIGURE 12.5. Sizing pertains to the width of the instrumented pedicle. Thus, it requires careful measurements, and it is recommended that 0.8 mm be added to the implant size for appropriate device selection.

Image courtesy of Alex Escobar, MD.

Parapedicular Approach

The transpedicular approach is standard for most of the lumbar and lower thoracic vertebrae, but it can be really challenging in the upper thoracic spine, where the reduced pedicle width and corresponding ribs preclude a transpedicular approach. The parapedicular approach used in the upper thoracic spine is also known as the transcostovertebral approach.[47] The needle trajectory is lateral to the pedicle instead of through it, thereby allowing for ipsilateral access to the center of the vertebral body. The risk of pedicle fracture is significantly reduced in this approach because the size of the needle or working cannula is not limited by the size or shape of the pedicle. This approach is also preferable for deploying devices into the vertebral body for augmentation. Chiras et al reported complication rates between 2.5% and 10% for the parapedicular approach in patients with benign and malignant spinal tumors.[49] In 2007, Beall et al published their seminal account of a safe and effective parapedicular technique that could reliably guide the needle tip in the center of

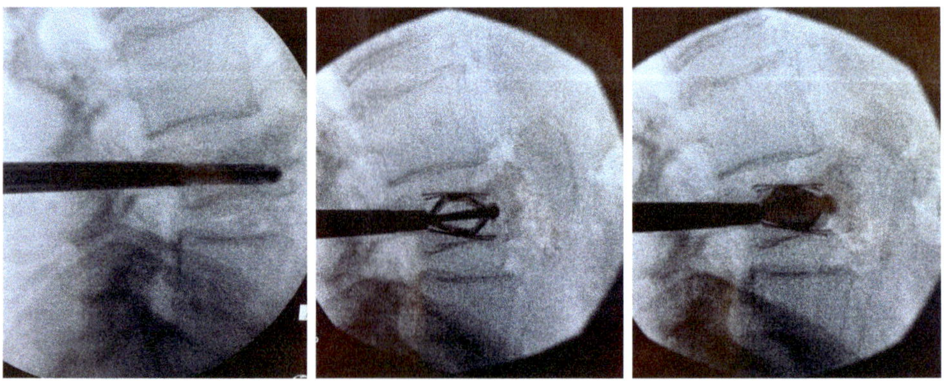

FIGURE 12.6. Fluoroscopy sequenced image: before deployment, after deployment, and TIVAD deployed with PMMA.

Image courtesy of Alex Escobar, MD.

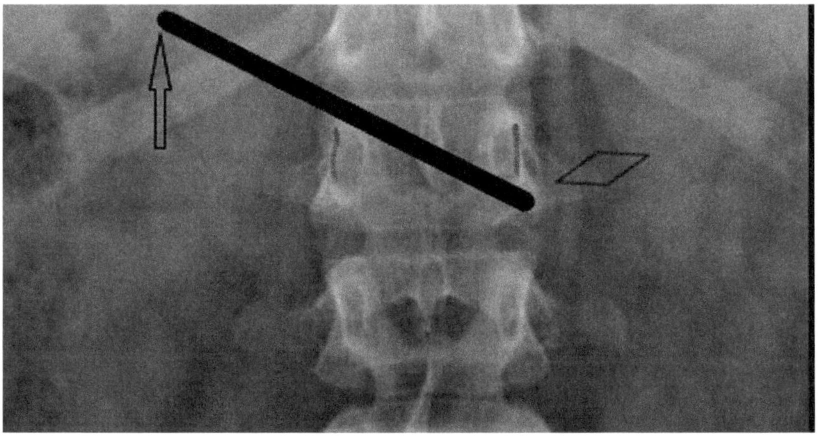

FIGURE 12.7. Parapedicular approach: AP view of L1 body, with a black line drawn from the contralateral inferior corner (diamond arrow) to the ipsilateral superior corner. The line extends the width of one vertebral body (distance between the blue lines) superior and lateral to a point of access in the skin (arrow).
Image courtesy of Hemant Kalia, MD, MPH.

the vertebrae.[50] Their approach starts with a line drawn between the ipsilateral superior corner and the contralateral inferior corner of the vertebral body. This line is extended superolaterally to identify a point that is approximately one vertebral body width beyond the lateral aspect of the vertebral body (Figure 12.7). An incision is made, and the needle is advanced at a 45° angle inferiorly toward the vertebral body. The needle should not breach the medial border of the pedicle in the AP view until the needle has crossed the posterior cortical wall in the lateral view (Figures 12.8 and 12.9).

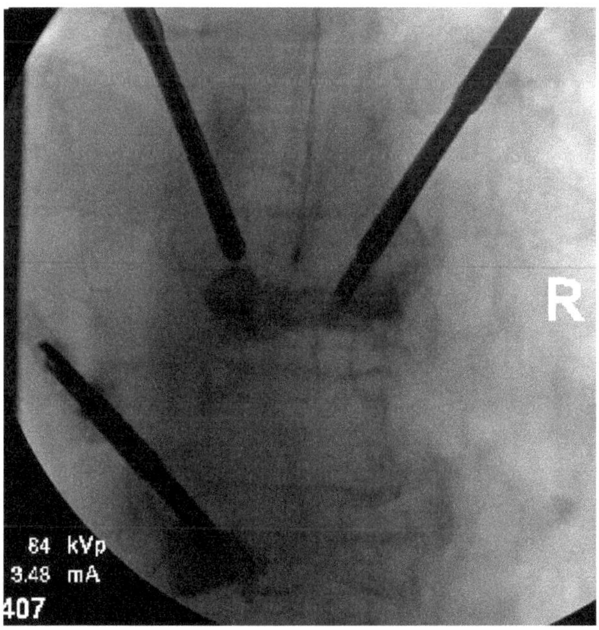

FIGURE 12.8. Parapedicular approach.
Image courtesy of Hemant Kalia, MD, MPH.

Extrapedicular Approach

Beall et al described a modified inferior endplate extrapedicular approach that is safe and effective and that is an ideal approach when access to the vertebral body is needed for devices that are larger than the size of the pedicle or in cases where there is significant compression of the superior endplate beyond the transverse pedicle line. The extrapedicular technique also allows for vertebral body access with preexisting spinal hardware. A total of 96 thoracic and lumbar VFs were treated using the extrapedicular modified inferior endplate approach without any significant complications.[51]

The technique described by Beall et al starts with the AP fluoroscope angle 45° off midline for the lumbar spine or 30° off midline for the thoracic spine to yield an oblique view (Figure 12.10). An incision is made anterior to the pedicle, just above the inferior endplate. The needle is inserted into the bone and subsequently docked. An AP view is obtained to confirm the lateral and medial location of the needle tip. A lateral view is obtained, and the needle is advanced between the middle to anterior third of the vertebral body. The needle should not breach the pedicle on the oblique view, to prevent injury to the descending ventral rami.[51]

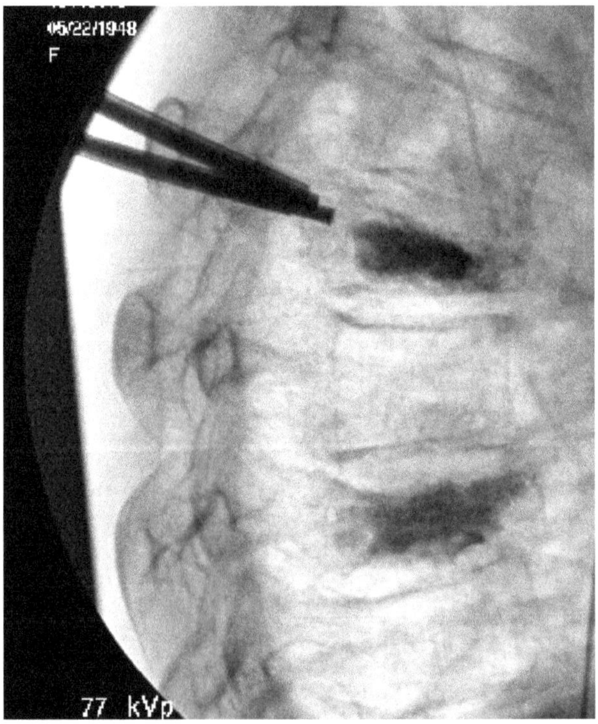

FIGURE 12.9. Parapedicular approach.
Image courtesy of Hemant Kalia, MD, MPH.

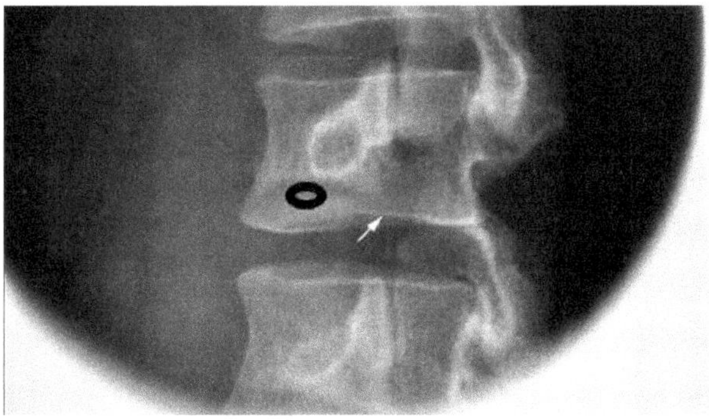

FIGURE 12.10. Extrapedicular approach: 45° oblique view of the vertebral body with entry point just anterior to the pedicle and above the inferior endplate.

Image courtesy of Hemant Kalia, MD, MPH.

Postoperative Management and Follow-up

Vertebral augmentation is mostly performed as an outpatient procedure, and patients are discharged home following standard postanesthesia care. Patients are monitored for neurologic deficits after the procedure. Postprocedure ambulation must be supervised carefully. Patients are advised to refrain from activities that can lead to additional or adjacent-level fractures. These include axial loading activities (primarily lifting more than 20 pounds), running, jumping, and exertional activities, especially pushing or pulling heavy objects against resistance. Standard postoperative infection prevention strategies should be instituted (e.g., no swimming or hot tub, pool, or sauna use for a minimum of 48 hours after the procedure). Incisions should be kept clean and dry for at least 3 to 4 days after the procedure.

Postoperative management includes a three-pronged approach for treating nonhealing osteoporotic VCFs: (1) percutaneous fracture stabilization, (2) treatment of the underlying metabolic bone disorder, and (3) exercise training for appropriate and adaptive posture and body mechanics. This comprehensive rehabilitation-focused approach to nonhealing osteoporotic VCFs improves the overall long-term outcomes in most patients. Only 25% of patients with osteoporotic compression fractures are prescribed pharmacological agents within the first year of their diagnosis for the treatment of underlying bone disorder.[52] An integrative multidisciplinary clinic or program that incorporates all specialties, including but not limited to rehabilitation medicine, interventional spine, radiology, pain medicine, and/or spine surgery, will improve long-term outcomes in this patient population.

Complications and Management

Overall, vertebral augmentation techniques are considered safe, with relatively low complication rates, and numerous studies support the procedure's net benefit and clinical/safety profile. In 2018, a review of numerous studies and guidelines concluded that both TIVAD and BKP are safe, with no increased risk of posttreatment refractures or adjacent-level fractures.[46] Reported complications included:

- Superficial/deep tissue infection
- Bleeding
- Pneumothorax
- Rib fracture
- Cement leakage to surrounding tissues
- Cord compression from acute spinal stenosis due to cement leakage
- Nerve root injury
- Pulmonary embolism from cement leakage

Kurra et al. reviewed mortality rates after BKP and VP for symptomatic VFs and concluded that mortality rates were lower in the BKP group.[53]

Conclusion

Although most patients with acute and painful VFs may be managed with NST, a subset (~40%) of VFs with persistent back pain, loss of vertebral height, and marked impact on QoL and function may benefit from vertebral augmentation, especially considering the substantial increase in bone loss and musculoskeletal debility associated with nonambulatory status after the acute onset of VFs.

The prognosis is poor if vertebral augmentation is not performed earlier than 6 months after injury, a finding that advocates for vertebral augmentation intervention early on. Furthermore, vertebral augmentation treatment for VFs provides a powerful mortality benefit.

Vertebral augmentation procedures have been studied extensively and have been found to be clinically effective and safe for patients with acute and painful VFs. The results of multiple studies, including systematic reviews and randomized controlled trials, favor the use of vertebral augmentation techniques, including BKP and TIVAD to improve pain, therefore facilitating ambulatory status, improving quality of life, and relieving back disability in patients with VFs. Studies seem to favor BKP use for improving acute pain, relieving vertebral stiffness to restore mechanics, reducing subsequent VFs and refractures, and improving pain and quality of life long term, but TIVAD has demonstrated noninferiority and potentially fewer adjacent-segment fractures compared to BKP. Since VFs have been associated with increased morbidity and mortality, multiple guidelines and medical societies favor and confidently advocate the use of vertebral augmentation, including BKP and TIVAD, in the treatment of acute and painful VFs nonresponsive to NST.

References

1. Garfin SR, Yuan HA, Reiley MA. New technologies in spine: kyphoplasty versus vertebroplasty for the treatment of painful osteoporosis compression fractures. *Spine*. 2001;26(14):1511–1515.

2. Ruiz Santiago F, Santiago CA, Guzman Alvarez L, et al. Comparative review of vertebroplasty and kyphoplasty. *World J Radiol.* 2014;6(6):329–343.
3. Jensen ME, Evans AJ, Mathis JM, et al. Percutaneous polymethylmethacrylate vertebroplasty in the treatment of osteoporotic vertebral body compression fractures: technical aspect. *AJNR Am J Neurol.* 1997;18(10):1897–1904.
4. Deramond H, Depriester C, Galibert P, et al. Percutaneous vertebroplasty with polymethylmethacrylate. Technique, indications and results. *Radiol Clin North Am.* 1998; 36(3):533–546.
5. Phillips FM, Wetzel FT, Lieberman I, et al. An in vivo comparison of the potential for extravertebral cement leak after vertebroplasty and kyphoplasty. *Spine.* 2002;27(19):2173–2179.
6. Khan M, Kushchayev SV. Percutaneous vertebral body augmentations: the state of the art. *Neuroimag Clin North Am.* 2020;29:495–513.
7. Zhu RS, Kan SL, Ning GZ, et al. Which is the best treatment of osteoporotic vertebral compression fractures: balloon kyphoplasty, percutaneous vertebroplasty, or non-surgical treatment? A Bayesian network meta-analysis. *Osteoporosis Int.* 2019;30(2):287–298.
8. Luo J, Adams MA, Dolan P. Vertebroplasty and kyphoplasty can restore normal spine mechanics following osteoporotic fracture. *J Osteoporosis.* 2010;729257.
9. Noriega DC, Ramajo RH, Lite IS, et al. Safety and clinical performance of kyphoplasty and Spine Jack procedures in the treatment of osteoporotic vertebral compression fractures: a pilot, monocentric, investigator-initiated study. *Osteoporosis Int.* 2016;27(6):2047–2055.
10. Noriega DC, Marcia S, Theumann N, et al. A prospective, international, randomized, noninferiority study comparing an implantable titanium vertebral augmentation device versus balloon kyphoplasty in the reduction of vertebral compression fractures (SALOS study). *Spine J.* 2019;19(11):1782–1795.
11. Goldstein CL, Chutkan NB, Choma TJ, Orr RD. Management of the elderly with vertebral compression fractures. *Neurosurgery.* 2015;77(4):S33–S45.
12. Epstein N. A comparison of kyphoplasty, vertebroplasty, or non-surgical treatment of traumatic of traumatic/atraumatic osteoporotic vertebral compression fractures: a short review. *Surg Neurol Int.* 2019;10(54):1–5.
13. Centers for Medicare & Medicaid Services (CMS). https://www.cms.gov/medicare-coverage-database/details/technology-assessments-details.aspx?TAId=25&bc=AAAQAAAAAAAAAA%253D%253D&.
14. Official Disability Guidelines (ODG). http://www.odg-twc.com.
15. Hirsch JA, Beall DP, Chambers MR, et al. Management of vertebral fragility fractures: a clinical care pathway developed by a multidisciplinary panel using the RAND/UCLA Appropriateness Method. *Spine J.* 2018;18:2152–2161.
16. American College of Radiologists (ACR). https://www.acr.org/-/media/ACR/Files/Practice-Parameters/VerebralAug.pdf.
17. Spine Interventional Society (SIS). https://cdn.ymaws.com/www.spineintervention.org/resource/resmgr/patient_safety/safety_practices/safetypractices_module6_vert.pdf.
18. Burton A, Rhines LD, Mendel E. Vertebroplasty and kyphoplasty: a comprehensive review. *Neurosurg Focus.* 2005;18(3):1–9.
19. McCall T, Cole C, Dailey A. Vertebroplasty and kyphoplasty: a comparative review of efficacy and adverse events. *Curr Rev Musculoskeletal Med.* 2008;1(1):17–23.
20. Kallmes DF, Comstock BA, Heagerty PJ, et al. A randomized trial of vertebroplasty for osteoporotic spinal fractures. *N Engl J Med.* 2009;361:569–579.
21. Buchbinder R, Osborne RH, Ebeling PR, et al. A randomized trial of vertebroplasty for painful osteoporotic vertebral fractures. *N Engl J Med.* 2009;361:557–568.
22. Jha RM, Yoo AJ, Hirsch AE, et al. Predictors of successful palliation of compression fractures with vertebral augmentation: single center experience of 535 cases. *J Vasc Intervent Radiol.* 2009; 20:760–768.
23. Wardlaw D, Cumming SR, Van Meirhaeghe J, et al. Efficacy and safety of balloon kyphoplasty compared with non-surgical care for vertebral compression (FREE): a randomised controlled trial. *Lancet.* 2009;373:1016–1024.
24. Clark W, Bird P, Gonski P, et al. Safety and efficacy of vertebroplasty for acute painful osteoporotic fractures (VAPOUR): a multicentre, randomised, double-blind, placebo-controlled trial. *Lancet.* 2016;388:1408–1416.

25. Firanescu CE, Vries J, Lodder P, et al. Vertebroplasty versus sham procedure for painful acute osteoporotic vertebral compression fractures (VERTOS IV): a randomised sham controlled clinical trial. *BMJ*. 2018;361:1551.
26. Ong KL, Beall DP, Frohbergh M, et al. Were VCF patients at higher risk of mortality following the 2009 publication of the vertebroplasty sham trials? *Osteoporosis Int*. 2018;29:375–383.
27. Hirsch JA, Chandra RV, Beall D, et al. Number needed to treat with vertebral augmentation to save a life. *Am J Neuroradiol*. 2019;10:317.
28. Wang F, Wang LF, Miao DC, Dong Z, Shen Y. Which one is more effective for the treatment of very severe osteoporotic vertebral compression fractures: PVP or PKP? *J Pain Res*. 2018;11:2625–2631.
29. Yuan WH, Hsu HC, Lai KL. Vertebroplasty and balloon kyphoplasty versus conservative treatment for osteoporotic vertebral compression fractures: A meta-analysis. *Medicine (Baltimore)*. 2016;95(31):4491.
30. Beall D, Lorio MP, Yun BM, Runa MJ, Ong KL, Warner CB. Review of vertebral augmentation: an updated meta-analysis of the effectiveness. *Int J Spine Surg*. 2018;12(3):295–321.
31. Buchbinder R, Johnson RV, Rischin KJ, et al. Percutaneous vertebroplasty for osteoporotic vertebral compression fracture. *Cochrane Database Syst Rev*. 2018;4(4).
32. Hoyt D, Urits I, Orhuru V, et al. Current concepts in the management of vertebral compression fractures. *Curr Pain Headache Rep*. 2020;20:24(5).
33. Gu CN, Brinjikji W, Evans AJ, et al. Outcomes of vertebroplasty compared with kyphoplasty: A systematic review and meta-analysis. *J Neurointervent Surg*. 2016;8:636–642.
34. Papanastassiou JV, Phillips FM, Meirhaeghe JV, et al. Comparing effects of kyphoplasty, vertebroplasty, and nonsurgical management in a systematic review of randomized and non-randomized controlled studies. *Eur Spine J*. 2012;21:1826–1843.
35. Anderson PA, Froyshteter AB, Tontz WL Jr. Meta-analysis of vertebral augmentation compared with conservative treatment for osteoporotic spinal fractures. *J Bone Miner Res*. 2013;28:372–382.
36. Boonen S, Van Meirhaeghe J, Bastian L, et al. Balloon kyphoplasty for the treatment of acute vertebral compression fractures: 2-year results from a randomized trial. *J Bone Miner Res*. 2011;26:1627–1637.
37. Berenson J, Pflugmacher R, Jarzem P, et al. Balloon kyphoplasty versus non-surgical fracture management for treatment of painful vertebral body compression fractures in patients with cancer: a multicenter, randomized controlled trial. *Lancet Oncol*. 2011;12:225–235.
38. Rousing R, Anderson MO, Jespersen SM, et al. Percutaneous vertebroplasty compared to conservative treatment in patient with painful acute or subacute osteoporotic vertebral fracture: three-months follow up in a clinical randomized study. *Spine*. 2009;34:134901354.
39. Beall DP, Chambers MF Thomas SM, et al. Prospective and multicenter evaluation of outcomes for quality of life and activities of daily living for balloon kyphoplasty in the treatment of vertebral compression fractures: the EVOLVE trial. *Neurosurgery*. 2019;84:169–178.
40. Shonnard NH, Berven S, Anderson PA, et al. Appropriate management of vertebral fragility fractures: development of a pathway based on a vertebral compression fracture registry. *Pain Physician*. 2020;23(4)343–352.
41. Rodriguez AJ, Fink HA, Mirigian L, et al. Pain, quality of life and safety outcomes of kyphoplasty for vertebral compression fractures: report of a task force of the American Society of Bone and Mineral Research. *J Bone Miner Res*. 2017;32(9):1935–1944.
42. Hoshino M, Takahashi S, Yasuda H, et al. Balloon kyphoplasty versus conservative treatment for acute osteoporotic vertebral fractures with poor prognostic factors: propensity score matched analysis-using data from two prospective multicenter studies. *Spine*. 2019;44(2):110–117.
43. Nairn RJ, Binkhamis S, Sheikh A. Current perspectives on percutaneous vertebroplasty: current evidence/controversies, patient selection and assessment, and technique and complications. *Radiol Res Pract*. 2011;2011:175079.
44. Denaro V, Longo UG, Maffulli N, Denaro L. Vertebroplasty and kyphoplasty. *Clin Cases Miner Bone Metab*. 2009;6(2):125–130.
45. Masala S, Fiori R, Massari F, Simonetti G. Kyphoplasty: indications, contraindications and technique. *Radiol Med*. 2005;110(1–2):97–105.
46. Marcia S, Muto M, Hirsch JA, et al. What is the role of vertebral augmentation for osteoporotic fractures? A review of the recent literature. *Neuroradiology*. 2018;60(8):777–783.

47. Predey T, Sewall L, Smith SJ. Percutaneous vertebroplasty: new treatment for vertebral compression fractures. *Am Fam Physician*. 2002;66(4):611–615.
48. Beall DP. *Vertebral Augmentation: The Comprehensive Guide to Vertebroplasty, Kyphoplasty, and Implant Augmentation*. 1st ed. Thieme; 2020.
49. Chiras J, Depriester C, et al. Percutaneous vertebral surgery. Technics and indications. *J Neuroradiol*. 1997;24:45–59.
50. Beall DP, Braswell JJ, Martin HD, et al. Technical strategies and anatomic considerations for parapedicular access to thoracic and lumbar vertebral bodies. *Skeletal Radiol*. 2007;36(1):47–52.
51. Beall DP, Pearsons B, Burner S. Technical strategies and anatomic considerations for an extrapedicular modified inferior endplate access to thoracic and lumbar vertebral bodies. *Pain Physician*. 2016;19:595–601.
52. Andrade SE, Majumdar SR, Arnold Chan K, et al. Low frequency of treatment of osteoporosis, among postmenopausal women following a fracture. *Arch Intern Med*. 2003;163(17):2052–2057.
53. Kurra S, Metkar U, Lieberman IH, et al. The effect of kyphoplasty on mortality in symptomatic vertebral compression fractures: a review. *Int J Spine Surg*. 2018;12(5):543–548.

13

Vertebral Augmentation with Osteotome

Christopher M. Lam and Nomen Azeem

Introduction

Osteotomy is a technique by which instruments (osteotomes) are used to either realign the axis of bone, allowing bone lengthening, or transport in efforts to promote healing and correction of any structural abnormalities.[1] First written in 415 BC by Hippocrates for humoral realignment after trauma, this technique has been adopted by orthopedic surgeons to promote healing and osteogenesis in long bone injuries. Osteotomy was later adopted by spine surgeons to correct debilitating spinal deformities; bone is remodeled utilizing several techniques, including the Smith-Petersen osteotomy, pedicle subtraction osteotomy, and vertebral column resection.[2] The result is the reestablishment of the normal spinal axis.

Osteotomes are utilized in minimally invasive spinal procedures by interventional proceduralists as well. These instruments are one of two commonly utilized modalities for performing vertebral augmentation procedures, which are important for management of debilitating vertebral compression fractures (VCF).

VCF impose a significant burden on those who develop them. For example, VCF often prevent patients from comfortably and safely performing activities of daily living. A study by Oleksik et al compared health-related quality of life in postmenopausal women who had low bone mineral density with and without vertebral fractures. The investigators found that the women without vertebral fractures had statistically significant ($P < .001$) lower scores (26 ± 14) on the Quality of Life Questionnaire of the European Foundation for Osteoporosis (QUALEFO, where a lower score means better quality of life) compared to the women with a vertebral fracture (36 ± 17).[3] Furthermore, QUALEFO scores were found to increase with increasing number of vertebral fractures.[3] A study by Tosteson et al evaluating the effects of hip and vertebral fractures on quality-adjusted life-years (QALY; in QALY, 1 represents perfect health and 0 represents death) found that the 114 women who had one or more vertebral fractures had a mean score of 0.82 (95% CI, 0.76, 0.87), while the mean score in the 201 women without fractures was 0.91 (95% CI, 0.88, 0.94).[4] Using multiple regression analysis, this difference in score was estimated to result in 20 to 58 days lost equated from Quality Adjusted Life Years per year for a vertebral fracture.[4]

Several sources, including the Nationwide Inpatient Sample,[5,6] the Centers for Medicare & Medicaid Services,[7,8] and the American College of Surgeons National Surgical Quality Improvement Program databases,[9] have provided insight into the morbidity associated with VCF. Regardless of treatment modalities, patients with VCF were found to have significant rates of deep vein thrombosis (0.7%–6.6%), pulmonary embolism (0.4%–1.9%), decubitus ulcers (1.1%–4.4%), and postoperative infections (0.1%–0.15%),[10] all of which are associated with significant healthcare costs. It was estimated in 2002 that the annual direct medical costs of osteoporotic fractures in the United States was $12.2 billion to $17.9 billion, with VCF contributing more than $1.07 billion of that cost, along with an estimated additional $6 billion from associated loss of productivity from the patient and caregiver.[11,12]

Vertebral augmentation has a unique role in the management of VCF because it is not a purely conservative means of management. Vertebroplasty is the process of placing cement in a vertebra, while kyphoplasty is a similar process except a balloon is inserted in the vertebral body to restore vertebral body height prior to the cement injection. Although it is an invasive means of VCF management, it is also not traditional surgery. Thus, vertebral augmentation may offer a means for management of VCF in patients who have refractory pain and significant hinderances in their activities of daily living while being treated via nonoperative measures. This chapter reviews the indications for, evidence for, and nuances of performing vertebral augmentation utilizing osteotomes.

Indications

Dr. Francis Denis, in his seminal 1983 retrospective review paper, proposed the three-column model of thoracolumbar spine stability after acute trauma. Denis revised the traditional two- column model to include a new segment (the middle column), which was deemed the critical component in maintaining spinal stability.[13,14] Denis defined the posterior column as the posterior arch and posterior ligamentous complex (supraspinous ligament, interspinous ligament, capsule, ligamentum flavum), while the anterior column was defined as the anterior longitudinal ligament, anterior annulus fibrosus, and anterior portion of the vertebral body. The middle column consisted of the posterior longitudinal ligament, posterior annulus fibrosus, and posterior vertebral body wall.[13]

While fractures of the posterior column do occur, constituting approximately 16.9% of acute spinal injuries, they are often classified as minor trauma (articular process fracture, transverse process fracture, spinous process fracture, and pars interarticularis fracture).[13] Major traumas are compression fractures, burst fractures, "seat-belt" injuries, and fracture

TABLE 13.1. Classification of Vertebral Burst Fractures[13]

Type	Incidence	Characteristics
A	23.7%	Fracture of both endplates
B	49.2%	Superior endplate fracture
C	6.8%	Inferior endplate fracture
D	15.2%	Burst with rotation of fragments
E	5.1%	Burst with lateral flexion (compression)

Data from Denis F. The three-column spine and its significance in the classification of acute thoracolumbar spinal injuries. Spine (Phila Pa 1976). 1983;8(8):817–831.

dislocations. The most common major spinal injuries are compression fractures (47.8%), followed by fracture dislocations (16.3%), burst fractures (14.3%), and seat-belt injuries (4.6%).[13] Both fracture dislocations and seat-belt injuries involve injuries to the posterior and middle column, with the main difference being preservation of the anterior column as a hinge point in seat-belt injuries. Burst and compression fractures also share similar characteristics, in that both involve anterior and/or lateral vertebral body wall fractures. However, burst fractures uniquely involve fractures of the posterior wall of the vertebral body.[14,15] Burst and compression fractures were further classified by Denis (Tables 13.1 and 13.2).

Visually, VCF can be classified by their morphology and degree of height loss. A system created by Genant et al (Table 13.3) proposed a four grades for categorizing the severity of compression fractures.[16] Sugita et al performed a retrospective review of VCF and clinical outcomes. In their study, VCF were classified as swelled-front, bow-shaped, projecting, concave, and dented. In their review of 73 patients, they found that swelled-front, bow-shaped, and projecting fractures had a poor prognosis, with late collapse resulting in a vacuum cleft.[17]

Although there are several classification systems for thoracolumbar injuries, the one that has gained traction is the AOSpine system.[18] Published in 2013, it is a three-component system that incorporates fracture grading, neurologic status, and patient modifiers to create a score (Table 13.4). While there is no formal consensus on management of spinal trauma, it has been proposed that AOSpine scores less than 3 should be treated first with conservative, nonoperative measures, while scores greater than 5 should be treated surgically.[19] Nonoperative measures include pharmacologic agents (NSAIDs, acetaminophen, lidocaine patch, calcitonin, muscle relaxants, narcotics), bracing, physical therapy, nerve blocks, and vertebral augmentation.[20] In

TABLE 13.2. Classification of Vertebral Compression Fractures[13]

Type	Incidence	Characteristics
A	16.2%	Fracture of both endplates
B	62.4%	Superior endplate fracture
C	6.09%	Inferior endplate fracture
D	15.2%	Anterior vertebral body wall fracture

Data from Denis F. The three-column spine and its significance in the classification of acute thoracolumbar spinal injuries. Spine (Phila Pa 1976). 1983;8(8):817–831.

TABLE 13.3. Genant Criteria for Grading of Vertebral Compression Fracture[16]

Grade	Description	Height Loss
0	Normal	N/A
1	Mild	20%–25%
2	Moderate	26%–40%
3	Severe	> 40%

Data from Genant HK, Wu CY, van Kuijk C, et al. Vertebral fracture assessment using a semiquantitative technique. J Bone Miner Res. 1993; 8(9):1137–1148.

general, the main clinical candidates for vertebral augmentation are patients with painful osteoporotic VCF that do not improve with 2 to 3 weeks of nonsurgical care, patients who are hospitalized due to a painful osteoporotic fracture, patients with pathologic fractures, patients with aggressive hemangiomas of the spine, and patients with Kümmell disease.[21]

TABLE 13.4. AOSpine Scoring System[14,18,19]

Morphology Type		
A: Compression Injuries		
Type	Description	Score
A0	Minor, nonstructural fractures	0
A1	Wedge compression	1
A2	Split	2
A3	Incomplete burst	3
A4	Complete burst	5
B: Distraction Injuries		
B1	Transosseous tension band disruption (Chance fracture)	5
B2	Posterior tension band disruption	6
B3	Hyperextension	7
C: Displacement or dislocation		8
N: Neurologic Status		
N0	Neurologically intact	0
N1	Transient neurologic deficit that is resolved	1
N2	Radicular symptoms	2
N3	Incomplete spinal cord injury; any cauda equina injury	4
N4	Complete spinal cord injury	4
NX	Neurologic status unknown due to patient state (sedation or head injury)	3
M: Patient Modifiers		
M1	Indeterminant injury to posterior tension band	1
M2	Patient-specific comorbidity that argues for or against surgery (e.g., burn injury overlying injured spine)	0

Data from references 14, 18, and 19

Evidence

Several studies have been performed to evaluate the safety and efficacy of vertebral augmentation in managing VCF. An early prospective, randomized controlled trial (RCT) to compare vertebroplasty and conservative measures was the VERTOS study, in which patients with subacute or chronic painful osteoporotic VCF were either medically managed or received percutaneous vertebroplasty. At 2-week follow-up, patients receiving vertebroplasty had greater pain reduction than patients receiving medical management, but the difference was not statistically significant. However, those receiving vertebroplasty had significantly improved QUALEFO and Roland Morris Disability (RMD) scores, along with reduced medication consumption.[22]

Many other early studies evaluating the efficacy of vertebroplasty for management of VCF did not show significant early improved outcomes compared to nonsurgical management.[23,24] Therefore, many organizations have argued against the use of vertebroplasty for treatment in neurologically intact patients. In fact, the 2011 American Academy of Orthopedic Surgeons (AAOS) guidelines on the treatment of symptomatic osteoporotic spinal compression fractures explicitly advised against (strong recommendation) vertebroplasty in neurologically intact patients who had developed osteoporotic VCF.[25] Meanwhile, in the same guidelines, the AAOS made a weak recommendation for kyphoplasty in neurologically intact patients with osteoporotic spinal compression fractures.[25]

Since 2011, several studies have further investigated the role of vertebral augmentation in management of VCF and have shown a benefit of vertebral augmentation in both improving pain relief and increasing functionality in patients. The VERTOS II trial evaluated patients with acute VCF (< 6 weeks) who received percutaneous vertebroplasty or nonoperative treatment. Of 431 patients with eligible VCF (from T5 or lower) with minimum height loss of 15%, 229 patients (53%) had spontaneous pain relief, while 202 had persistent pain and were randomized to conservative treatment or percutaneous vertebroplasty. The patients were followed for a year. Patients with percutaneous vertebroplasty were found to have greater Visual Analog Scale (VAS) score reduction than medically managed patients at 1-month follow-up (-5.2 vs. -2.7, $P < .0001$) and 1-year follow-up (-5.7 vs. -2.7, $P < .0001$).[26]

A 2012 review by Papanastassiou et al evaluated 27 articles on kyphoplasty and vertebroplasty that met the selection criteria of prospective multi-arm studies involving more than 20 patients. The review found that both kyphoplasty (-5.07/10) and vertebroplasty (-4.55/10) reduced pain scores more than nonsurgical management (-2.17/10), a difference that was statistically significant.[27] Patients receiving intervention within 7 weeks of injury were noted to have the greatest reduction in pain scores. Interestingly, it was found that subsequent fractures also occurred more frequently in patients managed nonsurgically (22%) than in those receiving vertebroplasty (11%, $P = .04$) or kyphoplasty (11%, $P = .01$).[27]

In 2013, Anderson et al performed a meta-analysis of RCTs evaluating conservative therapy and percutaneous vertebroplasty for management of osteoporotic spinal fractures. Six studies were included in the analysis, which found that the VAS score differences at early (2 to 12 weeks) and late (≥ 26 weeks) time points were statistically significant, favoring percutaneous vertebroplasty (0.73, CI 0.35-1.10, and 0.58, CI 0.19-0.97, respectively). Patients undergoing vertebroplasty also had a statistically significant improvement in health-related quality of life (on QUALEFO and EuroQol 5 Dimension (EQ-5D)) in comparison to patients receiving conservative management.[28]

Other studies have looked at the effects of balloon kyphoplasty (BKP) for the treatment of VCF. The earliest study to evaluate BKP in the management of VCF was the FREE trial by Wardlaw et al, which was an RCT across 8 countries and 21 study sites, in which 300 patients were placed in BKP or nonsurgical care treatment arms. Patients had a greater VAS score reduction after BKP compared to nonsurgical care at 1-week follow-up (2.2, CI 1.6-2.8; $P < .0001$) and at 12-month follow-up (0.9, CI 0.3-1.5; $P = .0034$). Furthermore, at 12 months, patients receiving BKP had a greater Short Form-36 (SF-36) score improvement than the nonsurgical group in body pain (9.2, CI 3.9-14.6, $P = .0008$), role physical (12.5, CI 4.8-20.2; $P = .0016$), vitality (5.2, CI 0.2-10.1; $P = .0399$), and social function (11.4, CI 4.0-18.9; $P = .0026$). There was also noted improved physical functioning in patients treated with BKP at 1 month (9.3, CI 2.4-16.2, $P = .0081$) and 12 months (1.9, CI -5.2 to 9.0; $P = .603$).[29]

Subsequently, Beall et al published the EVOLVE trial, an RCT evaluating outcomes for osteoporotic VCF and cancer-associated VCF among patients treated with BKP and nonsurgical care. A total of 354 patients with 350 kyphoplasties were included from 24 different study sites. At 3 months, patients who had recieved a BKP statistically significant decrease in numeric pain rating scale (NRS) (8.7 to 2.7, $P < .001$), improvement of their Oswestry Disability Index (ODI; 63.4 to 27.1, $P < .001$), improvement in their SF-36 PCS (24.2 to 36.6, $P < .001$), and improvement in their EQ-5D (0.383 to 0.746, $P < .001$).[30]

Subsequent meta-analysis of vertebral augmentation by Beall et al in 2018 reaffirmed many of the earlier findings. Twenty-five level 1 or level 2 prospective comparative studies of midthoracic to lumbar VCF with at least 20 patients were included. Overall, BKP and percutaneous vertebroplasty resulted in VAS score reductions (-4.05 and -3.88, respectively) after treatment of VCF. Though improved from nonsurgical management (-2.66), VP was not statistically different, while BKP was.[31] Hirsch et al, in a study of 10 years of sample data from the Medicare database, found that the adjusted number needed to treat (NNT) to save 1 life for nonsurgical management versus kyphoplasty in patients with VCF ranged from 14.8 at year 1 to 11.9 at year 5. Meanwhile, the adjusted NNT to save 1 life for nonsurgical management versus vertebroplasty in patients with VCF ranged from 22.8 at year 1 to 23.8 at year 5.[32] These studies and data highlight the importance of, and the significant improvement in morbidity and mortality yielded by, vertebral augmentation techniques for management of vertebral compression fractures.

Osteotomes are instruments utilized to create interosseous channels in the fractured vertebral body so either balloon or cement placement can reduce the fracture while providing stability. Classically, straight osteotomes have been used to create the channels. As sharp instruments entering the working cannula, they provide a linear channel. In a comparison of unipedicular and bipedicular access, Zhang et al showed that, when high-viscosity cement is used, there are no statistically significant differences in VAS score, ODI score, SF-36 score, cement leakage rate, or vertebral height restoration between the two access techniques.[33]

Further study by Chen et al evaluated the biomechanical strength changes in ex vivo thoracic vertebrae compression models undergoing unipedicular kyphoplasty with ipsilateral cement injection, unipedicular kyphoplasty with bilateral cement injection, and bipedicular kyphoplasty with bilateral cement injection. What their study found was that unipedicular and bipedicular kyphoplasty increased the total stiffness of the vertebral body. However, unipedicular kyphoplasty with cement injection to the ipsilateral side of the vertebral body increased the stiffness on the side of the cement injection, but the contralateral side had a significant decrease in relative stiffness, while unipedicular access with bilateral cement injection resulted in increased stiffness bilaterally.[34]

This paved the way for unipedicular access utilizing a single osteotome, which allowed for unilateral access with bilateral midline extension. One such technique utilizes a curved or steerable osteotome. With this instrument, the operator gains the ability to navigate in a curvilinear fashion. Therefore, steerable technology confers a few benefits. First, the articulating feature can be used to create channels in three dimensions for later introduction of cement, thereby ensuring more stable fixation. Second, the steerable osteotome is more accurate than fixed-shape devices for navigation, and certainly accuracy improves as the operator gains experience with making minor adjustments. Third, the articulation provides greater access to the entire vertebral body, thus making it more likely that a unipedicular approach will be sufficient for adequate cement spread. Fourth, procedure times may be shorter, which translates to a lower requirement for anesthesia and less time that the operator and patient are exposed to radiation from imaging.[35]

In a retrospective chart review of 104 vertebral augmentations (29 with the unipedicular approach and 75 with the bipedicular approach) over a 36-month period, the VAS and ODI were noted to have statistical improvement over their respective preoperative baselines but not between the unipedicular curved osteotome and the bipedicular approach groups. The amount of injected cement was the same between the two groups. However, the unipedicular group had a significantly shorter operation time, fewer fluoroscopic images, and lower cement leakage rates compared to the group with the bipedicular approach.[36] Furthermore, in a retrospective study by He et al that used propensity score matching, for the 63 patients who received vertebral augmentation by a steerable vertebral osteotome, postoperative VAS and ODI scores were lower than those in the control group.[37]

Patient Selection and Contraindications

Several organizations (e.g., AAOS and the Society of Interventional Radiology [SIR]) have published indications and contraindications for vertebral augmentation. As highlighted in the previous sections, the greatest benefits for pain relief and functional improvement in patients with VCF occur in patients who receive vertebral augmentation within the acute period. After 1 year, although there is notable difference between patients treated with nonsurgical care versus vertebral augmentation, it is not statistically significant. Thus, vertebral augmentation (kyphoplasty) should be offered only to patients with painful VCF who are refractory to conservative care, patients with painful VCF requiring hospitalization, patients with painful VCF and extensive osteolysis or invasion secondary to benign or malignant tumor, or patients with painful VCF associated with osteonecrosis.[21,38] Absolute contraindications include asymptomatic fractures, patients improving with medical therapy, history of vertebral body osteomyelitis, history of systemic infection, allergy to bone fillers or opacification agents, spinal canal compromise secondary to tumor resulting in myelopathy, asymptomatic tumor extension into the epidural space, and irreversible coagulopathy. Relative contraindications include presence of radiculopathy, bone retropulsion against neural structures, > 70% collapse of vertebral body height, multiple pathologic fractures, and lack of surgical backup to manage potential complications.[21,38] Interestingly, pharmacologic prophylaxis for osteoporosis is an absolute contraindication for some societies (SIR) but not for others (AAOS).

Perioperative Management

As with most advanced procedures in the neuraxial space, patients about to undergo vertebral augmentation need to have normal hematologic functioning. If patients have significant hepatic impairment or a history of coagulopathy, obtaining pre-procedure complete blood count, platelet levels, INR, or TEG is advised. The goal platelet level should be greater than 50,000.[39] Several organizations, such as the American Society of Regional Anesthesia (ASRA) and American Society of Interventional Pain Physicians (ASIPP), have published extensively on the recommended cessation periods for various antiplatelet and anticoagulant medications so that patients can safely receive various interventions, including vertebral augmentation.[40,41] Most vertebroplasty or BKP procedures for VCF can be performed with local anesthetic and light sedation. In patients requiring more anesthesia, conscious sedation may be an option. In uncooperative patients, general anesthesia may be necessary, but it is rarely utilized.[42] Because most of these procedures are performed without general anesthesia, neuromonitoring is not typically performed. Although infection after vertebral augmentation is rare, it could have catastrophic results. Therefore, pre-procedure antibiotic administration for management of skin flora is recommended.[43]

Technique

As with other forms of vertebral augmentation, percutaneous access to the vertebral body is through a transpedicular approach for lumbar segments and an intercostovertebral approach for thoracic segments.[44] Depending on the size of the fracture and degree of height loss, a bipedicular approach may be necessary. Planning for the procedure should include evaluation of advanced imaging to determine a safe approach. Traditionally, in a procedure with a nonsteerable osteotome, a transpedicular approach is used, because it avoids the radicular vessels, unlike the extrapedicular approach. Furthermore, a straight orientation through the pedicle reduces the risk of pedicle breach and epidural cement leakage

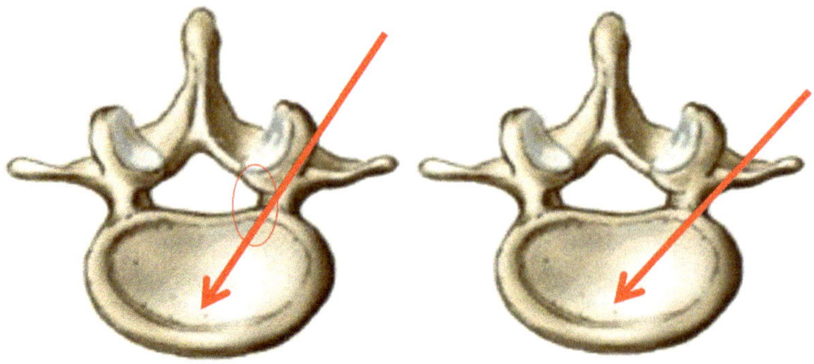

FIGURE 13.1. Left, Transpedicular approach (medial cortex circled). Right, Extrapedicular approach. Images reproduced with permission from Merit Medical (South Jordan, UT).

(Figure 13.1). Utilizing a steerable osteotome allows for adequate depth of insertion as well as a satisfactory degree of articulation, yielding safe access even in patients with suboptimal anatomy. In addition, it may allow targeted access, potentially decreasing the need for bipedicular access.

With CT or fluoroscopic guidance, a stab incision is made in the skin overlying the desired starting location and proposed tract, and the target periosteum is injected with local anesthetic. The working cannula is then aligned along the proposed trajectory and is gently hammered until it is introduced into the vertebral body. The inner cannula is removed, and under live imaging, the osteotome is redirected toward the anterior cortex (if a straight osteotome is used). If a curved osteotome is used, various views should be utilized to curve the osteotome toward the desired—often anterior or contralateral (Figure 13.2)—side of the vertebral body to increase the cavity size.

Once satisfactory cavity size has been obtained, depending on kyphoplasty preference (viscous cement or balloon), the cavity fracture is reduced. If a balloon is used, once the size is adequate within the pressure confines of the device (depending upon the manufacturer, but usually around 250 psi), the balloon is deflated and cement is injected under fluoroscopic guidance (Figure 13.3).

If viscous cement is used without a balloon, it is also injected under fluoroscopic guidance to evaluate fill. Once satisfactory fill is obtained (typically when the anterior two-thirds

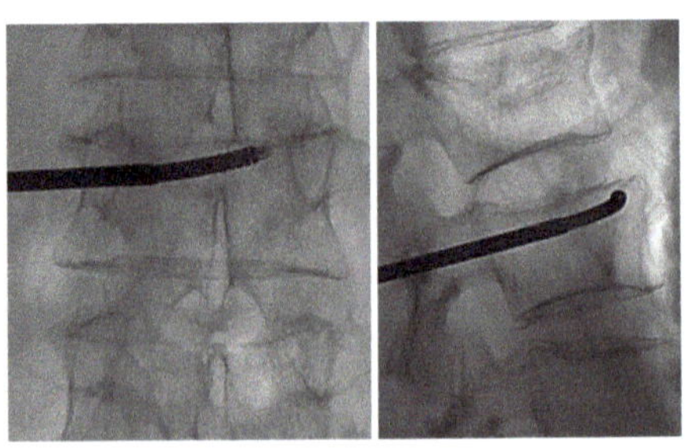

FIGURE 13.2. Curved deployment of steerable osteotome AP View (left), Lateral View (right). Images reproduced with permission from Merit Medical (South Jordan, Utah).

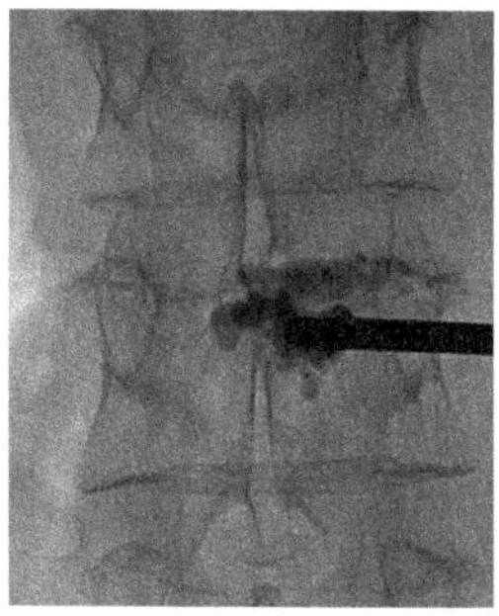

FIGURE 13.3. Cement fill of cavity, AP View. Images reproduced with permission from Merit Medical (South Jordan, Utah).

of the vertebral body is filled), the stylet is replaced in the working cannula. After the manufacturer's recommended period has elapsed for the cement, the cannulas are removed and fluoroscopy is used to evaluate for posterior leakage or retropulsion of cement.

If a steering osteotome is utilized, it is often possible to increase the cavity size after cement has been placed. Under careful observation, the steerable osteotome is reintroduced into the vertebral body to access other aspects of the vertebral body (Figure 13.4). Once the cavity has been increased in size, further cement is introduced (Figure 13.5). After satisfactory augmentation, the instruments are removed (Figure 13.6).

Postoperative Management and Follow-up

After the procedure, patients should remain flat for 1 hour to allow the cement to harden in place. Postoperative antibiotics are typically not needed. Patients may be sore for 3 days, and supplemental analgesics may be needed when patients are home. Standard restrictions on bathing (not submerging the wound until after the follow-up visit) are recommended. Patients may bathe, but water falling directly on the wound or submersion of the wound should be avoided. Patients are evaluated after the procedure and then follow up is 10–14 days afterwards.

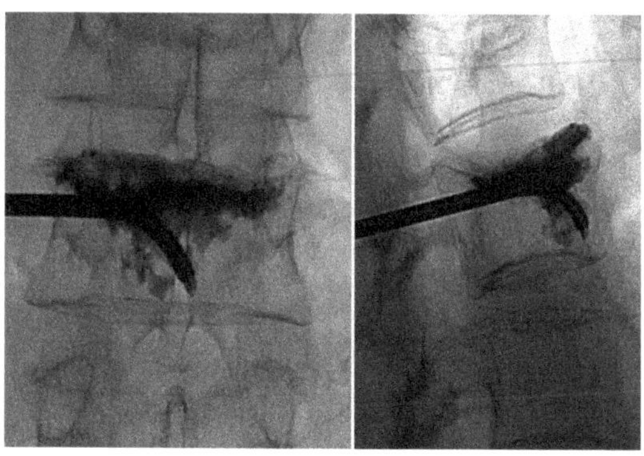

FIGURE 13.4. Curved osteotome directed cavity creation after interim cement fill AP View (left), Lateral View (right). Images reproduced with permission from Merit Medical (South Jordan, Utah).

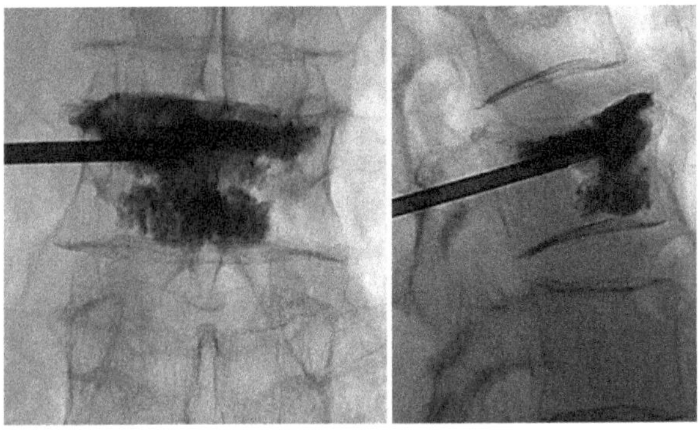

FIGURE 13.5. Cement fill after steerable osteotome cavity creation AP View (left), Lateral View (right). Images reproduced with permission from Merit Medical (South Jordan, Utah).

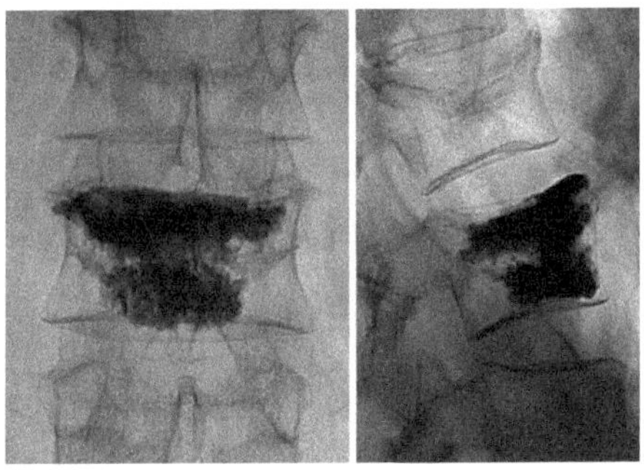

Cement filling compromised areas of bone

FIGURE 13.6. Final vertebral body fill AP View (left), Lateral View (right). Images reproduced with permission from Merit Medical (South Jordan, Utah).

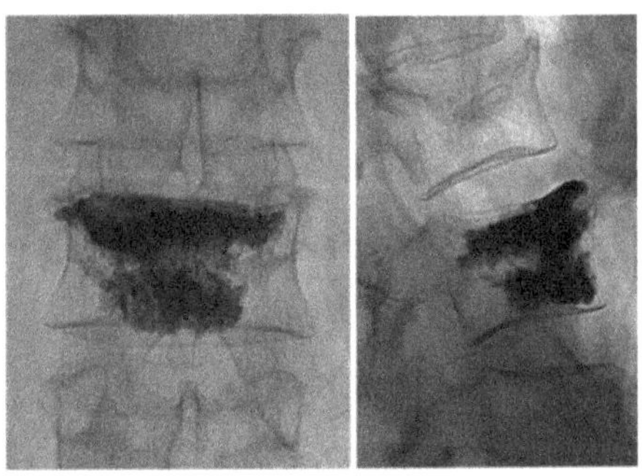

Optimal cement fill

FIGURE 13.7. Final vertebral body fill. Left, AP view. Right, Lateral view.Images reproduced with permission from Merit Medical (South Jordan, Utah).

Complications and Management

Complications of vertebral augmentation are rare. Major complications occur in < 1% of patients without neoplastic involvement of the vertebral body and in < 5% of those with neoplastic involvement.[38] Serious complications include spinal cord compression, nerve root compression, venous embolism, and pulmonary embolism (with possible cardiovascular collapse).[39] A review of the complications associated with vertebroplasty and kyphoplasty as reported to the Food and Drug Administration's device-related website was performed by Nussbaum et al in 2004. The review found that approximately 40,000 to 50,000 kyphoplasty procedures resulted in one death, five neurologic injuries from canal intrusion, one epidural hematoma that caused permanent weakness, 13 neurologic injuries from canal intrusion that resolved with surgery, one epidural hematoma with resolved symptoms after surgery, one cement-induced pulmonary embolism, one ileus, two infection-related events (discitis/osteomyelitis), one pneumothorax, one episode of hypotension, and six episodes of equipment breakage without clinical symptoms. In approximately 130,000 to 160,000 vertebroplasty procedures, three deaths occurred, one canal intrusion resulted in cord compression with paralysis, two cardiac arrests occurred with no clinical sequelae, one episode of anaphylaxis occurred without clinical sequelae, one cement embolus occurred without clinical sequelae, and five equipment breakages happened without clinical sequelae.[45]

A review of 1,100 vertebroplasty procedures in 616 patients found that the most common complication was polymethylmethacrylate (PMMA) cement leakage into surrounding tissues (20%). Patients also experienced cement leakage into a paravertebral vein (13%), intradiscal leakage (8.2%), and spinal canal leakage (0.8%).[46] Indeed, many of the complications associated with vertebral augmentation are associated with the deployment of cement. Cement leakage occurs in roughly 10% to 15% of cases, although many leakages are asymptomatic. Therefore, cement should be injected slowly and under direct radiographic visualization to evaluate for aberrant placement.[39] If PMMA leakage is clinically suspected, advanced imaging should be ordered for further evaluation of the extent of leakage, because surgical correction is needed to resolve the symptoms.

Adjacent-level fractures are also a possible complication. It was reported that new VCF may occur anywhere in 7% to 20% of cases within 1 year of follow-up, with refracture occurring sooner at adjacent levels.[47] Other studies have found that the fracture-free rate within 1 year was 93%, while the mean fracture-free period was 32 months. The rates of new VCF may reflect a patient population at higher risk of VCF, such as patients with significant osteoporosis, a history of VCF, or a history of organ transplant.[39] A meta-analysis of vertebral augmentation by Beall et al found that subsequent VCF was not statistically significant after BKP (32.7%; 95% CI, 8.8%-56.6%) or vertebroplasty (28.3%; 95% CI, 7.0%-49.7%) compared to nonsurgical management (15.9%; 95% CI, 5.2%-26.6%).[31] In a meta-analysis of seven trials by Guo et al, there was no difference in adverse event rates between the surgical treatment (BKP or percutaneous vertebroplasty) group and the sham and nonoperative group.

Conclusion

VCF are common, and they are often associated with significant morbidity and mortality. They contribute to significant healthcare costs and pose a great burden not only to patients but also to their caregivers. Vertebral augmentation can reduce pain and improve functioning in patients with VCF, and use of osteotomes helps improve the safety and efficiency of vertebral augmentation for VCF. Although data on long-term outcomes have been mixed, recent data indicate that vertebral augmentation is an effective means for immediate improvement of symptoms that has long-term benefit for the patient. Like many advanced spine procedures, vertebral augmentation has significant risks and complications, so vigilance when performing the procedure and monitoring patients afterward for complications are paramount in maintaining patient safety and ensuring the long-term success of the procedure.

References

1. Dabis J, Templeton-Ward O, Lacey AE, et al. The history, evolution and basic science of osteotomy techniques. *Strategies Trauma Limb Reconstr.* 2017;12(3):169–180.
2. Kim KT, Park KJ, Lee JH. Osteotomy of the spine to correct the spinal deformity. *Asian Spine J.* 2009;3(2):113–123.
3. Oleksik A, Lips P, Dawson A, et al. Health-related quality of life in postmenopausal women with low BMD with or without prevalent vertebral fractures. *J Bone Miner Res.* 2000;15(7):1384–1392.
4. Tosteson AN, Gabriel SE, Grove MR, et al. Impact of hip and vertebral fractures on quality-adjusted life years. *Osteoporosis Int.* 2001;12(12):1042–1049.
5. Goz V, Errico TJ, Weinreb JH, et al. Vertebroplasty and kyphoplasty: national outcomes and trends in utilization from 2005 through 2010. *Spine J.* 2015;15(5):959–965.
6. Zampini JM, White AP, McGuire KJ. Comparison of 5766 vertebral compression fractures treated with or without kyphoplasty. *Clin Orthop Relat Res.* 2010;468(7):1773–1780.
7. Chen AT, Cohen DB, Skolasky RL. Impact of nonoperative treatment, vertebroplasty, and kyphoplasty on survival and morbidity after vertebral compression fracture in the Medicare population. *J Bone Joint Surg Am.* 2013;95(19):1729–1736.
8. McCullough BJ, Comstock BA, Deyo RA, et al. Major medical outcomes with spinal augmentation vs conservative therapy. *JAMA Intern Med.* 2013;173(16):1514–1521.
9. Toy JO, Basques BA, Grauer JN. Morbidity, mortality, and readmission after vertebral augmentation: analysis of 850 patients from the American College of Surgeons National Surgical Quality Improvement Program database. *Spine (Phila Pa 1976).* 2014;39(23):1943–1949.
10. Goldstein CL, Chutkan NB, Choma TJ, et al. Management of the elderly with vertebral compression fractures. *Neurosurgery.* 2015;77(suppl 4):S33–S45.
11. Tosteson AN, Hammond CS. Quality-of-life assessment in osteoporosis: health-status and preference-based measures. *Pharmacoeconomics.* 2002;20(5):289–303.
12. Burge R, Dawson-Hughes B, Solomon DH, et al. Incidence and economic burden of osteoporosis-related fractures in the United States, 2005-2025. *J Bone Miner Res.* 2007;22(3):465–475.
13. Denis F. The three column spine and its significance in the classification of acute thoracolumbar spinal injuries. *Spine (Phila Pa 1976).* 1983;8(8):817–831.
14. Rosenthal BD, Boody BS, Jenkins TJ, et al. Thoracolumbar burst fractures. *Clin Spine Surg.* 2018;31(4):143–151.
15. Pateder DB, Khanna AJ, Lieberman IH. Vertebroplasty and kyphoplasty for the management of osteoporotic vertebral compression fractures. *Orthop Clin North Am.* 2007;38(3):409–418.

16. Genant HK, Wu CY, van Kuijk C, et al. Vertebral fracture assessment using a semiquantitative technique. *J Bone Miner Res.* 1993;8(9):1137–1148.
17. Sugita M, Watanabe N, Mikami Y, et al. Classification of vertebral compression fractures in the osteoporotic spine. *J Spinal Disord Tech.* 2005;18(4):376–381.
18. Vaccaro AR, Oner C, Kepler CK, et al. AOSpine thoracolumbar spine injury classification system: fracture description, neurological status, and key modifiers. *Spine (Phila Pa 1976).* 2013;38(23):2028–2037.
19. Vaccaro AR, Schroeder GD, Kepler CK, et al. The surgical algorithm for the AOSpine thoracolumbar spine injury classification system. *Eur Spine J.* 2016;25(4):1087–1094.
20. McCarthy J, Davis A. Diagnosis and management of vertebral compression fractures. *Am Fam Physician.* 2016;94(1):44–50.
21. Savage JW, Schroeder GD, Anderson PA. Vertebroplasty and kyphoplasty for the treatment of osteoporotic vertebral compression fractures. *J Am Acad Orthop Surg.* 2014;22(10):653–664.
22. Voormolen MH, Mali WP, Lohle PN, et al. Percutaneous vertebroplasty compared with optimal pain medication treatment: short-term clinical outcome of patients with subacute or chronic painful osteoporotic vertebral compression fractures. The VERTOS study. *AJNR Am J Neuroradiol.* 2007;28(3):555–560.
23. Kallmes DF, Comstock BA, Heagerty PJ, et al. A randomized trial of vertebroplasty for osteoporotic spinal fractures. *N Engl J Med.* 2009;361(6):569–579.
24. Buchbinder R, Osborne RH, Ebeling PR, et al. A randomized trial of vertebroplasty for painful osteoporotic vertebral fractures. *N Engl J Med.* 2009;361(6):557–568.
25. Esses SI, McGuire R, Jenkins J, et al. The treatment of symptomatic osteoporotic spinal compression fractures. *J Am Acad Orthop Surg.* 2011;19(3):176–182.
26. Klazen CA, Lohle PN, de Vries J, et al. Vertebroplasty versus conservative treatment in acute osteoporotic vertebral compression fractures (Vertos II): an open-label randomised trial. *Lancet.* 2010;376(9746):1085–1092.
27. Papanastassiou ID, Phillips FM, Van Meirhaeghe J, et al. Comparing effects of kyphoplasty, vertebroplasty, and non-surgical management in a systematic review of randomized and non-randomized controlled studies. *Eur Spine J.* 2012;21(9):1826–1843.
28. Anderson PA, Froyshteter AB, Tontz WL Jr. Meta-analysis of vertebral augmentation compared with conservative treatment for osteoporotic spinal fractures. *J Bone Miner Res.* 2013;28(2):372–382.
29. Wardlaw D, Cummings SR, Van Meirhaeghe J, et al. Efficacy and safety of balloon kyphoplasty compared with non-surgical care for vertebral compression fracture (FREE): a randomised controlled trial. *Lancet.* 2009;373(9668):1016–1024.
30. Beall DP, Chambers MR, Thomas S, et al. Prospective and multicenter evaluation of outcomes for quality of life and activities of daily living for balloon kyphoplasty in the treatment of vertebral compression fractures: the EVOLVE trial. *Neurosurgery.* 2019;84(1):169–178.
31. Beall D, Lorio MP, Yun BM, et al. Review of vertebral augmentation: an updated meta-analysis of the effectiveness. *Int J Spine Surg.* 2018;12(3):295–321.
32. Hirsch JA, Chandra RV, Carter NS, et al. Number needed to treat with vertebral augmentation to save a life. *AJNR Am J Neuroradiol.* 2020;41(1):178–182.
33. Zhang L, Liu Z, Wang J, et al. Unipedicular versus bipedicular percutaneous vertebroplasty for osteoporotic vertebral compression fractures: a prospective randomized study. *BMC Musculoskelet Disord.* 2015;16:145.
34. Chen B, Li Y, Xie D, et al. Comparison of unipedicular and bipedicular kyphoplasty on the stiffness and biomechanical balance of compression fractured vertebrae. *Eur Spine J.* 2011;20(8):1272–1280.
35. Brower J. Interventional news: a new course. *Radiology Today.* 2020; 21 (1): 6–7.
36. Zhong R, Liu J, Wang R, et al. Unilateral curved versus bipedicular vertebroplasty in the treatment of osteoporotic vertebral compression fractures. *BMC Surg.* 2019;19(1):193.
37. He X, Liu Y, Zhang J, et al. An innovative technique for osteoporotic vertebral compression fractures—vertebral osteotome with side-opening cannula. *J Pain Res.* 2018;11:1905–1913.
38. McGraw JK, Cardella J, Barr JD, et al. Society of Interventional Radiology quality improvement guidelines for percutaneous vertebroplasty. *J Vasc Intervent Radiol.* 2003;14(9 part 2):S311–S315.

39. Burton AW. Vertebroplasty and kyphoplasty: case presentation, complications, and their prevention. *Pain Med.* 2008;9:S58–S64.
40. Narouze S, Benzon HT, Provenzano D, et al. Interventional spine and pain procedures in patients on antiplatelet and anticoagulant medications (second edition): guidelines from the American Society of Regional Anesthesia and Pain Medicine, the European Society of Regional Anaesthesia and Pain Therapy, the American Academy of Pain Medicine, the International Neuromodulation Society, the North American Neuromodulation Society, and the World Institute of Pain. *Reg Anesth Pain Med.* 2018;43(3):225–262.
41. Kaye AD, Manchikanti L, Novitch MB, et al. Responsible, safe, and effective use of antithrombotics and anticoagulants in patients undergoing interventional techniques: American Society of Interventional Pain Physicians (ASIPP) guidelines. *Pain Physician.* 2019;22(1S):S75–S128.
42. White SM. Anaesthesia for percutaneous vertebroplasty. *Anaesthesia.* 2002;57(12):1229–1230.
43. Moon E, Tam MD, Kikano RN, et al. Prophylactic antibiotic guidelines in modern interventional radiology practice. *Semin Intervent Radiol.* 2010;27(4):327–337.
44. Denaro V, Longo UG, Maffulli N, et al. Vertebroplasty and kyphoplasty. *Clin Cases Miner Bone Metab.* 2009;6(2):125–130.
45. Nussbaum DA, Gailloud P, Murphy K. A review of complications associated with vertebroplasty and kyphoplasty as reported to the Food and Drug Administration medical device related web site. *J Vasc Intervent Radiol.* 2004;15(11):1185–1192.
46. Saracen A, Kotwica Z. Complications of percutaneous vertebroplasty: an analysis of 1100 procedures performed in 616 patients. *Medicine (Baltimore).* 2016;95(24):e3850.
47. Trout AT, Kallmes DF, Kaufmann TJ. New fractures after vertebroplasty: adjacent fractures occur significantly sooner. *AJNR Am J Neuroradiol.* 2006;27(1):217–223.

14

Spinal Tumor Ablation

Andrew Sack and Harry Sukumaran

Introduction

It was estimated that, in 2020, 1.8 million Americans would be diagnosed with cancer.[1] About 70% of the cases were expected to develop metastases, and 30% to 70% of the metastases were expected to involve the spine.[2,3] The vertebral column is the most common site of metastasis due to the vascular red marrow and the venous communication with thoracic and pelvic vessels.[4] The thoracic spine accounts for 65% of vertebral metastases, followed by the lumbosacral spine (25%) and the cervical spine (10%).[5] Spinal pain is the presenting symptom in 90% of vertebral metastases.[6] However, vertebral metastases can also cause vertebral fracture, instability, or neurologic deficits due to compression of the spinal cord or spinal nerves.[7] The consequences of vertebral metastases include declines in functional status and quality of life.[5]

For decades, external beam radiation therapy (EBRT) has been the standard treatment for vertebral metastases.[8] However, EBRT has important limitations. A 2006 meta-analysis of EBRT for vertebral metastases found that less than half of patients achieved a 50% reduction in pain 1 month after completion of treatment.[9] Some tumors are resistant to EBRT, such as melanoma, sarcoma, renal cell carcinoma, and non-small-cell lung carcinoma.[10] The poor radiation tolerance of the spinal cord limits EBRT retreatment of recurrent tumors or adjacent-level metastases.[11]

Stereotactic body radiotherapy (SBRT) is a subtype of EBRT that uses focused beams of radiation to target small vertebral tumors. It has been shown to have improved outcomes for pain and tumor control in comparison to conventional EBRT. However, SBRT has up to a 5% risk of radiation-induced myelopathy and up to a 39% risk of vertebral compression fracture.[12] Like EBRT, SBRT is administered in fractionated doses over several appointments, which can be prohibitive for patients who have transportation challenges.

Surgical treatment of vertebral metastases includes tumor resection, corpectomy, and hardware stabilization of the spine. Many patients with vertebral metastases have poor functional status or limited life expectancy, which can preclude a surgical procedure with prolonged recovery and significant morbidity. Therefore, surgery is typically limited to patients who experience neurologic compromise or instability.[6]

Radiofrequency (RF) ablation is a common treatment modality that uses needle electrodes to carry high-frequency alternating current into tissue, causing a focused zone of heating and necrosis.[13] For many years, it was primarily used for the treatment of osteoid osteomas and spinal pain due facet arthropathy. However, in 2000, Dupuy et al published the first two cases of using RF ablation to treat metastases to the vertebral body.[14] This marked the beginning of spinal tumor ablation (STA). STA utilizes a percutaneous, minimally invasive approach whereby one or more electrodes are inserted into an affected vertebra. STA requires only a single outpatient treatment, with mild-to-moderate sedation and local anesthetic. Minimal ionizing radiation is required for image guidance with fluoroscopy or CT, in contrast to the high radiation doses used during EBRT. Many patients undergoing STA also require biopsy or vertebral augmentation for the stabilization or prevention of fracture; STA facilitates these simultaneous procedures since all necessary vertebral access is already in place. Although RF is the most common modality used for vertebral tumor ablation, cryoablation and microwave ablation have also been described.[13]

Indications

The most common indication for STA is palliation of painful tumors of the vertebral body or pedicles involving the thoracic, lumbar, and sacral regions.[15] It is indicated for primary or metastatic tumors, with or without pathologic vertebral fracture. However, STA has other notable indications. It is used to decrease tumor burden and the risk of tumor extension into neural structures. It can also be used with a curative intent for small benign bone tumors, such as osteoblastomas or osteoid osteomas.[16]

In 2015, the Metastatic Spine Disease Multidisciplinary Working Group developed guidelines for the treatment of spinal metastases. The guidelines recommend standard analgesics and bisphosphonates as first-line treatment for any vertebral metastatic disease in the absence of an unstable fracture.[17,18] Bisphosphonates reduce both pain and the risk of compression fractures.[19] The group also included EBRT or its subtypes as first-line treatment for painful spinal metastases without any unstable fracture. Regarding STA, they state, "Percutaneous tumor ablation may be considered when spinal metastases do not respond to radiation therapy, the cumulative tolerance of the spinal cord to radiation has been reached, or inclusion criteria in clinical trials preclude radiation therapy."[17] The second-line designation of STA was due to the paucity of high-quality prospective evidence at the time of guideline publication rather than clinical evidence of inferiority.

STA should also be considered for patients who have a problem that would preclude successful EBRT treatment. Patients generally must be able to lie flat and motionless for 30 to 60 minutes during each of several EBRT sessions. They must also have transportation to and from each of these appointments, which can be challenging due to distance or social situations. STA can often be performed in 15 to 30 minutes in a single appointment.

Evidence

The earliest evidence for STA was a 2000 report written by Dupuy et al. Interestingly, this single publication simultaneously described an in vivo study of vertebral ablation in pigs, an ex vivo study in excised pig vertebrae, and two human cases.[14] For the in vivo pig study, saline-cooled RF ablation was carried out in lumbar vertebrae for 12 minutes, while temperature was measured in vertebral bone and in the anterior spinal canal. The maximum achievable current within the vertebral body without increasing impedance was 220 ± 35 mA (in muscle it was 326 ± 42 mA). The maximum temperature measured in the anterior epidural space was 44°C, and the maximum bone temperature was 48°C. Yamane et al had previously shown that spinal cord injury occurs at 45°C or greater,[20] so the new temperature data suggested that STA could be safely carried out without spinal cord injury. Dupuy et al also described two human cases: a 54-year-old woman with a painful L2 vertebral body metastasis due to hemangiopericytoma, and a 14-year-old male with a painful osteoid osteoma of T11. Both patients were treated with RF STA and were reported to have from “remarkable” to complete pain relief and no neurologic deficits.

Shortly after the Dupuy et al publication, a porcine model demonstrated several instances of paraplegia and radiculitis after vertebral and pedicular ablation.[21] Therefore, a retrospective study was developed by Hillen et al to determine the safety of STA for posterior vertebral body lesions of the thoracic and lumbar spine.[15] Data were collected from 26 patients who had 47 spinal tumors that underwent STA using an articulating bipolar RF electrode with a proximal thermocouple. Manufacturer data were used to determine the size of the ablation, based on the distance of the thermocouple from the electrode tip, and the electrode was placed a concordant distance from the anterior spinal canal. Ablation was carried out until the thermocouple registered 50°C in each case. Of the 26 patients, there were no cases of permanent neurologic injury. Four patients developed transient radiculitis; all four had undergone intentional pedicular ablation due to tumor involvement. Mean pain score on the Visual Analog Scale (VAS) decreased from 7.82 at baseline to 2.82 at 1 week and 3.30 at 1 month ($P < .001$). Fifty percent of patients were able to decrease their use of pain medications.

The first prospective study evaluating RF STA was published by Goetz et al in 2004.[22] This was a single-arm, multicenter study designed to evaluate the pain relief provided by ablation of bone metastases. All patients either had previously received EBRT or were deemed poor candidates for radiation by a radiation oncologist. Although the study included subjects with nonvertebral bone metastases, 16 of the 43 patients did have vertebral involvement and underwent STA. Ablation was carried out for an average of 49.5 minutes per patient at a temperature of 100°C. The results demonstrated significant and progressive reductions in peak pain, average pain, and pain interference at weeks 1, 4, 8, 12, and 24. One patient developed a second-degree burn at the grounding pad site, and another developed transient bowel and bladder incontinence following an upper sacral ablation.

In 2010, Dupuy et al published their own prospective study of the effect of RF ablation on pain related to osseous metastatic disease.[8] There was no requirement for previous EBRT for this study. Like the trial conducted by Goetz et al, this study was not limited to vertebral metastases, and only 8 of the 55 patients had vertebral metastases treated. Ablation was carried out for 4 to 12 minutes at a target temperature of 60°C and was repeated at other locations if the initial ablation zone was estimated not to cover the entire tumor. The results demonstrated reductions in pain of 26.9 and 14.2 at 1 month and 3 months, respectively (on a 0 to 100 scale). Mood also improved by 19.9 and 14.9 at the same respective time points (also on a 100-point scale). Complications included transient neuropathic pain in two patients, foot drop in one patient, and one burn at the grounding pad site. The study did not specify whether the complications occurred during vertebral or nonvertebral ablation.

A larger, retrospective, multicenter analysis of 92 patients with 96 lesions was published in 2014 by Anchala et al.[23] All patients had vertebral metastases and were treated with RF STA using a navigational bipolar ablation probe. Prior EBRT had occurred in 43% of patients. Ablation was carried out for an average of 361 seconds per lesion, with an average of 4.3 lesions created per patient. The target temperature was a reading of 50°C at the proximal thermocouple of the probe. Of the 96 lesions treated, 92 were treated with simultaneous cement augmentation. Pain significantly reduced from a baseline score of 7.51 to 1.73 at 1 week, 2.25 at 1 month, and 1.75 at 6 months. The only complications noted were two instances of vertebral fractures, both in patients who did not undergo vertebral augmentation during STA.

Another retrospective trial published in 2015 showed similar results.[24] Wallace et al reviewed 72 patients who underwent RF STA with or without prior EBRT. The same navigational bipolar probe was used as in the Anchala et al study, with the same target temperature of 50°C at the proximal thermocouple. Vertebral augmentation was performed immediately after STA in 95% of treatments. Pain scores significantly reduced from a baseline of 8.0 to 3.9 at 1 week and 2.9 at 4 weeks. At 4 weeks, pain medication use decreased in 31% of patients and activity level increased in 50% of patients. Transient radiculitis developed in four patients who had pedicular ablations. There were no permanent neurologic deficits reported. Three out of 5 vertebrae that were not treated with immediate vertebral augmentation developed fractures within 12 months.

The most robust study of STA to date was published in 2016 by Bagla et al.[25] This was a multicenter prospective study that evaluated pain, disability, and quality of life following RF STA. Fifty subjects were enrolled, and 69 tumors were treated. Vertebral augmentation was performed in 96% of the affected vertebrae. The Numeric Rating Scale pain score decreased from 5.9 at baseline to 3.5 at week 1 and 2.1 at month 3 ($P < .001$ for both time points). The Modified Oswestry Disability Index score decreased from 52.9 at baseline to 45.9 at week 1 and 37.0 at month 3 ($P < .01$ for both time points). The Functional Assessment of Cancer Therapy Quality-of-Life Measurement in Patients with Bone Pain (FACT-BP) score increased from 22.6 at baseline to 35.6 at week 1 and 38.9 at month 3 ($P < .0001$ for both time points). One patient developed post-STA pain related to an adjacent herniated disk that was herniated prior to STA. Another patient reported syncope. No other complications occurred that were related to the procedure.

A single retrospective study by Tomasian et al provided insight into tumor control with RF STA.[6] The authors reviewed 27 patients with 33 tumors who underwent RF STA combined with vertebral augmentation. At 16 weeks after the procedure, radiographic tumor control was evident in 96% of the tumors treated, despite systemic metastatic progression in 77% of the patients. Pain relief was not reported. No complications were noted.

Cryoablation is an alternative ablative modality that delivers nitrogen or argon gas through probes to cool tissue to approximately -40°C. This technique requires CT guidance rather than fluoroscopy, but it has the advantage of a CT-visible "ice ball" that clearly delineates the margins of the lesion. There is evidence demonstrating the safety and efficacy of cryoablation for several types of tumors, but evidence specific to vertebral tumors is lacking.[26,27] The utility of vertebral cryoablation as a pain treatment is questionable due to the lack of CT guidance in most interventional pain practices.

Patient Selection and Contraindications

Patient selection is critical in STA to maximize patient benefit and minimize risk. Table 14.1 lists clinical features of ideal candidates for STA.

The relative contraindications to STA must be considered on a case-by-case basis, with an analysis of risks and benefits. Body mass index over 40, especially with comorbid osteoporosis, can severely limit fluoroscopic image quality and impair procedural image guidance. Metastatic epidural involvement (where tumor has breached the posterior cortex of the vertebral body) can result in altered heat transfer into the spinal canal due to a lack of insulating osseous cortex and can increase risk of neurologic injury. Poor baseline performance status, visceral metastatic involvement, and life expectancy of less than 3 months are associated with reduced benefit after STA.[16] Presence of an implanted pacemaker or cardiac defibrillator is generally safe but requires consultation with the patient's cardiologist and compliance with manufacturer recommendations.[28]

Absolute contraindications to STA are cervical vertebral tumors, spinal instability, focal neurologic deficits, local or systemic infection, and irreversible coagulopathy.

TABLE 14.1. Characteristics of Candidates for Spinal Tumor Ablation

One or more painful vertebral metastases, with or without pathologic fracture
Systemic analgesics with poor pain relief or poor tolerance
Moderate performance status or better
Life expectancy ≥ 3 months
Poor response to EBRT or not a candidate
Body mass index < 40

Perioperative Management

Prior to scheduling the procedure, a basic set of preoperative laboratory studies should be obtained to screen for infection, coagulopathy, and any potential metabolic abnormality. The oncologic patient can be immunocompromised due to the disease state and chemotherapy, and radiation treatment can cause further compromise. For optimum timing and planning, working in conjunction with the oncologist and radiation oncologist in a team model is recommended.

The cancer patient can also be at increased risk for surgical-site infections (SSI). A review of the literature reveals that there are a few case reports of infection after vertebroplasty or kyphoplasty. While infectious complications are rare, they can have a devastating outcome and can be difficult to effectively treat. Preoperative intravenous antibiotic administration is recommended, along with meticulous attention to aseptic technique. Antibiotic prophylaxis is usually guided by weight-based dosing of cefazolin or clindamycin, because the common organisms associated with infection are skin flora, namely staphylococci and streptococci.[29] If the patient cannot receive either cefazolin or clindamycin, vancomycin is recommended. It is always good practice to check with your facility regarding antibiotic susceptibility/resistance and choose an agent accordingly. Antibiotics should be administered 1 hour prior to surgical incision.

Imaging of the spine should be performed to identify tumor level, to determine if a fracture is present and to what degree, and to aid in procedural planning. MRI and CT scans should be reviewed and used for planning of STA. The presence of an acute fracture can be determined by using short tau inversion recovery (STIR) sequences on MRI, which identify areas of increased signal and bone marrow edema, indicating an acute fracture.

Anesthesia is typically required in the form of local anesthesia with moderate conscious sedation or monitored anesthesia care (MAC). Standard ASA monitoring—blood pressure measurement, pulse oximetry, and electrocardiogram—should be utilized. General anesthesia is sometimes needed in patients unable to tolerate the prone position or those having increased analgesic requirements making MAC unsafe.

Technique

There are currently two commercially available systems for percutaneous STA: OsteoCool™ Radiofrequency Ablation System by Medtronic (Figure 14.1) and the STAR™ Tumor Ablation System by Merit Medical (Figure 14.2). Both systems use bipolar RF to ablate vertebral body tumor and provide pain relief. The STAR system utilizes conventional RF ablation, at 50°C, and a steerable tip that allows a unipedicular approach while still treating the entire vertebral body. The OsteoCool system utilizes water-cooled technology, at 70°C, in a uni- or bipedicular fashion. The water-cooled technology continuously cools the active probe tip, allowing better maintenance of tissue temperature and less char formation.

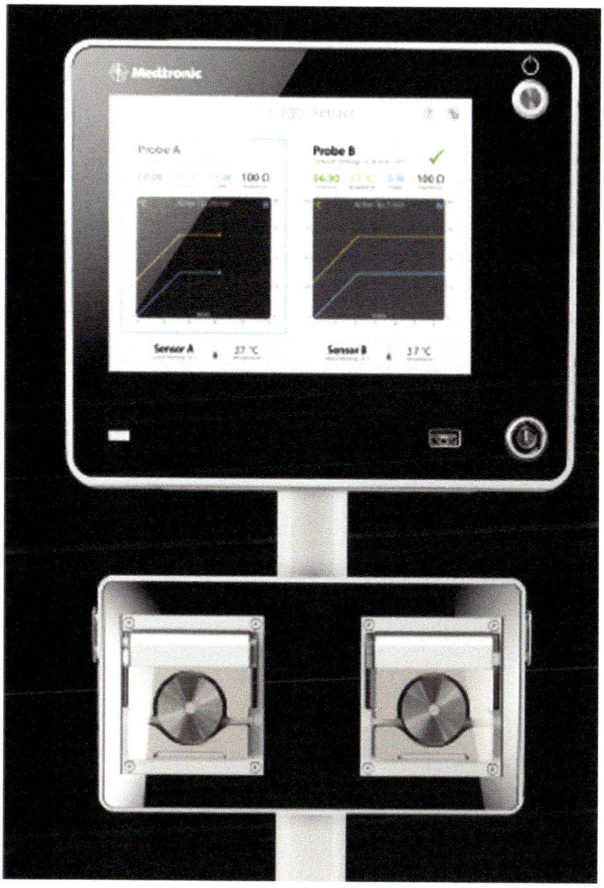

FIGURE 14.1. Medtronic OsteoCool Radiofrequency Generator.[30]

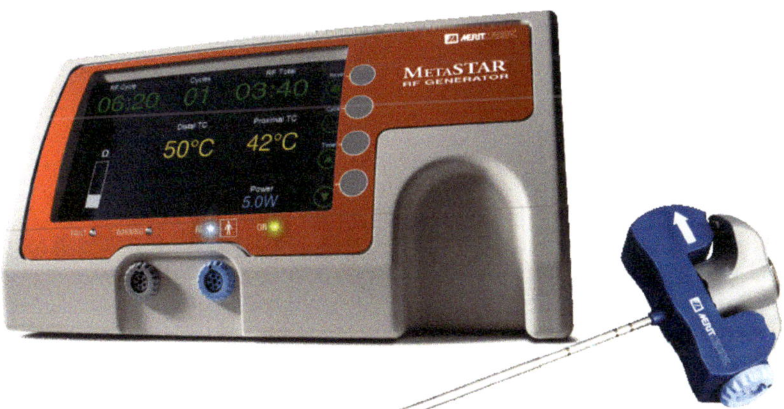

FIGURE 14.2. STAR Tumor Ablation System.[31]

Vertebral Body Access

Placement of the needle to achieve vertebral body access is similar for both systems and is approached in the same manner as for vertebroplasty or kyphoplasty.

Transpedicular Approach

- After confirming the level(s) for treatment, utilize cephalocaudad tilt to align the inferior endplate of the target vertebral body.
- Utilize ipsilateral oblique so that the pedicle is superimposed on the vertebral body and the superior articulating process (SAP) is approximately in the lateral one-third of the vertebral body.
- Using an *en face* or barrel view, place a 22-gauge spinal needle on the pedicle. This serves two purposes: local anesthesia and trajectory planning in an AP and lateral view.
- Place the access needle (working cannula) along the same trajectory, considering tumor/fracture location and the area to be treated (Figure 14.3). Dock the needle within the periosteum with a few gentle taps of the mallet.
- Superior (10 or 2 o'clock on pedicle)
- Middle
- Inferior (5 or 7 o'clock on pedicle)
- Rotate the image back to an AP view and carefully advance the needle through the pedicle. The needle is advanced until it is through the pedicle and the tip rests in the posterior portion of the vertebral body. It is particularly important to stay lateral to the medial border of the pedicle while staying within the superior, inferior, and lateral borders of the pedicle. This ensures safe needle placement, avoiding the spinal cord medially and the nerve roots superiorly and inferiorly, as well as preventing pneumothorax (in thoracic locations). For this reason, until the needle has entered the vertebral body,

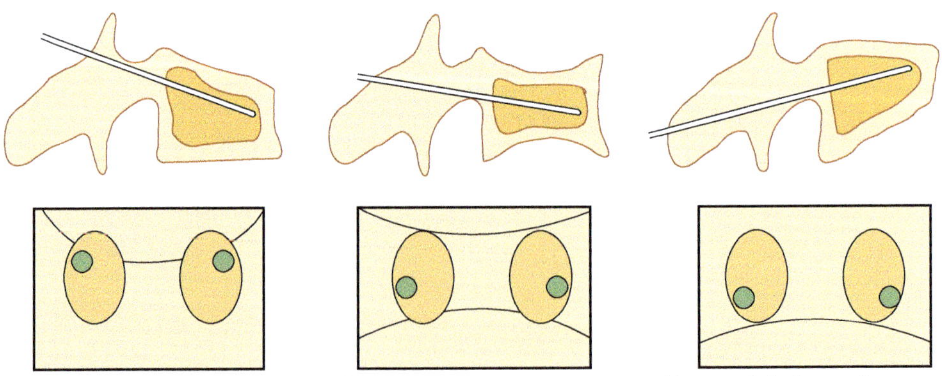

(a) Superior wedge (b) Biconcave (c) Inferior wedge

FIGURE 14.3. Pedicle entry points and trajectories.[32]

needle advancement should be done in an AP view. Frequent image checks in AP and lateral views can ensure proper trajectory. Once the needle has entered the vertebral body, advancement should be done utilizing a lateral view. Biplanar fluoroscopy, if available, can be used to help with efficiency.

- A bone biopsy can be taken and sent to pathology for tissue confirmation and diagnosis.

Radiofrequency Ablation of the Tumor

OsteoCool Radiofrequency Ablation System

- Once the working cannula (8-, 10-, or 13-gauge) is positioned in the posterior one-third of the vertebral body, the stylet is removed, leaving the working cannula in place. Repeat on the contralateral side if utilizing bipedicular access.
- The precision color-coded hand drill is inserted through the working cannula and is advanced in a lateral view to the desired location based on previously identified treatment areas (Figure 14.4). It is important to drill through the tumor so that the drill aligns with, or extends slightly past, the tumor margin. Placement of the probe tips 8 to 10 mm apart yields the largest ablation zone. The drill is color-coded to correspond to the different sizes of 17-gauge RF probes (7 mm, 10 mm, 15 mm, and 20 mm; Figure 14.5). The appropriate probe is chosen based on the drill markings on the proximal end as well as the desired lesion size, based on previously identified treatment areas.

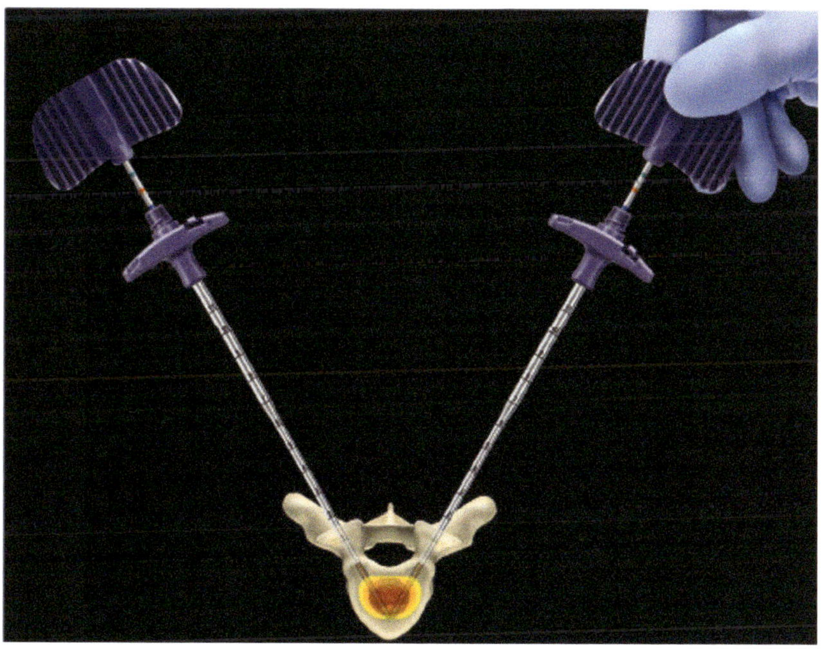

FIGURE 14.4. Placement of precision color-coded hand drill.[30]

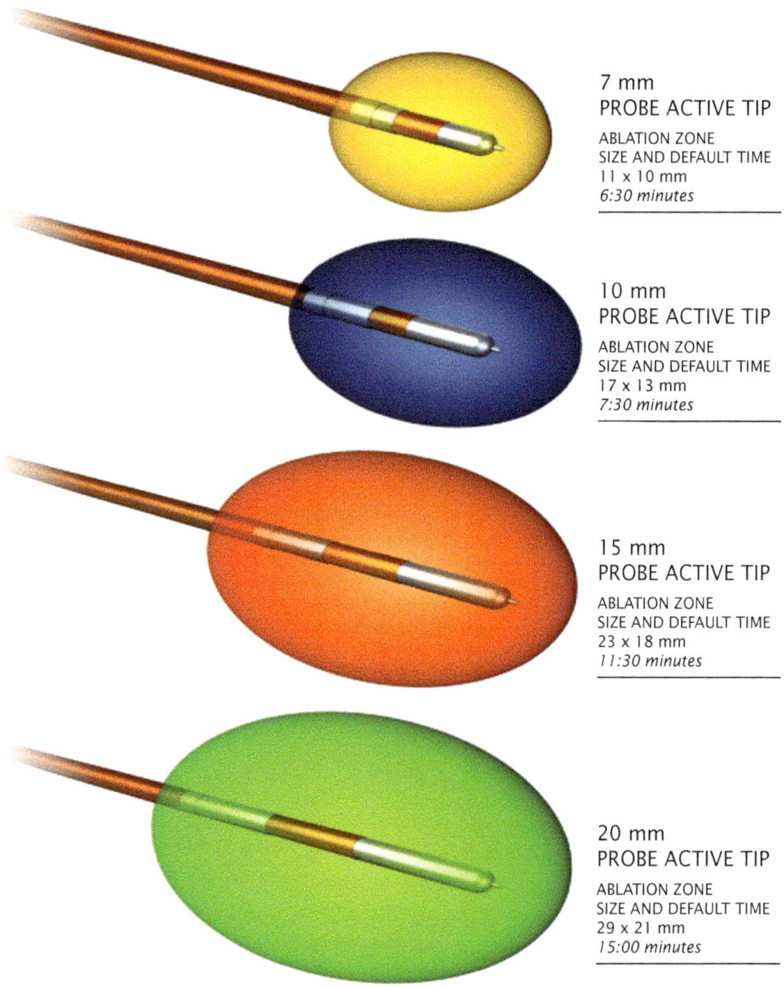

FIGURE 14.5. OsteoCool RF ablation probes.[30]

- Probe placement can be unipedicular or bipedicular, based on the area needed to be treated.
- The RF probes are placed, and the lesion is started for the corresponding time. RF lesioning can be painful, so communication with nursing staff or the anesthesia provider is critical.
- If additional temperature monitoring of tissue is required, an independent thermocouple can be placed.
- The retract feature allows for manual extension of the RF ablation zone, if necessary, back toward the pedicle as the probe is removed.
- Once the RF treatment is complete, the RF probes can be removed, the stylet replaced, and the instrument removed, if vertebral augmentation is not necessary. Otherwise, vertebral augmentation is undertaken as described elsewhere in this text.

STAR Tumor Ablation System

- Once the 10-gauge working cannula is positioned in the posterior third of the vertebral body, the stylet is removed, leaving the working cannula in place.
- The SpineSTAR® bipolar RF ablation instrument is then inserted through the working cannula into the vertebral body, with caution taken to ensure that the electrode is fully retracted.
- Under image guidance, the gray articulating handle (Figure 14.2) is rotated to steer the articulating segment and to navigate the instrument to the previously identified treatment areas (Figure 14.6).
- Once in the proper location, the electrode is extended by rotating clockwise the white electrode on the ablation instrument.
- The SpineSTAR instrument has two different configurations (Figure 14.7), with the choice of configuration depending on the ablation size.

SpineSTAR 5 | 10

- Distal thermocouple at 5 mm
- Proximal thermocouple at 10 mm
- RF energy is terminated when proximal thermocouple registers 50°C.
- Maximum ablation zone is ~2 cm × 1.5 cm.

SpineSTAR 10 | 15

- Distal thermocouple at 10 mm
- Proximal thermocouple at 15 mm

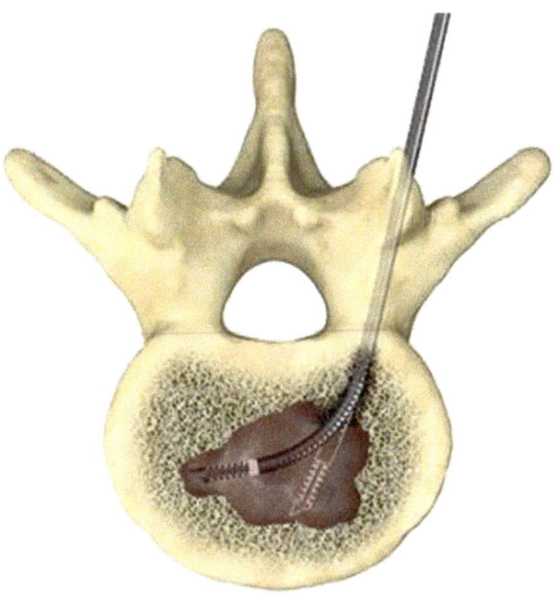

FIGURE 14.6. SpineSTAR articulating instrument.[31]

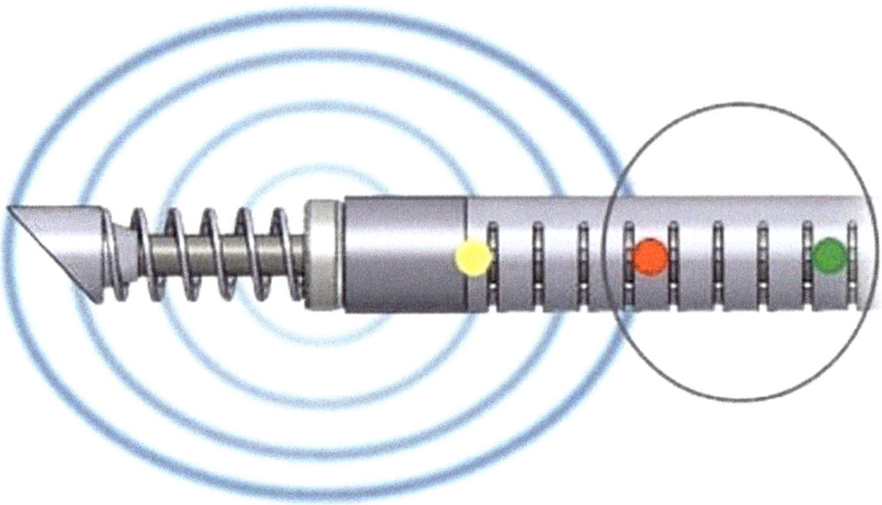

FIGURE 14.7. SpineSTAR configurations.[31]

- RF energy is terminated when proximal thermocouple registers 50°C.
- Maximum ablation zone is ~3 cm × 2 cm.
  - The electrode is then connected to the MetaSTAR RF generator (Figure 14.2). The RF ablation is manually controlled by the physician using the hand switch on the generator. The total amount of ablation time is determined by the tumor size and vascularization and is adjusted by the physician to create the desired size of ablation while the physician monitors the thermocouple temperatures on the generator screen. Once the temperature at the distal thermocouple reaches 50°C, the delivery of energy is stopped.
  - To further influence lesion size, the MetaSTAR RF generator has four different power settings: 3, 5, 7.5, and 10 W.
  - Once the ablation zone has been created, the SpineSTAR instrument can be repositioned under image guidance to create a larger lesion if desired.
  - Once the ablation has been completed, the electrode is retracted by turning the white knob counterclockwise.
  - The SpineSTAR instrument is then removed, with the working cannula left in place.
  - The stylet can be replaced, and the instrument can be removed if vertebral augmentation is not necessary. Otherwise, the physician can proceed with vertebral augmentation as described elsewhere in this text.

Kyphoplasty

After RF ablation of the tumor has been completed, vertebral augmentation utilizing vertebroplasty or kyphoplasty can follow. There are numerous advantages to vertebral augmentation after RF ablation. It can strengthen the vertebral body and restore height, enhancing spinal stability and preventing a pathological fracture induced by RF ablation. The delivery of cement can work synergistically with RF ablation to destroy sensory nerve fibers and increase pain relief. If vertebral augmentation is desired, the provider can proceed as described elsewhere in this text.

Postoperative Management and Follow-up

Patients should be observed and should maintain bedrest for 1 to 2 hours as deemed appropriate by the provider. During that time, routine vital signs as well as neurologic function should be monitored, with particular attention paid to the lower extremities. If there are any concerns about new deficits or decline in neurologic function, imaging and appropriate management are necessary.[33] Patients can often be discharged home the same day.

Complications and Management

The most common reported complication of STA is thermal nerve injury, which occurs in approximately 10% to 16% of cases.[34] In a case series of 10 patients reported by Nakatsuka et al, one patient experienced transient thermal nerve injury during RF ablation.[35] Symptoms resolved in 2 days after conservative care and intravenous administration of systemic steroids.

Posterior leakage of cement is a known complication. It is most concerning when cement migrates toward the neural foramen or spinal canal. Prevention is the first step, accomplished by delivering cement in a lateral view with attention to posterior leakage. If there is any concern about spread into the posterior third of the vertebral body, cement delivery should be stopped and images should be reviewed.

Vascular injury can occur directly via needle placement or indirectly though vascular uptake of cement. Extrapedicular approaches should be carefully considered, especially with a left-sided thoracolumbar approach, due to potential injury to radicular feeding arteries (particularly the artery of Adamkiewicz). Injury to radicular feeding arteries could cause interruption of blood supply to the anterior portion of the spinal cord, leading to irreversible infarct.

Pneumothorax or hemothorax is a risk when needle placement above the T12 vertebral body level is indicated. Maintaining the needle trajectory medial to the lateral border of the pedicle during a transpedicular approach can avoid this complication.

Conclusion

Spinal metastases are a common and serious source of pain and disability in patients with cancer. Conventional treatment with systemic analgesics and radiation therapy can be inadequate, intolerable, or otherwise infeasible. Spinal tumor ablation is a safe, effective, and efficient treatment option to reduce pain and restore function in this important patient population.

References

1. *Cancer Facts & Figures 2020*. American Cancer Society. https://www.cancer.org/content/dam/cancer-org/research/cancer-facts-and-statistics/annual-cancer-facts-and-figures/2020/cancer-facts-and-figures-2020.pdf.
2. Witham TF, Khavkin YA, Gallia GL, Wolinsky JP, Gokaslan ZL. Surgery insight: current management of epidural spinal cord compression from metastatic spine disease. *Nat Clin Pract Neurol*. 2006;2:87–94.
3. Klimo P Jr, Schmidt MH. Surgical management of spinal metastases. *Oncologist*. 2004;9:188–196.
4. Coleman RE. Clinical features of metastatic bone disease and risk of skeletal morbidity. *Clin Cancer Res*. 2006;12:6243s–6249s.
5. Kim JM, Losina E, Bono CM, et al. Clinical outcome of metastatic spinal cord compression treated with surgical excision ± radiation versus radiation therapy alone: a systematic review of literature. *Spine (Phila Pa 1976)*. 2012;37:78–84.
6. Tomasian A, Hillen TJ, Chang RO, Jennings JW. Simultaneous bipedicular radiofrequency ablation combined with vertebral augmentation for local tumor control of spinal metastases. *AJNR Am J Neuroradiol*. 2018;39:1768–1773.
7. Bayley A, Milosevic M, Blend R, et al. A prospective study of factors predicting clinically occult spinal cord compression in patients with metastatic prostate carcinoma. *Cancer*. 2001;92:303–310.
8. Dupuy DE, Liu D, Hartfeil D, et al. Percutaneous radiofrequency ablation of painful osseous metastases: a multicenter American College of Radiology Imaging Network trial. *Cancer*. 2010;116:989–997.
9. Agarawal JP, Swangsilpa T, van der Linden Y, Rades D, Jeremic B, Hoskin PJ. The role of external beam radiotherapy in the management of bone metastases. *Clin Oncol (R Coll Radiol)*. 2006;18:747–760.
10. Gerszten PC, Mendel E, Yamada Y. Radiotherapy and radiosurgery for metastatic spine disease: what are the options, indications, and outcomes? *Spine (Phila Pa 1976)*. 2009;34:S78–S92.
11. Masucci GL, Yu E, Ma L, et al. Stereotactic body radiotherapy is an effective treatment in reirradiating spinal metastases: current status and practical considerations for safe practice. *Expert Rev Anticancer Ther*. 2011;11:1923–1933.
12. Sahgal A, Whyne CM, Ma L, Larson DA, Fehlings MG. Vertebral compression fracture after stereotactic body radiotherapy for spinal metastases. *Lancet Oncol*. 2013;14:e310–e320.
13. Rybak LD. Fire and ice: thermal ablation of musculoskeletal tumors. *Radiol Clin North Am*. 2009;47:455–469.
14. Dupuy DE, Hong R, Oliver B, Goldberg SN. Radiofrequency ablation of spinal tumors: temperature distribution in the spinal canal. *AJR Am J Roentgenol*. 2000;175:1263–1266.
15. Hillen TJ, Anchala P, Friedman MV, Jennings JW. Treatment of metastatic posterior vertebral body osseous tumors by using a targeted bipolar radiofrequency ablation device: technical note. *Radiology*. 2014;273:261–267.
16. Cazzato RL, Auloge P, De Marini P, et al. Spinal tumor ablation: indications, techniques, and clinical management. *Tech Vasc Intervent Radiol*. 2020;23:100677.
17. Wallace AN, Robinson CG, Meyer J, et al. The Metastatic Spine Disease Multidisciplinary Working Group algorithms. *Oncologist*. 2015;20:1205–1215.
18. Burton AW, Fanciullo GJ, Beasley RD, Fisch MJ. Chronic pain in the cancer survivor: a new frontier. *Pain Med*. 2007;8:189–198.
19. Lopez-Olivo MA, Shah NA, Pratt G, Risser JM, Symanski E, Suarez-Almazor ME. Bisphosphonates in the treatment of patients with lung cancer and metastatic bone disease: a systematic review and meta-analysis. *Support Care Cancer*. 2012;20:2985–2998.
20. Yamane T, Tateishi A, Cho S, et al. The effects of hyperthermia on the spinal cord. *Spine (Phila Pa 1976)*. 1992;17:1386–1391.
21. Nour SG, Aschoff AJ, Mitchell IC, Emancipator SN, Duerk JL, Lewin JS. MR imaging-guided radiofrequency thermal ablation of the lumbar vertebrae in porcine models. *Radiology*. 2002;224:452–462.
22. Goetz MP, Callstrom MR, Charboneau JW, et al. Percutaneous image-guided radiofrequency ablation of painful metastases involving bone: a multicenter study. *J Clin Oncol*. 2004;22:300–306.

23. Anchala PR, Irving WD, Hillen TJ, et al. Treatment of metastatic spinal lesions with a navigational bipolar radiofrequency ablation device: a multicenter retrospective study. *Pain Physician.* 2014;17:317–327.
24. Wallace AN, Greenwood TJ, Jennings JW. Radiofrequency ablation and vertebral augmentation for palliation of painful spinal metastases. *J Neurooncol.* 2015;124:111–118.
25. Bagla S, Sayed D, Smirniotopoulos J, et al. Multicenter prospective clinical series evaluating radiofrequency ablation in the treatment of painful spine metastases. *Cardiovasc Intervent Radiol.* 2016;39:1289–1297.
26. Callstrom MR, Dupuy DE, Solomon SB, et al. Percutaneous image-guided cryoablation of painful metastases involving bone: multicenter trial. *Cancer.* 2013;119:1033–1041.
27. Gallusser N, Goetti P, Becce F, et al. Percutaneous image-guided cryoablation of painful bone metastases: a single institution experience. *Orthop Traumatol Surg Res.* 2019;105:369–374.
28. Skonieczki BD, Wells C, Wasser EJ, Dupuy DE. Radiofrequency and microwave tumor ablation in patients with implanted cardiac devices: is it safe? *Eur J Radiol.* 2011;79:343–346.
29. Deer TR, Provenzano DA, Hanes M, et al. The Neurostimulation Appropriateness Consensus Committee (NACC) recommendations for infection prevention and management. *Neuromodulation.* 2017;20:31–50.
30. *OsteoCool New Technology Reference Guide.* Medtronic.
31. *SpineSTAR Product Card.* Merit Medical.
32. Furman MB, ed. *Atlas of Image-Guided Spinal Procedures.* 2nd ed. Philadelphia, PA: Elsevier; 2018.

15

Basivertebral Nerve Ablation

Anthony Giuffrida and Benjamin D. Westerhaus

Introduction

The basivertebral nerve (BVN) and its role in chronic low back pain has been the subject of much clinical excitement in recent years. As the literature on the topic has swelled since it was first described, opportunities to intervene on this pain generator have greatly improved.

Embryology of the spinal column is a complex and tightly coordinated process that largely remains outside the scope of this chapter, but a cursory review of embryology of the spine is offered here to serve as a basis for understanding the anatomy of the BVN. First, it is important to recall that the development of the spinal column is a function of somites, which are each made up of a dermatomyotome and a sclerotome. The dermatomyotome becomes the overlying muscles and skin of the spine, and the sclerotome becomes the vertebral column. Around the fourth week of gestation, the sclerotomal cells migrate toward the notochord and neural tube to surround them. Once the notochord and neural tube are enveloped by sclerotomal cells, each level separates into a cranial section of loosely packed cells and a caudal section with densely packed cells, while the area in between is called a "cell-free space."[1] This cell-free space will develop into the intervertebral disk with cellular contributions from the densely packed sclerotomal cells that form the annulus fibrosus, while the notochord becomes the nucleus pulposus. Meanwhile, as the loosely packed cells fuse with the densely packed cells, they form the centrum and eventually the vertebral body.[1] Between these two layers, a neurovascular bundle enters and supplies the vertebral body; this bundle has several different names, including the basivertebral foramen (BVF), the nutrient canal, and Hahn's cleft.[2]

The sinuvertebral nerve was first described in 1850 by Hubert von Luschka of Germany. This nerve arises bilaterally from the ventral ramus of each spinal nerve just distal to the dorsal root ganglia and supplies both proprioceptive and nociceptive fibers. Upon separation from the ventral ramus, the nerve travels approximately 3 mm and

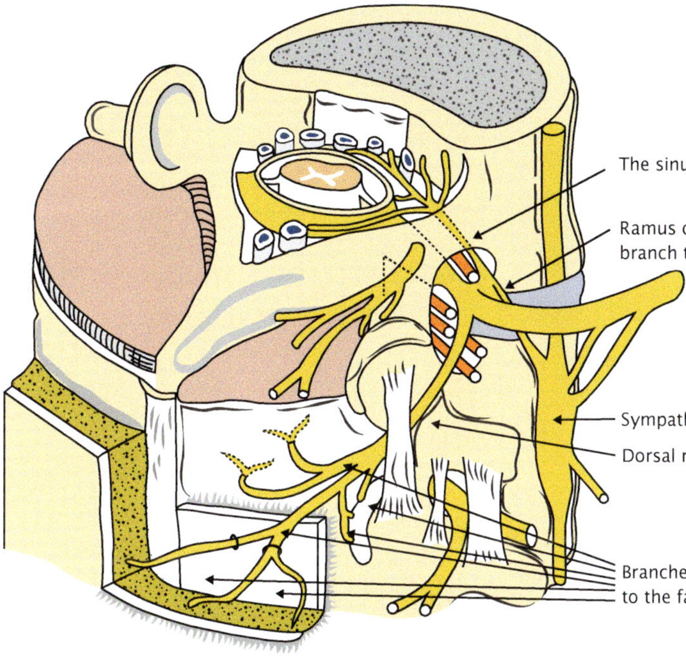

FIGURE 15.1. The separation of the nerve fibers from the ventral ramus joins with a branch of the gray ramus communicans, which contributes sympathetic neurons to the nerve fibers, at which point it then becomes the sinuvertebral nerve and starts as it completes its recurrent course back into the spinal canal.

is then joined by a branch of the gray ramus communicans, which contributes sympathetic neurons to the sinuvertebral nerve. The nerve then takes a recurrent course and reenters the spinal canal through the osteofibrous foramen formed by the deep anterior intraforaminal ligament located just caudal to the pedicle. Once in the midline, the fibers then dive into the posterior aspect of the vertebral body through the BVF and become the BVN (see Figures 15.1, 15.2 and 15.3).[3–10]

The transition from the sinuvertebral nerve to the BVN was first described in 1963 by Sherman, who observed a "large solitary nerve trunk" entering the vertebral body through a bony tunnel in the posterior cortex (now known as the BVF), with its entry at midline and slightly above equidistant from the superior and inferior endplate. Once in the BVF, the BVN traverses from posterior to anterior approximately 30% to 50% into the vertebral body (measuring posterior to anterior) into the vertebral body. At this point, the BVN bifurcates to the superior and inferior endplate. This bifurcation, or just proximal to it, is the target for the BVN ablative procedure. After the bifurcation, the nerve continues to arborize, culminating at the endplate/disk junction. The arborized nerve endings have been shown to have an increased density in regions of vertebral endplate microdamage.[3–10]

In the sacrum, and more importantly S1, the course of the sinuvertebral nerve into the vertebral body is slightly altered. At this level, a large plexus of nerves emanate from both the left and right anterior sacral nerves. These nerves penetrate the lateral border of S1 as they pass through their respective left and right anterior sacral foramen. They continue

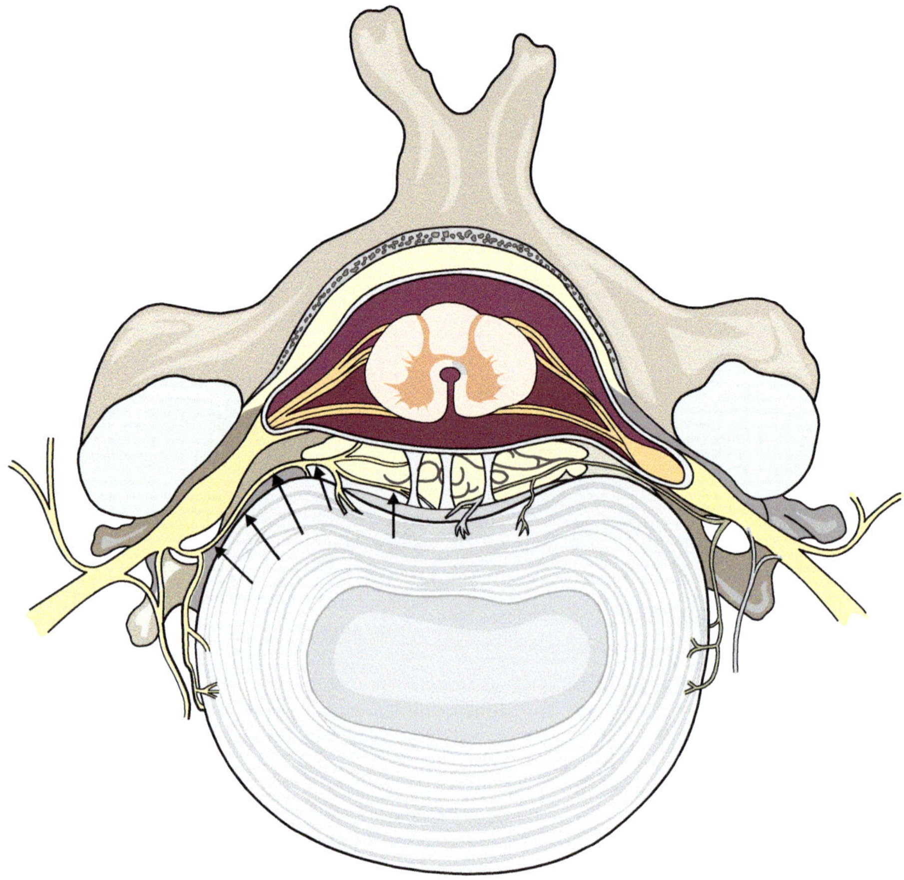

FIGURE 15.2. Axial view of the sinuvertebral nerve (indicated by black arrows) on its recurrent course into the spinal canal and crossing the midline.

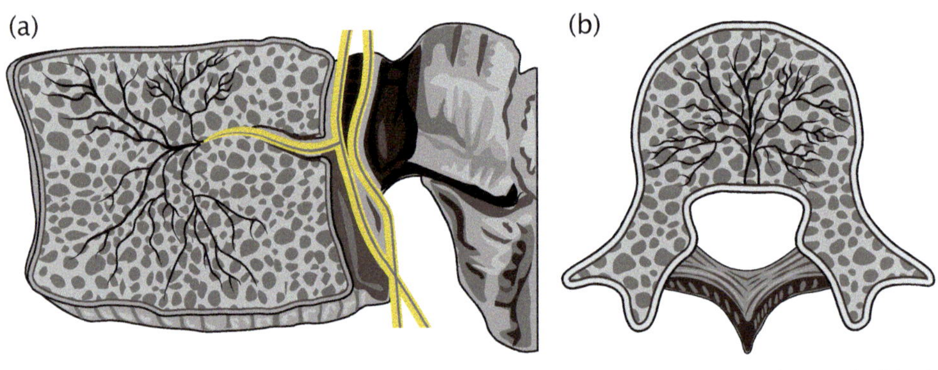

FIGURE 15.3. A, sagittal and, B, axial view of the sinuvertebral nerve as it enters the vertebral body through the basivertebral foramen, becoming the basivertebral nerve. Note that the basivertebral foramen is located slightly superior to the midline, between the superior and inferior endplate, and exactly midline in the axial view. Once it is approximately 30% to 50% from posterior to anterior, the basivertebral nerve splits cranially and caudally and begins to arborize to the superior and inferior endplates of the respective vertebral body.

toward the center, running just above the equator (25% to 40% down from the superior endplate at S1). This location will be the target for the ablation of the BVN at S1. Once the two sides converge, the nerves form a large cluster in the center of the vertebra, bifurcate, and arborize cranially and caudally to their respective endplates in a fashion similar to that seen in the lumbar vertebral bodies.[11] In both the lumbar and sacral vertebrae, the BVN loses its myelin sheath shortly after entering the VB vertebral body, which effectively prevents the nerve from regenerating with thermal or mechanical destruction.

Indications

It has long been known that degeneration of the vertebral endplate and intervertebral disk complex is a common cause of low back pain (LBP). The native, healthy disk is avascular and aneural, excluding some small nerves and blood vessels surrounding the periphery of the annulus.[12,13] The adjacent endplate and vertebral bodies, however, are highly vascularized and innervated. It is these vessels that supply most of the disk with the necessary nutrition to maintain healthy cells in the nucleus pulposus.[14–16] As the disk degenerates, the vertebral endplate also starts to degenerate, causing fissuring and microfractures within the endplate.[17] Microscopic studies have shown that with an increase in endplate degeneration, there is an upregulation of nerve fibers, giving evidence that endplate damage is a significant source of LBP. The density of pain fibers was compared between normal endplates and damaged endplates, and it was noted that the density of the BVN is significantly higher in patients with degenerated endplates.[18,19] This is consistent with the understanding of "nerve sprouting" as a response to nonhealed fractures, as described by Chartier et al, who examined the nerve structures of nonhealed fractures and noted exuberant sensory and sympathetic nerve sprouting, an increase in density of nerve fibers, and formation of neuroma-like structures near fracture sites.[20] The nociceptive nature of these nerves was established by immunohistochemical analysis that showed the nerves contain substance P, CGRP Calcitonin gene-related peptide, and PGP P-glycoprotein 9.5.[21–23] This concept was further supported by imaging studies correlating endplate abnormalities with pain.[24] This understanding built upon previously described and well-established research regarding Modic changes on MRI, which are signs of inflammation and edema.[25] Furthermore, intraoperative reports have described that the endplate is painful when touched, and clinical data have demonstrated that back pain resolves after the destruction of the BVN and its branches during vertebral augmentation procedures.[26–28]

Because Modic changes on MRI represent the pathophysiology of the degenerative endplates, which is fundamental to the rationale for BVN ablation, their definitions are briefly discussed here. Modic first described changes in the vertebral body marrow seen on MRI in 1988.[25] He and his colleagues reviewed 474 consecutive MRIs of the lumbar spine and described two types of changes, seen in 4% and 16% of patients, respectively. In type I changes, the vertebral marrow had decreased signal on T1 and increased signal on T2, whereas in type II changes, the marrow showed increased signal on T1 and T2 images. Since that first description, a third type of Modic change, type III, has been described that is isointense or has decreased intensity on T1 and decreased intensity on T2. Type

I Modic changes represent active inflammation, whereas type II Modic changes represent fatty marrow infiltration, an indicator of subacute to chronic inflammation.[25]

The microbiological cellular mechanisms of injury that manifest as Modic changes have been studied by many researchers. As with most inflammation, cytokines play an important role. The disk adjacent to Modic changes has been shown to produce higher amounts of cytokines and osteoclastic factors than are produced by disks without adjacent Modic changes.[29,30] As osteoclasts increase, so does bone absorption, which can alter or weaken the trabecular bone of the vertebral body. Another proposed mechanism is Toll-like receptor (TLR) stimulation of the disk and marrow cells, which leads to enhanced transcription of NF-κB, which is a pathway involved in osteoarthritis and degenerative disk disease. TLRs can also induce hypertrophy of adipocytes within the vertebral body, further compromising its integrity.[31,32]

The typical patient who requires BVN ablation will present with axial chronic low back pain (CLBP) caused by degenerative endplate changes that manifest on MRI as Modic changes. In order for the back pain to be considered chronic and for the patient to be a candidate for the procedure, the patient must have experienced the pain for more than 6 months, must have failed to respond to 6 months of conservative therapy, and must have degenerative endplate changes seen on MRI in at least one vertebral endplate at one or more levels from L3 to S1. The patient's pain will usually worsen with activities, such as bending forward, running, twisting, and lifting items off the ground. The pain can be relieved with lying flat and resting. The pain must originate from degenerative endplate changes and not be radicular. Originally, the indications for BVN ablation included only patients with Modic type I or type II changes, but they have expanded to include endplates that demonstrate inflammation; edema; vertebral endplate changes; disruption and fissuring of the endplate; vascularized fibrous tissues within the adjacent marrow; hypointense signals in, and changes to, the vertebral body marrow, including replacement of normal bone marrow by fat; and hyperintense signals.

Evidence

The evidence for BVN ablation is robust and is supported by two Level 1 randomized clinical trials (RCTs). Both the SMART trial and the Intracept study demonstrated statistically and clinically significant results compared to both standard care and a sham procedure. There was consistent improvement in both pain and function across both trials, and patients had durable results more than 5 years after their procedure.

In 2017, Becker et al published the first results of BVN ablation; their study was a single-arm, open-label, first-in-humans pilot study that sought to establish the efficacy and safety of the procedure in patients with CLBP.[33] The study enrolled 17 patients with > 6 months of LBP and with type I or type II Modic changes on MRI. Discography was performed to establish the level of pathology, and radiofrequency (RF) was used to ablate the BVN in the vertebral bodies adjacent to the disk. Sixteen patients were successfully treated with the described method. Oswestry Disability Index (ODI) and Visual Analog Scale

(VAS) scores were obtained at baseline and at 3 months. A statistically significant reduction of ODI (by an average of 29 points) was achieved at 3-month follow-up. The improvement in ODI persisted through 12-month follow-up, and statistically significant improvements were noted in all outcome measures at 3 months.[33]

The first Level 1 RCT, the Surgical Multi-center Assessment of RF Ablation for the Treatment of Vertebrogenic Back Pain (SMART trial), was designed to evaluate the safety and effectiveness of BVN ablation, in a Food and Drug Administration approved Investigational Device Exemption (IDE) trial. The study was a randomized, double-blind, sham-controlled trial conducted at 18 centers (15 in the United States and 3 in Europe), and 225 patients were enrolled, with 147 randomized to the treatment arm, while 78 received a sham procedure that consisted of docking on the pedicle without accessing the BVN or ablation. The patients were regularly evaluated postoperatively at 2 and 6 weeks and 3, 6, 12, and 24 months using the ODI, Short Form 36 (SF-36), and VAS. All patients were skeletally mature individuals with chronic (≥ 6 months), isolated axial lumbar pain who had not responded to at least 6 months of nonoperative management, and all patients had type I or II Modic changes in up to three vertebral bodies between L3 and S1.[28]

Initial results at 24 months showed clinical improvements in the ODI, VAS, and the Medical Outcomes Trust Short-Form Health Survey Physical Component Summary that were statistically significant compared to baseline. The mean percentage improvements in ODI and VAS compared to baseline at 2 years were 53.7% and 52.9%, respectively. Responder rates for ODI and VAS were sustained at 2 years, with patients showing clinically meaningful improvements in both, with ODI ≥ 10-point improvement in 76.4% of patients and ODI ≥ 20-point improvement in 57.5%, as well as VAS ≥ 1.5-point improvement in 70.2% of patients.[28]

The SMART trial was then continued to 5 years, with the results showing that of the 117 US-treated patients, 100 (85%) were available to follow-up within a mean time of 6.4 years since procedure (5.4–7.8 years). In this group, the mean ODI score showed a reduction of 25.95 points, from 42.81 to 16.86 ($P < .001$). Mean reduction in VAS pain score was 4.38 points from a baseline 6.74 ($P < .001$). Overall, 66% of patients reported a greater than 50% reduction in pain, 47% reported a greater than 75% reduction in pain, and 34% of patients reported 100% pain reduction. This study concluded that BVN ablation is a durable, minimally invasive treatment for vertebrogenic CLBP.[28,34,35]

The second Level 1 RCT, the Intracept study, aimed to compare the effectiveness of the BVN ablation to standard care for the treatment of vertebrogenic CLBP. The study design was prospective, randomized, and multicenter (across 20 sites), with 104 patients randomized to two groups. The Intracept group included 51 patients who received the ablation, and the standard care group included 53 patients who received conservative care measures for axial LBP. Patients were evaluated at baseline and at 3, 6, 9, and 12 months after treatment using VAS and ODI scores. Baseline ODI was 46.1, VAS was 6.67, and mean patient age was 50 years. Inclusion criteria were skeletally mature patients with LBP ≥ 6 months who had not responded to at least 6 months of conservative care, and all patients had type I or type II Modic changes in up to 4 vertebral bodies between L3 and S1.[36]

Early results in the study (3 months) showed clear statistical superiority ($P < .001$) in the RF ablation arm compared with the standard care arm. These early results prompted a data management committee recommendation to halt enrollment in the study and to offer early crossover to the control arm after 3 months. Therefore, the primary endpoint was moved to 3 months. At the time the study was halted, the mean decrease in ODI was 25.3 points in the procedure arm versus 4.4 points the conservative care arm. The mean decrease in VAS was 3.46 in the procedure arm versus 1.02 in the conservative care arm. Of note in the BVN ablation arm, 74.5% of patients achieved a ≥ 10-point improvement in ODI, compared with 32.7% in the standard care arm ($P < .001$). The study concluded that BVN ablation led to significant improvement of pain and function at 3 months in patients with vertebrogenic CLBP.[36]

Adding to the evidence was a case series published by Truumees et al that examined the effectiveness of the BVN ablation procedure in a prospective, single-arm, multicenter, open-label fashion.[39] This series had more liberal inclusion criteria that were more representative of typical CLBP patients, including prior discectomy and current use of opioids. The primary outcome for the series was patient-reported change in ODI at 3 months after the procedure. Secondary outcomes included change in VAS, SF-36, and EQ-5D-5L scores and responder rates. The 28 patients enrolled in the study had LBP symptoms for > 5 years, and 25% were actively using opioids, while 61% had been previously treated with injections. At the 3-month primary endpoint, there were clinically and statistically significant improvements demonstrated in all outcome measures. ODI improvement at 3 months was a decrease of 30 ± 14.5 points, and mean improvement in VAS was a decrease of 3.50 ± 2.33 points. When the minimal clinically important difference of ≥ 10-point improvement in ODI was considered, 93% of patients were responders; and when criteria were tightened to ≥ 20-point improvement in ODI, 75% of patients were responders. It was also noted that in this patient population, which included working-age individuals (mean age of 45), 83% subjectively reported improved work function. This nonrandomized, consecutive series of 28 patients with vertebrogenic CLBP showed that RF ablation of the BVN significantly improved pain and function at 3-month endpoints.[37]

Finally, Markman et al recently added to the growing body of evidence with a useful study that specifically looked at opioid use and its correlation with BVN ablation success as determined by patient-reported outcomes.[38] The data were derived from secondary analysis of the SMART trial (with 225 patients randomized 2:1 to treatment versus sham groups, in a double-blind fashion). Two external reviewers, blinded to patient outcomes and study arms, determined if patient opioid use had "increased" (> 10 morphine milligram equivalent [MME] increase), had "decreased" (> 10 MME decrease), or was "unchanged." Opioid change was correlated with ODI and VAS scores. Patients who received the BVN ablation and who decreased their opioid use had significantly improved ODI and VAS scores (24.9 ± 16.0 and 3.3 ± 2.5, respectively), in contrast to patients who increased their opioid use after the procedure (7.3 ± 9.8 and 0.6 ± 1.8, respectively).[38] Although the results may seem subtle nuanced, the study underscores a paramount goal of pain management today: namely, a treatment option that leads to improvements in ODI and VAS scores combined with decreased opioid use.

In all the studies, there were no device- or procedure-related patient deaths, no unanticipated adverse device effects, and no device-related serious adverse events.[28,36]

One limitation of all the Level 1 RCTs is their industry funding sources, which could be a source of bias in the available data reviewed. The limited number of studies and their inherent short-term follow-up for most of the patients to date are other potential limitations of the evidence. Finally, the effect of the RF energy on the primary degenerative process is unknown.[39] These are relatively common limitations of studies of novel devices or procedures.

Patient Selection

There are many different possible sources of CLBP, but the main sources are the muscles, fascial structures, vertebral endplates, nerve roots, facet joints, and intervertebral disks. This discussion focuses on correct diagnosis of CLBP caused by irritation of the sinuverterbal/basivertebral nerve due to degeneration of the complex vertebral endplate/disk junction.[40,41]

The diagnostic evaluation of patients with CLBP can be very challenging and requires complex clinical decision-making. However, the correct identification of the source of the patient's pain is paramount in providing a therapeutic plan and providing pain relief. The physician's first job is to get a thorough history of the patient's pain. This must include the pain's onset, duration, location, characterization, severity, and alleviating and aggravating factors, as well as whether the pain radiates. Next, a full-body and comprehensive physical exam must be performed, which will also help pinpoint the patient's pain generator. Furthermore, the physician may need to order x-rays and advanced imaging, such as MRI and/or CT scans.[42,43]

All the information from the history, exam, and imaging can be used to identify which patients will benefit from ablation of the basivertebral/sinuvertebral nerve. First, pain from an irritated endplate is purely axial and somatic; therefore, patients with mainly radicular pain and/or neurogenic claudication can be ruled out. In brief, radicular pain is pain that radiates from the back into the leg in a dermatomal distribution and can cause weakness in a myotome congruent with the impinged nerve root. Disk herniation is the most common cause, and inflammation or compression of the adjacent nerve is the most common pathophysiological process. Neurogenic claudication is caused by lumbar spinal stenosis due to venous congestion and hypertension around the lumbar nerve roots. The pain is exacerbated by lumbar extension and is relieved by lumbar flexion.

Next to be considered are the CLBP generators that most commonly cause axial pain. The main culprits are facet joint syndrome, sacroiliac joint (SIJ) pain, discogenic pain, and the focus of this chapter, vertebrogenic pain. Although vertebrogenic pain is not a diagnosis by exclusion, the other causes of axial back pain are discussed briefly to distinguish them from each other.

Facet Joint Syndrome

Pain from facet joint syndrome is nonradicular and tends to be off-center. Unlike vertebrogenic pain, facetogenic pain increases with hyperextension, rotation, lateral bending, and walking uphill.[45,46] Facetogenic pain is also more prevalent in the elderly, whereas vertebrogenic pain is more likely in patients age 35 to 65.

Lumbar x-rays are very helpful in ruling in or ruling out facet joint syndrome.[45] Dynamic x-rays (flexion/extension views) are particularly valuable because they may show column instability (spondylolisthesis), which causes an overloaded and painful facet joint. It is challenging to diagnose lumbar facet syndrome using advanced radiologic images since there are no pathognomonic findings. On MRI, there are nonspecific signs of osteophyte formation, fluid in the joint, and hypertrophy of the joint complex. CT is the preferred imaging modality due to an increased clarity of the osseous structures. The final diagnosis can be made by performing medial branch blocks or facet joint injections. A finding is considered positive if the patient gets > 80% relief after two separate injections.[46,47]

SIJ Pain

The SIJ is another leading source of pain in many patients who present with CLBP. During the physical examination, it is important to examine the patient for pain with movement of this joint. The pain is normally located over the buttocks just lateral to the sacrum and may radiate down the leg, but rarely below the knee.[48] There are many SIJ provocative tests, which are not discussed in this chapter, and unfortunately SIJ provocative tests in isolation have been show to lack sensitivity and specificity (positive SIJ provocative testing in 3 of 5 tests increases specificity drastically). In most patients, advanced imaging will do little to help guide the diagnosis, but if a rheumatologic cause of the patient's pain is suspected, one could consider an MRI to look for articular effusion and inflammation. To further rule in/out the SIJ as the source of the patient's LBP, an SIJ diagnostic injection can be performed to see if the patient receives substantial (> 50%) relief.[48,49]

After facet joint syndrome and SIJ pain are ruled out, the causes of axial CLBP that are left are discogenic and vertebrogenic causes. Differentiating between the two can be difficult, but there are some subtle distinctions that will help with the diagnosis.

Discogenic versus Vertebrogenic Pain

Vertebrogenic and discogenic back pain have been estimated to account for 39% of CLBP.[30] Discogenic pain is caused by the degradation of the vertebral disk, with dehydration of the nucleus pulposus and accompanying radial/concentric fissures in the surrounding annulus fibrosus. Vertebrogenic pain is caused by the degeneration of the smooth endplate adjacent to the disk that serves as the nutrient-porous barrier between the disk and the vertebral body. Vertebrogenic pain is what is carried by the fibers of the BVN, which is the target of the ablation.

Both etiologies will present with central axial pain that radiates across the lumbar region. During physical exam, the patient may have increased pain with forward flexion, especially while seated. Pain is most severe when the patient tries to lift weight from the floor while in a seated position. Pain may be relieved with extension.

The main difference between the etiologies is seen with advanced imaging, mainly MRI. With vertebrogenic pain, changes in the endplates, such as invaginations, and edema in the vertebral bodies (Modic type I-II) can be seen (see Figure 15.4). In patients with isolated discogenic pain, the endplate will still be intact, but there can be a high-intensity zone (HIZ) within the annulus of the disk (see Figure 15.5).

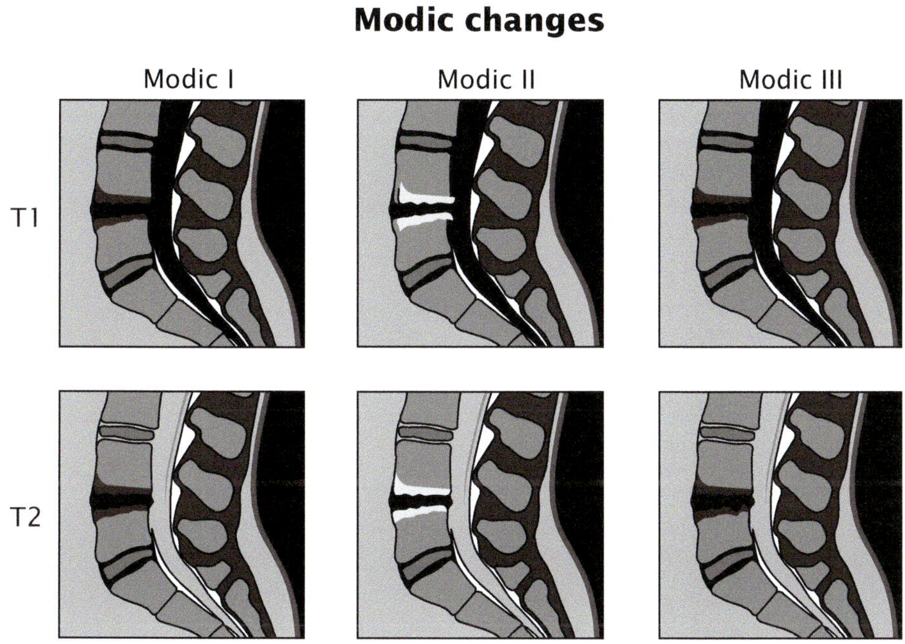

FIGURE 15.4. Representation of how Modic changes present on T1- and T2-weighted MRI. Modic type I change will be dark on T1 and bright on T2. Modic type II change will be bright on both T1 and T2. Modic type III change will be dark on both T1 and T2.

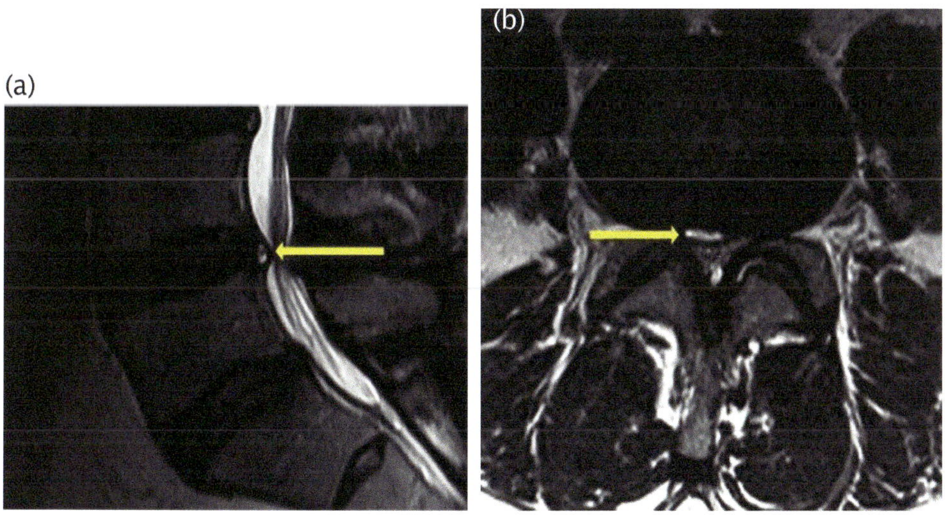

FIGURE 15.5. The presence of a high-intensity zone (HIZ) within the annulus of the disk, as indicated by the yellow arrow on MRI T2-weighted images in both (A) lateral and (B) axial views.

In conclusion, if a patient presents with axial CLBP without radicular symptoms, the facet joint and the SIJ have been ruled out as the pain generator, and the patient has degenerative endplate changes on MRI, it would be prudent to consider BVN ablation as the next course of action to help alleviate the patient's debilitating pain.

Contraindications

BVN ablation is contraindicated in:

- Patients with severe cardiac or pulmonary compromise
- Patients in whom the targeted ablation zone is < 10 mm away from a sensitive structure not intended to be ablated, including the vertebral foramen (spinal canal)
- Patients with active systemic infection or local infection in the area to be treated
- Patients who are pregnant
- Skeletally immature patients (generally < 18 years old)
- Patients with implantable pulse generators (e.g., pacemakers, defibrillators) or other electronic implants
- Situations where unintended tissue damage may result, based on the clinical assessment by the physician

Perioperative Management

Currently, there is no consensus on perioperative management for the BVN ablation procedure, but most physicians practice patient management similar to what they do with any other minimally invasive spine procedure.

Preoperatively, the physician should obtain blood tests to rule out any infections, profound anemia, or metabolic disorders that may prevent the patient from having a safe minimally invasive outpatient procedure. It is also imperative to follow American Society of Regional Anesthesia and Pain Medicine (ASRA) guidelines for discontinuing anticoagulants.

Perioperatively, patients should receive IV antibiotics, but there is no need to give a postoperative course of antibiotics. Based on the patient's comorbidities, the ablation procedure is done under general anesthesia, monitored anesthesia care (MAC), or, less likely, conscious sedation. Most procedures performed to date have been initiated under MAC sedation. Assume that the procedure will take roughly 30 minutes per vertebral level being treated. There is no concrete need for neuromonitoring, so its use is left to the physician's judgment.

Technique

The procedure is performed unilaterally with the patient in a prone position. The patient is placed under either general anesthesia or conscious sedation. Using fluoroscopy and standard anatomic landmarks, the location of the entry pedicle is determined and marked.

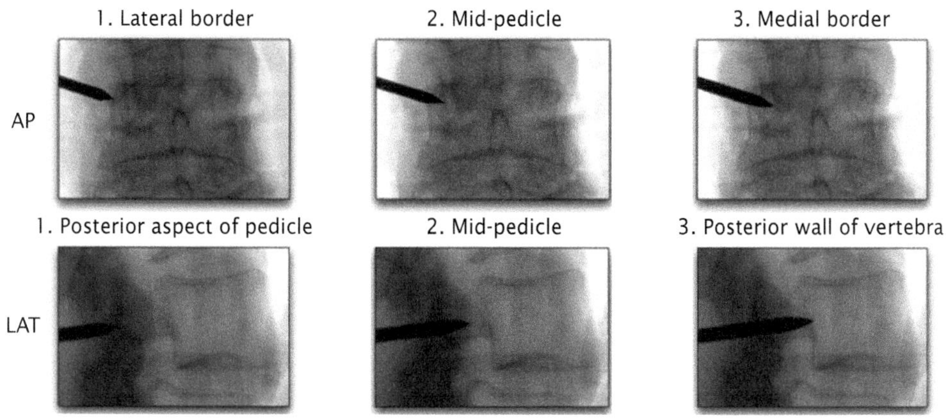

FIGURE 15.6. AP and lateral fluoroscopic images during safe descent and traverse through the pedicle. Note that the starting position is in the superolateral aspect of the pedicle, heading in an inferior medial direction.

Note that a single C-arm or a biplaner approach can be used. Because the procedure requires multiple AP and lateral images, for the sake of saving time, biplaner imaging may be preferred. To begin the procedure, the skin is anesthetized and a small puncture is made with a scalpel. The introducer cannula is advanced and docked on the superolateral aspect of the pedicle. Once proper positioning on the posterior aspect of the pedicle is confirmed in both AP and lateral views, the trocar is slowly descended through the pedicle until the trocar just breaches the posterior vertebral wall. The descent through the pedicle is made from superior lateral to inferior medial in order to obtain an optimal starting position for the curved cannula (Figure 15.6). The introducer trocar is replaced by a smaller plastic cannula/curved nitinol stylet assembly. This curved cutting tool facilitates the creation of a curved path from the posterior wall to the predetermined target located at the terminus of the BVN. The endpoint of the channel is in the midline of the vertebral body in the AP view and between 25% to 40% posterior to lateral in the lateral view (Figure 15.7). Finally, the curved nitinol stylet is removed, and the RF probe is introduced into the created channel

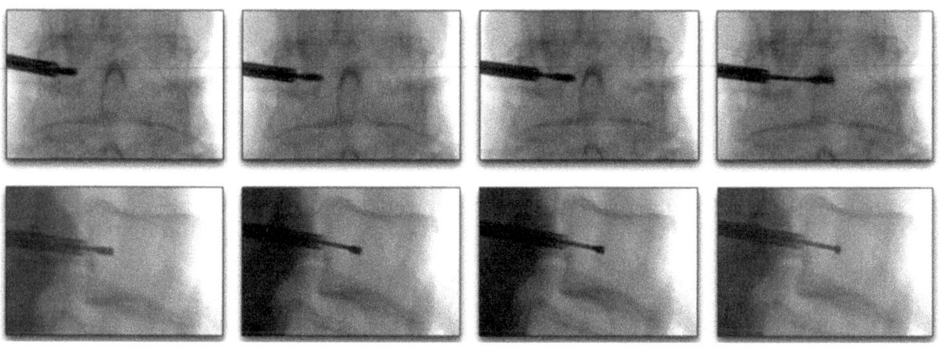

FIGURE 15.7. AP and lateral views of the meticulous advancement of the curved stylet. The final placement is shown in the right-most images, with the stylet ending at the midline in the AP view and 25% to 40% between the posterior and anterior walls in the lateral view.

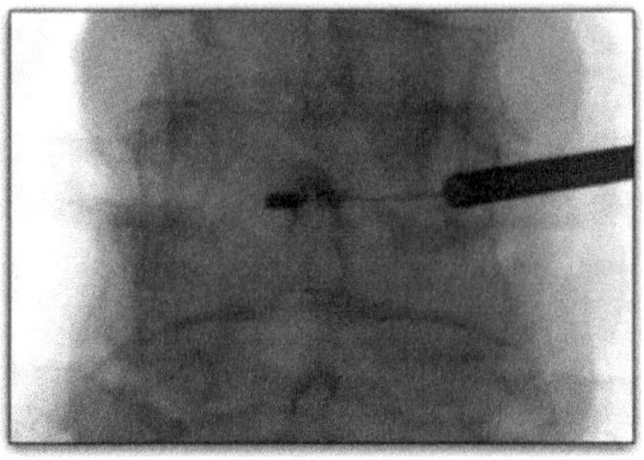

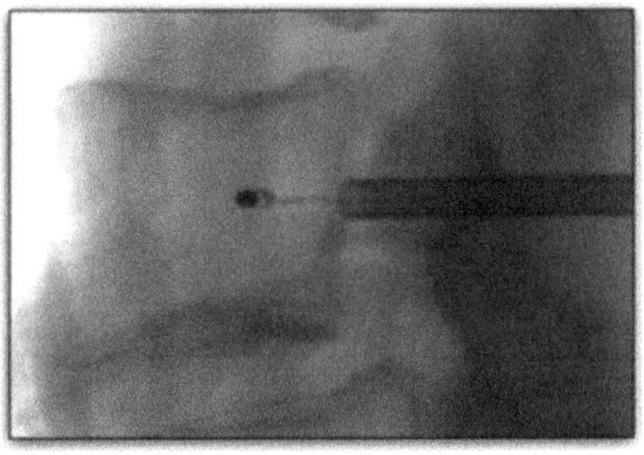

FIGURE 15.8. The final position of the radiofrequency probe within the created curved channel. Once this position has been obtained and confirmed, ablation can commence.

and positioned at the terminus of the BVN. Once the position of the probe is confirmed in both the AP and lateral views (Figure 15.8), the wire is connected to the RF generator. Last, the bipolar RF probe is activated, and the temperature at the tip is maintained at a constant 85°C for 7 or 15 minutes, in order to create an approximately 1-cm spherical lesion within the vertebral body at the site of the BVN. Once the 15 minutes prescribed time have passed, the RF probe is removed, the straight and curved cannulas are removed, and the patient is ready for postoperative management.[28]

Postoperative Management and Follow-up

Postoperatively, the puncture site(s) usually does not require sutures and/or staples for closure. The puncture site can be secured with Steri-Strips and a pressure dressing to ensure there is no bleeding or oozing from the site. If there has been no bleeding through the dressing, the patient may remove the bandage after 48 hours and replace it with a simple Band Aid. The patient is not to submerge in water for 48 hours after the procedure. Also, it is not required, but some physicians may instruct the patient to avoid bending, twisting, or lifting items weighing more than 15 pounds until the follow-up 7 to 10 days postoperatively.

At the postoperative visit, the puncture site should be checked for any signs of infection. The site is normally closed, if not healed completely, by this time. If there is any concern about infection, the site should be cultured and redressed with antibiotic ointment and occlusive dressing. If the patient has any signs of systemic infection, empiric oral antibiotics should be initiated immediately, and the patient should be monitored closely. If there are no adverse effects found at the postoperative visit, the patient may return to full activity (if there were any restrictions) and may begin the process of strengthening their lumbar spine now that they are likely pain free. Of note, it may take up to 6 weeks for the patient to feel the full relief from the BVN ablation. Full return to activity is always based on physician discretion.

Complications and Management

Clinical Study Safety Reporting Safety data have been collected for 473 patients treated with BVN ablation. In the 473 patients, one serious device- or procedure-related event was reported, and 25 nonserious device- or procedure-related events were reported. The one serious event was a vertebral compression fracture in a patient with osteoporosis that was treated successfully with vertebral augmentation, which resolved the issue. The nonserious events were related to postoperative acute radiculitis. The exact etiology of the radiculitis is unknown. Patients were treated with oral steroids and most recovered within 7 to 14 days, with the longest period being 62 days.

During commercial use of BVN ablation, there were two reported medical device- or procedure-related events. One vertebral fracture was noted on MRI at 2 months after the procedure. Once again, the patient was treated with vertebral augmentation and the event resolved without further sequelae. Also, there was one report of a retroperitoneal hematoma at L5 due to the introducer's being advanced superolaterally to the pedicle target. The patient was treated with transfusion and the event resolved without further sequelae.

Conclusion

RF ablation of the BVN is a relatively new minimally invasive procedure for relief of vertebrogenic CLBP diagnosed using clinical and radiologic findings. BVN ablation is supported by a growing body of literature that includes Level 1 evidence from two RCTs. The evidence demonstrates a statistically and clinically significant durable improvement in pain and function, with studies showing relief lasting more than 5 years. Treating CLBP has been proven to be one of the most challenging and one of the most expensive endeavors in the world of interventional pain management. The studies and outcomes presented in this chapter show very promising evidence that BVN ablation can provide an integral treatment modality in the algorithm of axial LBP management.

References

1. Kaplan KM, Spivak JM, Bendo JA. Embryology of the spine and associated congenital abnormalities. *Spine J*. 2005;5(5):564–576. doi:10.1016/j.spinee.2004.10.044.
2. Lotz JC, Fields AJ, Liebenberg EC. The role of the vertebral end plate in low back pain. *Global Spine J*. 2013 Jun;3(3):153–63.
3. Bailey JF, Liebenberg E, Degmetich S, Lotz JC. Innervation patterns of PGP 9.5-positive nerve fibers within the human lumbar vertebra. *J Anat*. 2011;218(3):263–270. doi:10.1111/j.1469-7580.2010.01332.x.
4. Bogduk N. The innervation of the lumbar spine. *Spine (Phila Pa 1976)*. 1983;8:286–293.
5. Edgar MA. The nerve supply of the lumbar intervertebral disc. *J Bone Joint Surg Br*. 2007;89:1135–1139.
6. Bogduk N, Tynan W, Wilson AS. The nerve supply to the human lumbar intervertebral discs. *J Anat*. 1981;132:39–56.
7. Adams MA, Dolan P. Intervertebral disc degeneration: evidence for two distinct phenotypes. *J Anat*. 2012. 221(6): 497–506.
8. Bogduk N, Windsor M, Inglis A. The innervation of the cervical intervertebral discs. *Spine (Phila Pa 1976)*. 1988;13:2–8.

9. Bailey JF, Liebenberg E, Degmetich S, Lotz JC. Innervation patterns of PGP 9.5-positive nerve fibers within the human lumbar vertebra. *J Anat*. 2011;218(3):263–270. doi:10.1111/j.1469-7580.2010.01332.x.
10. Kojima Y, Maeda T, Arai R, Shichikawa K. Nerve supply to the posterior longitudinal ligament and the intervertebral disc of the rat vertebral column as studied by acetylcholinesterase histochemistry. II. Regional differences in the distribution of the nerve fibres and their origins. *J Anat*. 1990;169:247–255.
11. Groen GJ, Baljet B, Drukker J. The innervation of the spinal dura mater: anatomy and clinical implications. *Acta Neurochir (Wien)*. 1988;92:39–46.
12. Shayota B, Wong TL, Fru D, et al. A comprehensive review of the sinuvertebral nerve with clinical applications. *Anat Cell Biol*. 2019;52(2):128–133. doi:10.5115/acb.2019.52.2.128.
13. Degmetich S, Bailey JF, Liebenberg E, Lotz JC. Neural innervation patterns in the sacral vertebral body. *Eur Spine J*. 2016;25(6):1932–1938. doi:10.1007/s00586-015-4037-4.
14. Malinsky J. The ontogenetic development of nerve terminations in the intervertebral discs of man. (Histology of intervertebral discs, 11th communication.) *Acta Anat (Basel)*. 1959;38:96–113
15. Humzah MD, Soames RW. Human intervertebral disc: structure and function. *Anat Rec*. 1988;220:337–356.
16. Urban JP, Smith S, Fairbank JC. Nutrition of the intervertebral disc. *Spine (Phila Pa 1976)*. 2004;29(23):2700–2709. doi:10.1097/01.brs.0000146499.97948.52. PMID:15564919.
17. Holm S, Maroudas A, Urban JP, Selstam G, Nachemson A. Nutrition of the intervertebral disc: solute transport and metabolism. *Connect Tissue Res*. 1981;8(2):101–119. doi:10.3109/03008208109152130. PMID: 6453689.
18. Ogata K, Whiteside LA. Nutritional pathways of the intervertebral disc. An experimental study using hydrogen washout technique. 1980 Volvo Award winner in basic science. *Spine (Phila Pa 1976)*. 1981;6(3):211–216. PMID:7268543.
19. Antonacci MD, Hanson DS, Leblanc A, et al. Regional variation in vertebral bone density and trabecular architecture are influenced by osteoarthritic change and osteoporosis. *Spine (Phila Pa 1976)*. 1997;22:2393–2401
20. Freemont AJ, Watkins A, Le Maitre C, et al. Nerve growth factor expression and innervation of the painful intervertebral disc. *J Pathol*. 2002;197:286–292.
21. Brown MF, Hukkanen MV, McCarthy ID, et al. Sensory and sympathetic innervation of the vertebral endplate in patients with degenerative disc disease. *J Bone Joint Surg Br*. 1997;79:147–153.
22. Chartier S, Thompson M, Longo G, et al. Exuberant sprouting of sensory and sympathetic nerve fibers in nonhealed bone fractures and the generation and maintenance of chronic skeletal pain. *Pain*. 2014;155(11):2323–2336.
23. Fagan A, Moore R, Vernon Roberts B, Blumbergs P, Fraser R. ISSLS prize winner: the innervation of the intervertebral disc: a quantitative analysis. *Spine (Phila Pa 1976)*. 2003;28(23):2570–2576.
24. Bailey JF, Liebenberg E, Degmetich S, Lotz JC. Innervation patterns of PGP 9.5-positive nerve fibers within the human lumbar vertebra. *J Anat*. 2011;218(3):263–270
25. Fras C, Kravetz P, Mody DR, Heggeness MH. Substance P-containing nerves within the human vertebral body: an immunohistochemical study of the basivertebral nerve. *Spine J*. 2003;3(1):63–67.
26. Weishaupt D, Zanetti M, Hodler J, et al. Painful lumbar disk derangement: relevance of endplate abnormalities at MR imaging. *Radiology*. 2001;218:420–427.
27. Modic MT, Masaryk TJ, Ross JS, Carter JR. Imaging of degenerative disk disease. *Radiology*. 1988;168(1):177–186.
28. Kuslich SD, Ulstrom CL, Michael CJ. The tissue origin of low back pain and sciatica: a report of pain response to tissue stimulation during operations on the lumbar spine using local anesthesia. *Orthop Clin North Am*. 1991;22:181–187.
29. Niv D, Gofeld M, Devor M. Causes of pain in degenerative bone and joint disease: a lesson from vertebroplasty. *Pain*. 2003; 105(3): 387–92.
30. Fischgrund JS, Rhyne A, Franke J, et al. Intraosseous basivertebral nerve ablation for the treatment of chronic low back pain: a prospective randomized double-blind sham-controlled multi-center study. *Eur Spine J*. 2018;27(5):1146–1156.
31. Dudli S, Fields AJ, Samartzis D, Karppinen J, Lotz JC. Pathobiology of Modic changes. *Eur Spine J*. 2016;25(11):3723–3734.

32. Torkki M, Majuri M-L, Wolff H, et al. Osteoclast activators are elevated in intervertebral disks with Modic changes among patients operated for herniated nucleus pulposus. *Eur Spine J.* 2016;25(1):207–216.
33. Thomas GPL, Hemmrich K, Abberton KM, et al. Zymosan-induced inflammation stimulates neo-adipogenesis. *Int J Obes (Lond).* 2008;32(2):239–248.
34. Monden M, Koyama H, Otsuka Y, et al. Receptor for advanced glycation end products regulates adipocyte hypertrophy and insulin sensitivity in mice: involvement of Toll-like receptor 2. *Diabetes.* 2013;62(2):478–489.
35. Becker S, Hadjipavlou A, Heggeness MH. Ablation of the basivertebral nerve for treatment of back pain: a clinical study. *Spine J.* 2017;17:218–223.
36. Fischgrund JS, Rhyne A, Franke J, et al. Intraosseous basivertebral nerve ablation for the treatment of chronic low back pain: 2-year results from a prospective randomized double-blind sham-controlled multicenter study. *Int J Spine Surg.* 2019;13(2):1–10.
37. Fischgrund JS, Rhyne A, Macadaeg K, et al. Long-term outcomes following intraosseous basivertebral nerve ablation for the treatment of chronic low back pain: 5-year treatment arm results from a prospective randomized double-blind sham-controlled multi-center study. *Eur Spine J.* 2020;29(8):1925–1934.
38. Khalil J, Smuck M, Koreckij T, et al. A prospective, randomized, multi-center study of intraosseous basivertebral nerve ablation for the treatment of chronic low back pain. *Spine J.* 2019; 19(10):1620–32.
39. Truumees E, Macadaeg K, Pena E, et al. A prospective, open-label, single arm, multi-center study of intraosseous basivertebral nerve ablation for the treatment of chronic low back pain. *Eur Spine J.* 2019; 28:1594–602. doi:10.1007/s00586-019-05995-2.
40. Markman JD, Rhyne AL, Sasso RC, et al. Association between opioid use and patient-reported outcomes in a randomized trial evaluating basivertebral nerve ablation for the relief of chronic low back pain. *Neurosurgery.* 2020;86(3):343–347.
41. Lorio M, Clerk-Lamalice O, Beall DP, Julien T. International Society for the Advancement of Spine Surgery guideline—intraosseous ablation of the basivertebral nerve for the relief of chronic low back pain. *Int J Spine Surg.* 2020;14(1):18.
42. Balagué F, Mannion AF, Pellisé F, et al. Non-specific low back pain. *Lancet.* 2012;379(9814):482–491. doi:10.1016/S0140-6736(11)60610-7.
43. Allegri M, Montella S, Salici F, et al. Mechanisms of low back pain: a guide for diagnosis and therapy. *F1000Res.* 2016;5:F1000 Faculty Rev-1530. doi:10.12688/f1000research.8105.2.
44. Amirdelfan K, McRoberts P, Deer TR. The differential diagnosis of low back pain: a primer on the evolving paradigm. *Neuromodulation.* 2014;17(suppl 2):11–17. doi:10.1111/ner.12173.
45. Minkalis AL, Vining RD. What is the pain source? A case report of a patient with low back pain and bilateral hip osteonecrosis. *J Can Chiropr Assoc.* 2015;59(3):300–310
46. Peh W. Image-guided facet joint injection. *Biomed Imaging Intervent J.* 2011;7(1):e4.
47. Beresford ZM, Kendall RW, Willick SE. Lumbar facet syndromes. *Curr Sports Med Rep.* 2010;9(1):50–56. doi:10.1249/JSR.0b013e3181caba05.
48. Jackson RP, Jacobs RR, Montesano PX. 1988 Volvo Award in clinical sciences. Facet joint injection in low-back pain: a prospective statistical study. *Spine (Phila Pa 1976).* 1988;13(9):966–971.
49. Manchikanti L, Singh V, Pampati V. Evaluation of the relative contributions of various structures in chronic low back pain. *Pain Physician.* 2001;4(4):308–316.
50. Dreyfuss P, Dreyer SJ, Cole A, et al. Sacroiliac joint pain. *J Am Acad Orthop Surg.* 2004;12(4):255–265.
51. Helm S II, Deer TR, Manchikanti L, et al. Effectiveness of thermal annular procedures in treating discogenic low back pain. *Pain Physician.* 2012; 15(3): E279–304.

PART 5

Sacroiliac Joint Therapies

16

Sacroiliac Joint Fusion—Posterior Approach

Patrick Buchanan and Jack Diep

Introduction

Low back pain (LBP) is one of the most common health problems and creates a substantial burden globally. An estimated 70% to 85% of the Western population will develop LBP at least once during their lifetime.[1] Sacroiliac joint (SIJ) pain is one of the most common causes of LBP, accounting for 15% to 30% of all cases.[2] The SIJ is the most likely source of LBP in patients having undergone either lumbar or lumbosacral fusion surgery.[3] The incidence of SIJ degeneration in patients who have undergone lumbar fusion surgery is 75% at 5 years after surgery, based on imaging.[4] Although SIJ dysfunction contributes to a large portion of chronic LBP, it can often be overlooked and underdiagnosed.

The SIJ is a large diarthrodial joint that connects the sacrum with the pelvis. It acts as a shock absorber by dissipating the vertical forces of the spine and transmitting them to the hips and lower extremities. The SIJ becomes unstable when ligament laxity occurs, especially in the interosseous and posterior ligaments. Most of the time, SIJ degeneration starts with the failure of the anterior ligament, which is an extension of the anterior joint capsule.

The etiology of SIJ pain can be classified into two categories: traumatic and atraumatic. Traumatic causes can involve sudden events, such as motor vehicle accidents, falls, and lifting. Atraumatic causes can include infections, cumulative injury, and inflammatory arthropathies. Risk factors that cause stress on the SIJ include prior lumbar fusion,[5] obesity, pregnancy,[6] leg length discrepancy,[7] gait abnormalities,[8] and scoliosis.[9]

Conservative treatment options, including intra-articular steroid injections and radiofrequency ablation, focus on decreasing inflammation and blocking the pain. These interventions have been shown to have limited success in the short term. Surgical fusion of the SIJ aims to correct the mechanics by stabilizing the joint, which prevents inflammation and laxity.

SIJ fusion can be performed using either a lateral or a posterior approach. The current literature supports the lateral approach, with limited studies supporting the posterior approach. Recently, minimally invasive techniques have been designed to stabilize the SIJ posteriorly. These techniques utilize one or two cortical allografts that can be placed along the joint by a surgeon or an interventional pain physician. There can be many advantages to fusing the joint posteriorly. Posterior fusion minimizes the risk of neurological complications by avoiding the sacral foramen. The posterior approach passes through less soft tissue, including the gluteal musculature, and decreases postoperative recovery time. The lateral approach typically requires the patient to undergo general sedation, while the posterior approach can be performed under conscious sedation.

Indications

SIJ pain typically presents as an aching pain below the L5 dermatomal level, without burning or numbness/tingling. It can be differentiated from other forms of LBP by taking a thorough history and physical exam. SIJ pain is diagnosed when three out of five provocative maneuvers are positive (the five tests are the FABER, compression, distraction, thigh thrust, and Gaenslen's maneuvers). By performing these provocative maneuvers, there is an 85% pretest probability that an intra-articular joint injection will be successful.[10] A diagnostic intra-articular SIJ block is considered the gold standard for diagnosing SIJ pain. Fluoroscopic guidance has been shown to be more accurate than ultrasound guidance (98.2% versus 87.3%).[11] The International Association for the Study of Pain (IASP) criteria for diagnosis of SIJ dysfunction include pain in the area of the SIJ that is reproducible with provocative maneuvers and that must be relieved with local anesthetic injection into the SIJ or the lateral branch nerves.[12]

Posterior SIJ fusion is indicated once all conservative therapies have been exhausted. The patient must have undergone and failed a minimum of 6 months of intensive nonoperative treatment, including medication optimization, activity modification, and physical therapy. The patient also must have positive results on three out of the five provocative maneuvers and benefit from two SIJ blocks. Finally, destructive lesions (e.g., tumor, infection) or inflammatory arthropathy must be excluded, because they would not be properly addressed by percutaneous SIJ fusion.

Evidence

Conventional interventions, such as intra-articular injections and radiofrequency ablation, have been mainstay therapies for SIJ dysfunction. The evidence for these treatment options is limited, with most studies showing short-term to intermediate-term relief.[13] (The substantial Level 1 evidence studies on the long-term success of lateral SIJ fusion are discussed in Chapter 17, on the lateral approach.) Multicenter prospective studies on posterior fusion are currently being conducted.

Patient Selection and Contraindications

Patient selection is critical to the success of SIJ fusion. Patients who are candidates for this procedure are required to undergo at least 6 months of conservative therapy, including medications, physical therapy, and injections. Figure 16.1 provides an algorithm for determining whether a patient is a good candidate for SIJ fusion.

SIJ fusion can complement other treatments of the spine. Three areas to consider are patients with prior lumbar fusions, salvage therapy after spinal cord stimulation (SCS), and incomplete resolution of LBP after lumbar radiofrequency (RF) ablation. As mentioned above, SIJ pain is very common after lumbar surgery due to adjacent-segment disease, because more pressure gets displaced onto the SIJ after lumbar fixation. SIJ pain should also be considered in patients who continue to have low back pain after SCS therapy. Substantial evidence shows that SCS therapy is effective for neuropathic pain but not for joint pain. Finally, it is important to look for SIJ pain in patients who continue to have LBP despite lumbar RF ablation. The lumbar facet joints are close to the SIJ and tend to refer pain into the buttock area. One way to differentiate facet pain from SIJ pain is to perform facet-loading maneuvers and to compare the results to the results of SIJ provocative maneuvers.

It is also important to determine who is not a candidate for SIJ fusion. It is essential to rule out causes of SIJ pain that require medical treatment, including infection, tumor, or any treatable inflammatory arthropathy. Furthermore, because patient compliance is crucial to the success of SIJ fusion, patients who are resistant to following postoperative restrictions, especially in athletic or strenuous occupational activities, may have a difficult time allowing proper fusion of the joint to take place. Also, patients must have proper SIJ anatomy, because congenital abnormalities may inhibit posterior access to the joint. Osteoporosis is a relative contraindication, because it may limit the degree of obtainable correction, stabilization, and/or mechanical fixation. Finally, the patient should be willing to comply with advice not to smoke or to consume alcohol during the bone graft healing process.

Perioperative Management

A pain table is the preferred procedural table; it can be a flattop procedure table to a Jackson table that is radiolucent, given the different views (AP, oblique, and lateral) required for the procedure. There should be no metal rails along the sides or metal support structures underneath the table that would obscure the fluoroscopic image.

The patient is positioned prone, with a bump or roll under the iliac crest in order to remove as much lumbar lordosis as possible. The hips should have 15 to 20 degrees of flexion, to level off the pelvis.

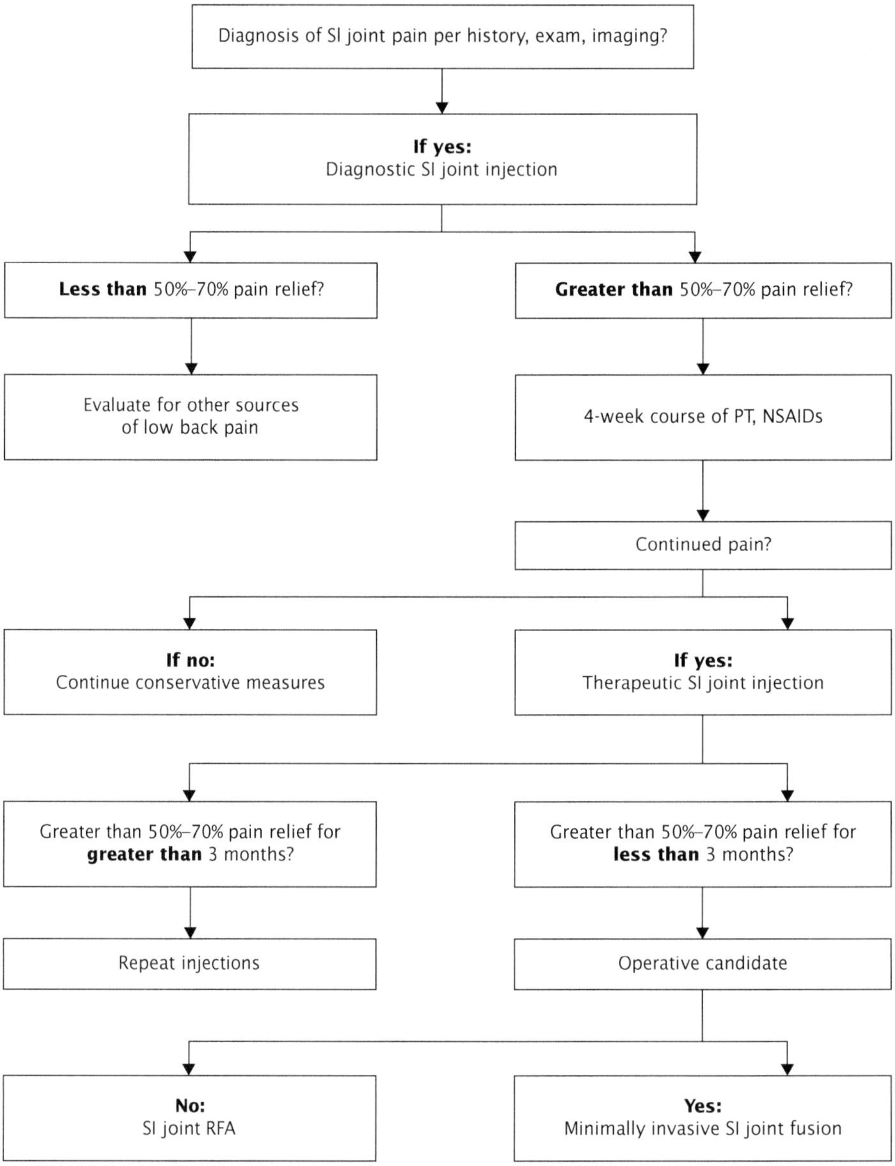

FIGURE 16.1. Algorithmic approach to sacroiliac joint fusion.[164]

Technique

A 22-gauge 3.5-inch or 5-inch spinal needle is used to infiltrate the working site with local anesthesia. This can help to reduce the amount of intravenous sedation needed and the recovery time after the procedure. Additionally, the needle can be used to access the joint prior to incision or to guide pin placement.

A long sponge clamp is used to hold the guide pin during fluoroscopy to reduce the amount of radiation exposure to the interventionist. Another option is to wear lead gloves.

Standard antibiotic prophylaxis to prevent surgical site infection is recommended. Antibiotics based on weight are given within 1 hour before incision.

Hair at the site of incision should be clipped.

The procedure can be performed under local anesthesia only, local anesthesia with sedation, or even general anesthesia.

Begin by obtaining an AP view of the SIJ. Identify the sacrum, ilium, posterior superior iliac spine, anterior joint line, and posterior joint line. Next, oblique the C-arm contralaterally until the joint lines are superimposed. This typically occurs between 10° and 35°. The medial and lateral cortical lines of the ilium will sharpen as the joint lines are superimposed.

Unilateral Single-Implant Technique

Locate the bifurcation of the anterior and posterior SIJ line, which will be the insertion point for the Steinman/K-wire/guide pin. Localize the skin and subcutaneous tissue. Consider inserting and advancing a 22-gauge spinal needle into the joint to localize the working site. With a scalpel, make a stab incision at the insertion point that is parallel to the joint. Remove the spinal needle, insert the guide pin, and slowly advance the guide pin into the joint. The guide pin can have a superior to inferior angle, allowing for a perpendicular trajectory into the joint. Rotate the C-arm to the lateral position upon entry of the joint and advance the guide pin to the anterior cortical line of the sacrum. The guide pin can be gently tapped with a mallet to advance it to the anterior cortical line. This will allow for good purchase and prevent the pin from backing out as the dilators are advanced. The optimal target area is under the posterior superior iliac spine near the S2 foramen (Figure 16.2).

Once correct guide pin placement has been confirmed in the lateral view (Figure 16.3), place the outside dilator/working channel around the pin and parallel to the joint. The surgeon can draw a line from tong to tong on the outside dilator to mark the incision (Figure 16.4). After the skin has been anesthetized, a #10 blade scalpel is used to make an incision that is long enough to accommodate the width of the outside dilator. The tendons and ligaments are cleared by running the blade along the caudal and cephalic sides of the guide pin all the way to the joint.

Next, depending on the system, advance the inside dilator (finder) or combined internal/external dilators (retraction guide) over the guide pin to the posterior cortical line of the sacrum while in the lateral view (Figure 16.5). Return to the oblique view and tilt the C-arm cephalad to visualize the upper tong. Ensure that the tong is medial to the medial cortical wall of the ilium (Figure 16.6). Next, tilt the C-arm caudally until the bottom tong is visualized. Ensure that the bottom tong is aligned with the posterior joint line (Figure 16.7). Once alignment is confirmed, return to lateral view and advance the dilators by gently tapping on the handle with a mallet until the hard stop on the outer dilator meets the posterior cortical line of the sacrum. Once the dilators are fully seated on the sacrum, remove the internal dilator and guide pin. Rotate the C-arm around to an AP view. Obtain a "barrel shot" to confirm that the outer dilator is in the joint. Sometimes it is not possible to visualize the joint within the dilator. At this point,

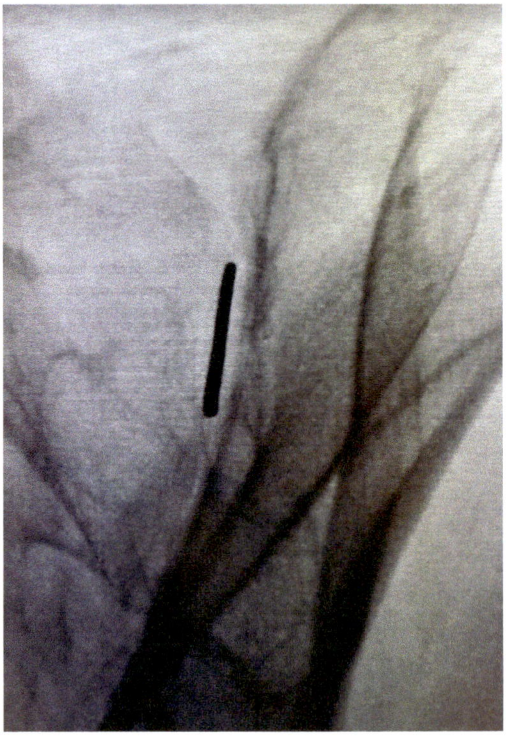

FIGURE 16.2. Optimal placement of guide pin in the contralateral oblique view. Redraw.

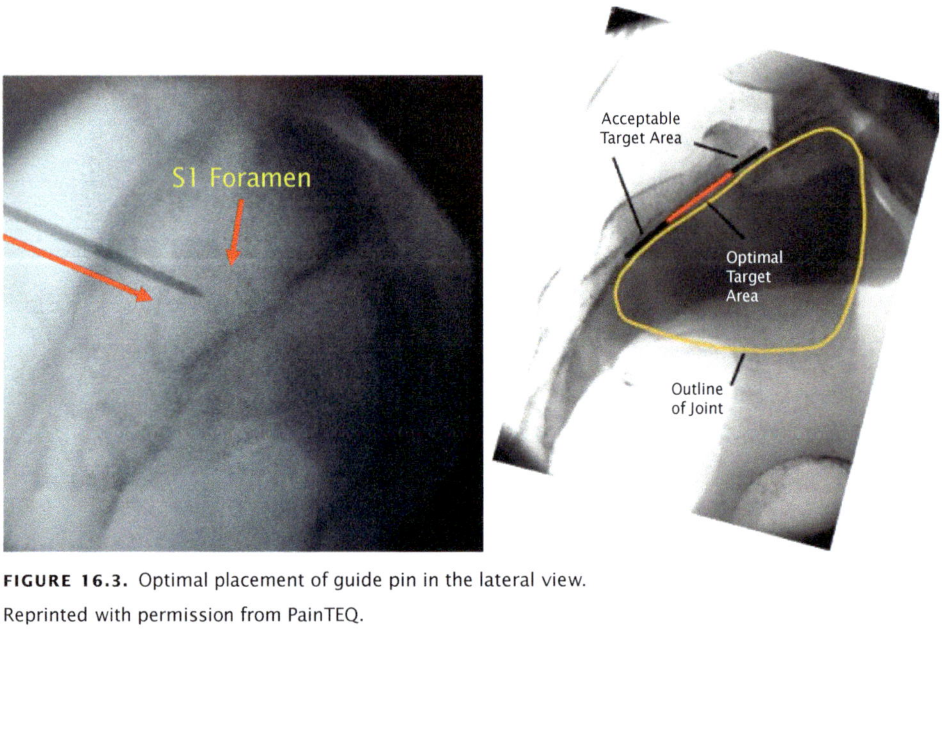

FIGURE 16.3. Optimal placement of guide pin in the lateral view.

Reprinted with permission from PainTEQ.

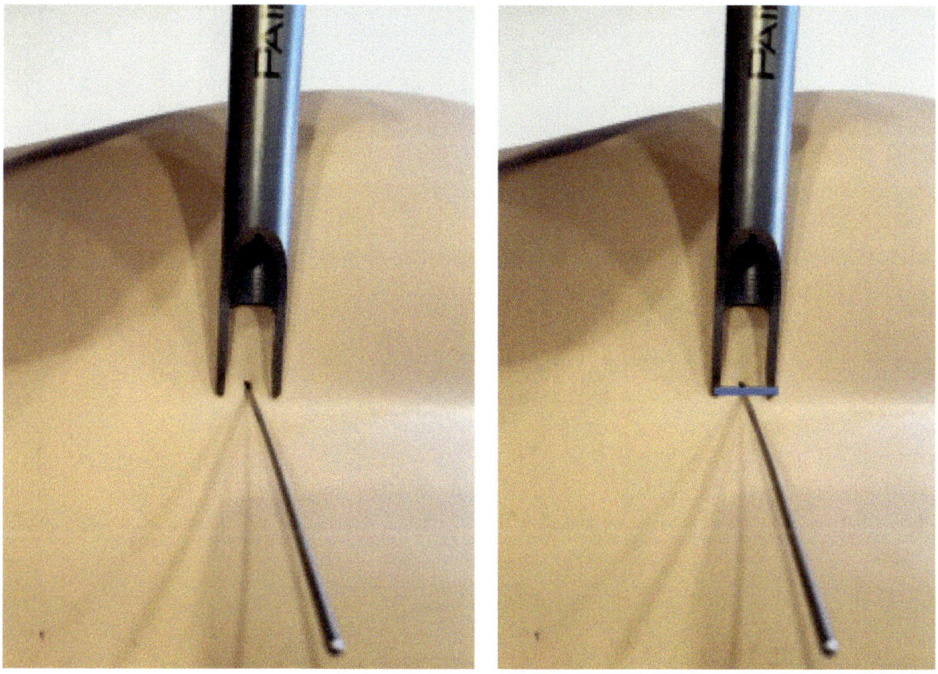

FIGURE 16.4. Line drawn from tong to tong on the outer dilator to mark the incision.
Reprinted with permission from PainTEQ.

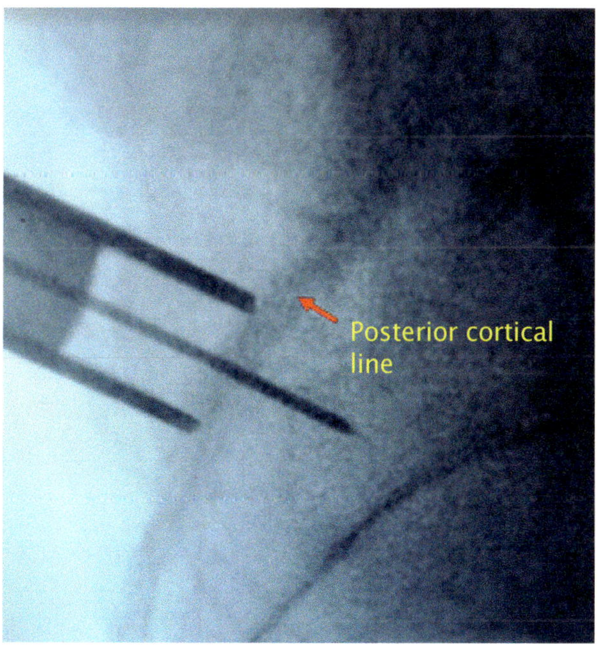

FIGURE 16.5. External dilator at the posterior cortical line in the lateral view.
Reprinted with permission from PainTEQ.

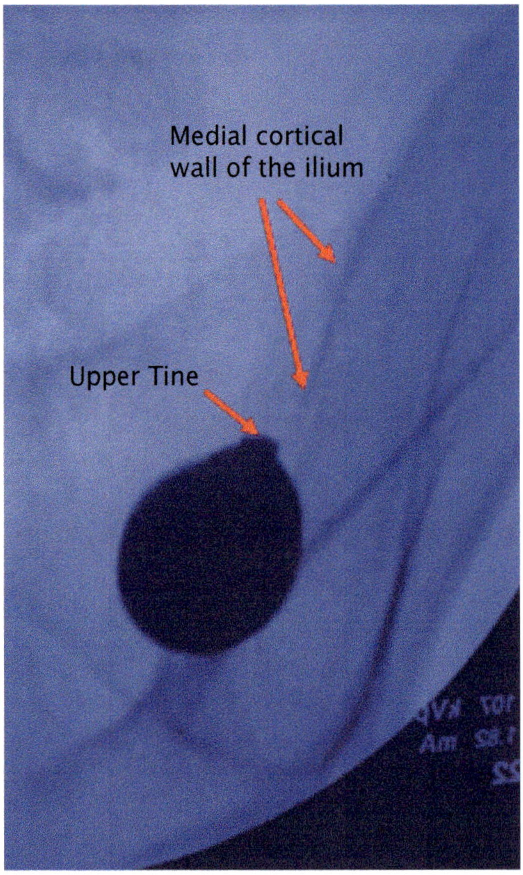

FIGURE 16.6. Optimal position of upper tong in oblique view.
Reprinted with permission from PainTEQ.

the surgeon will need to consider the orientation and trajectory in the oblique view. The surgeon should also consider if minimal malleting was performed. Once the surgeon is satisfied, they can proceed with decortication and/or drilling. The joint decorticator and/or surgical drill is advanced until it reaches the anterior cortical line of the sacrum, and then it is removed. The broach is advanced to prepare the graft site and then it is removed. The cortical allograft with demineralized bone matrix is inserted via an inserter. If the system has a final impactor, it is inserted and then removed. Finally, the outer dilator/working channel is removed.

Unilateral Double-Implant Technique

The double-implant technique requires the use of two guide pins and two entry points. The first guide pin is placed in the superior third of the SIJ lateral to the L5–S1 facet joint, while the second guide pin is placed in the inferior third of the SIJ inferior to the posterior superior iliac spine. The two pins should be in intersecting planes at 70° to 90° to each other in the AP plane as seen from the lateral view (Figure 16.8).

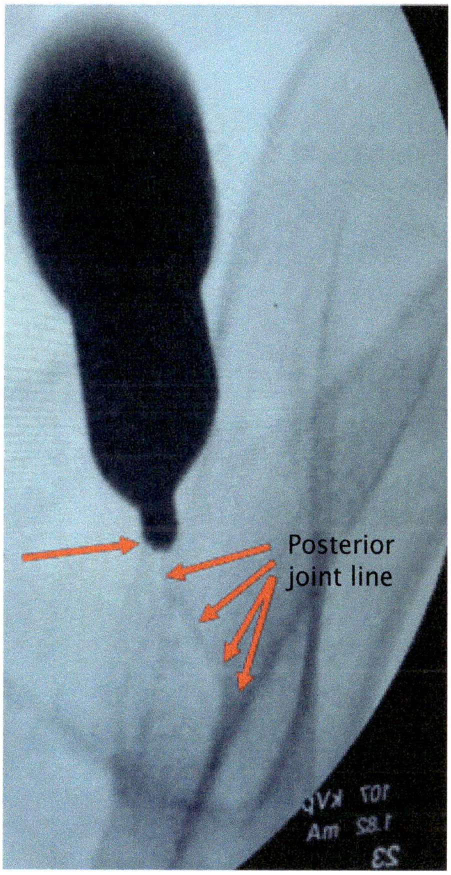

FIGURE 16.7. Optimal position of bottom tong in oblique view.
Reprinted with permission from PainTEQ.

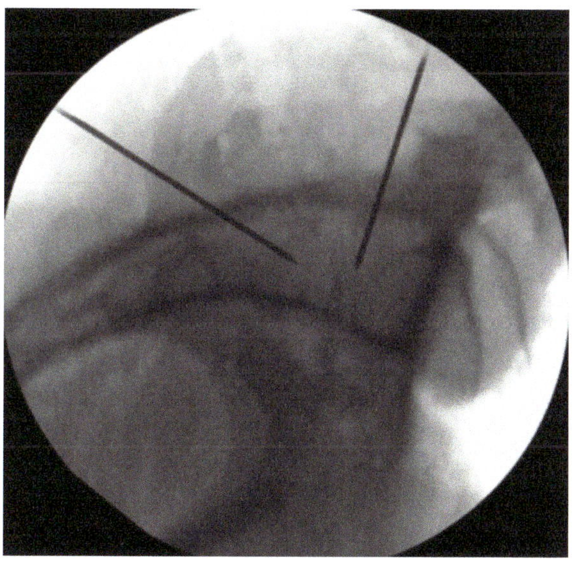

FIGURE 16.8. Optimal position of guide pins in lateral view.
Reprinted with permission from PainTEQ.

Postoperative Management and Follow-up

Patients should avoid twisting, bending, and lifting for 6 to 12 weeks to allow proper fusion to take place. Patients can be weight bearing as tolerated right after the procedure. Patients may take sponge baths or brief showers up to 2 weeks.

Complications and Management

Adequate hemostasis is ensured utilizing Bovie electrocautery. If there is postoperative bleeding, given the small but deep incision(s), a Weitlaner or Gelpi retractor is used to allow visualization of the soft tissue. The surgeon may consider using absorbable hemostatic agents or extending the incision to look for the source of bleeding.

Abscess(es), depending on whether they are superficial or deep, may require drainage, irrigation, and antibiotics. Cultures should be taken prior to administration of antibiotics.

Conclusion

SIJ pathology can account for 15% to 30% of LBP. Posterior SIJ arthrodesis is a minimally invasive approach that reduces tissue trauma, allows for faster recovery time, and provides a safe and effective treatment for SIJ pain. Patients must be selected carefully to ensure

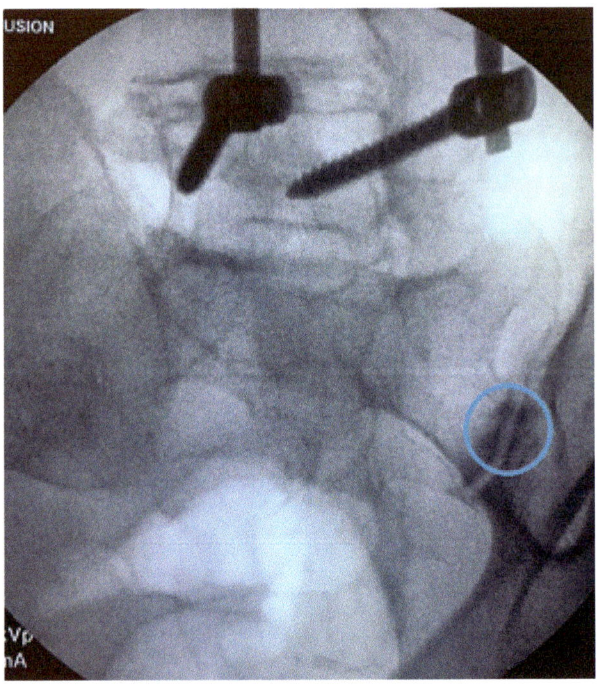

FIGURE 16.9. SIJ implant in the oblique view.

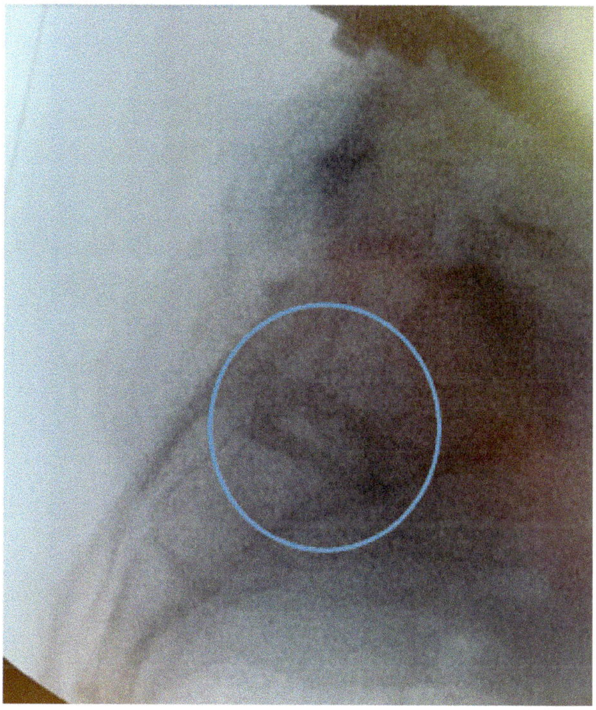

FIGURE 16.10. SIJ implant in the lateral view.

excellent outcomes. Given that posterior SIJ arthrodesis is a new approach, further studies are required to evaluate its long-term outcomes and safety profile.

References

1. Andersson GB. Epidemiological features of chronic low-back pain. *Lancet.* 1999;354(9178):581–585. doi:10.1016/S0140-6736(99)01312-4. PMID:10470716.
2. Cohen SP, Chen Y, Neufeld NJ. Sacroiliac joint pain: a comprehensive review of epidemiology, diagnosis and treatment. *Expert Rev Neurother.* 2013;13(1):99–116. doi:10.1586/ern.12.148. PMID:23253394.
3. DePalma MJ, Ketchum JM, Saullo TR. Etiology of chronic low back pain in patients having undergone lumbar fusion. *Pain Med.* 2011;12(5):732–739. doi:10.1111/j.1526-4637.2011.01098.x. PMID:21481166.
4. Ha KY, Lee JS, Kim KW. Degeneration of sacroiliac joint after instrumented lumbar or lumbosacral fusion: a prospective cohort study over five-year follow-up. *Spine (Phila Pa 1976).* 2008;33(11):1192–1198. doi:10.1097/BRS.0b013e318170fd35. PMID:18469692.
5. Katz V, Schofferman J, Reynolds J. The sacroiliac joint: a potential cause of pain after lumbar fusion to the sacrum. *J Spinal Disord Tech.* 2003;16(1):96–99. doi:10.1097/00024720-200302000-00015. PMID:12571491.
6. Albert H, Godskesen M, Westergaard J. Prognosis in four syndromes of pregnancy-related pelvic pain. *Acta Obstet Gynecol Scand.* 2001;80(6):505–510. PMID:11380285.
7. Schuit D, McPoil TG, Mulesa P. Incidence of sacroiliac joint malalignment in leg length discrepancies. *J Am Podiatr Med Assoc.* 1989;79(8):380–383. doi:10.7547/87507315-79-8-380. PMID:2810074.
8. Kiapour A, Joukar A, Elgafy H, Erbulut DU, Agarwal AK, Goel VK. Biomechanics of the sacroiliac joint: anatomy, function, biomechanics, sexual dimorphism, and causes of pain. *Int J Spine Surg.* 2020;14(suppl 1):3–13. doi:10.14444/6077. PMID:32123652. PMCID:PMC7041664.

9. Szadek KM, van der Wurff P, van Tulder MW, Zuurmond WW, Perez RS. Diagnostic validity of criteria for sacroiliac joint pain: a systematic review. *J Pain.* 2009;10(4):354–368. doi:10.1016/j.jpain.2008.09.014. PMID:19101212.
10. Jee H, Lee JH, Park KD, Ahn J, Park Y. Ultrasound-guided versus fluoroscopy-guided sacroiliac joint intra-articular injections in the noninflammatory sacroiliac joint dysfunction: a prospective, randomized, single-blinded study. *Arch Phys Med Rehabil.* 2014;95(2):330–337. doi:10.1016/j.apmr.2013.09.021. PMID:24121083.
11. Treede RD. The International Association for the Study of Pain definition of pain: as valid in 2018 as in 1979, but in need of regularly updated footnotes. Pain Rep. 2018 Mar 5;3(2):e643. doi: 10.1097/PR9.0000000000000643. PMID: 29756089; PMCID: PMC5902252.
12. Buchanan P, Mehta A, Gerstman B. Interventional treatments for sacroiliac joint pain. *Curr Phys Med Rehabil Rep.* 2014;2:66–69. https://doi.org/10.1007/s40141-014-0042-5.
13. Falowski S, Sayed D, Pope J, et al. A review and algorithm in the diagnosis and treatment of sacroiliac joint pain. *J Pain Res.* 2020;13:3337–3348. doi:10.2147/JPR.S279390. PMID:33335420. PMCID: PMC7737553.6.

17

Sacroiliac Joint Fusion—Lateral Approach

Steven M. Falowski

Introduction

Low back pain (LBP) has an overall prevalence of 9.4% and is a significant contributor to disability, making it one of the most common health problems worldwide.[1] The sacroiliac joint (SIJ) is part of the mobility of the lower spine and lower extremities and may factor in as a pain generator, with SIJ pain often mimicking hip and lumbar spine pathologies. SIJ pathology may quite often be a missed diagnosis, causing patients to undergo unnecessary lumbar surgeries.[2] This underscores the importance of a correct and accurate diagnosis to implement a proper treatment strategy. The SIJ has been found to contribute to LBP in as many as 10% to 38% of cases, and SIJ pain is commonly missed, undertreated, and misdiagnosed.[2–4]

Presentation and Diagnosis

SIJ pain commonly presents with pain below the belt line, with radiation into the groin and lower extremity, infrequently with radiation below the knee in the L5-S1 Dermatomal distribution extending down the posterior lower extremity.[5] The pain is largely isolated over the SIJ on the respective side and can be sharp or aching in quality.[6] Movement often exacerbates the pain, and the pain can radiate into the ipsilateral groin.[7]

Physical exam includes provocative maneuvers: the distraction test, FABER maneuver, Gaenslen's test, thigh thrust, and compression test.[7] The highest validity and predictive value have been found when three or more of the provocative tests are positive,[7] with the FABER maneuver having the highest sensitivity.

Imaging has low sensitivity for the diagnosis of SIJ pain or pathology.[8] Imaging modalities, such as x-ray, CT, and MRI, may offer some indication of abnormalities, but they are not specific by themselves. A telling sign that could lead to SIJ pain is sacroiliitis, with MRI being the most sensitive in detecting it.[9]

Risk factors for, and associations with, SIJ pain include scoliosis, lumbar fusion, pregnancy, repetitive athletic activity, and leg length discrepancies.[6] The most commonly recognized risk factors are pregnancy and prior lumbar surgery. Multilevel lumbar surgery and fusion may yield a higher incidence of SIJ pain than discectomy alone.[10]

The International Association for the Study of Pain diagnostic criteria[11] for SIJ pain include pain in the area of the SIJ that is reproducible with provocative maneuvers and that is relieved with local anesthetic injection into the SIJ. It has been demonstrated that patients who do well with surgical treatment have a response to local anesthetic injection of 75% relief or greater for at least 30 to 60 minutes.[12,13]

Surgical Fixation of the SIJ

Surgical fusion of the SIJ for stabilization can be done by either a lateral approach and/or a posterior and posterior oblique approach. Publications have demonstrated that minimally invasive modalities for SIJ fusion can improve pain and increase function.[14–18] The current medical literature supports the lateral approach, but there are limited studies that support the posterior and posterior lateral oblique approach.

Lateral Approach

SIJ fusion was originally performed via an open approach, until the lateral approach to SIJ fusion was initiated in 2008 with FDA 510(k) approval for the first minimally invasive system using the lateral approach (iFuse Implant System, SI Bone). Many other systems have come on the market that use variations of the lateral approach. The benefits of the minimally invasive systems using the lateral approach, compared to an open approach, were limited blood loss, decreased tissue dissection, and shorter recovery times.[19] SIJ fusion with the lateral approach is still largely performed by surgeons, but it has replaced surgery via open approaches.

Surgical Technique

The procedure is usually performed under general anesthesia with the use of fluoroscopic guidance. Due to the risk of damage to the lumbosacral nerve roots, intraoperative neuromonitoring may be utilized.[20] Although there are variations based on the system that is being used, it is most common to place guidewires at the presumed locations for graft placement. With the commonly used iFuse Implant System, the three guidewires are placed at the superior, middle, and inferior aspects of the SIJ. Cannulas can be used over the guidewires for dilation and tissue separation. Drilling is then performed over the guidewires inside the dilators. Most systems then utilize titanium screws packed with allograft to promote arthrodesis. The use of graft material, such as allograft, is crucial to promote bony

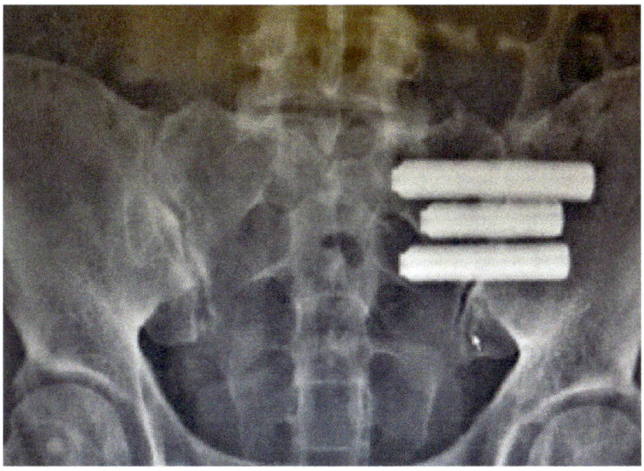

FIGURE 17.1. Three titanium screws used in fixation of the sacroiliac joint via a lateral approach.

fusion beyond the immediate fixation from the hardware. Figure 17.1 shows fluoroscopy of an implanted system.

Outcomes

The lateral approach has proven efficacious in reducing back pain and in improving functional outcomes. In a 2-year randomized controlled study comparing the lateral surgical approach to conservative management, there was significant improvement in back pain and Oswestry Disability Index (ODI) score with the lateral approach. Those undergoing the lateral approach had an improvement of 55.4 points on the 100-point Visual Analog Scale (VAS), compared to 12.2 points with conservative management, and 68% of surgical patients had a greater than 15-point improvement on the ODI at 24 months, compared to 7.5% in the conservative arm.[13] A published comprehensive review of the literature with a pooled analysis was able to demonstrate surgical patients had a mean decrease of 80.3 to 32.2 on the VAS, as well as a decrease in ODI of 56.2 to 34.4.[21]

Safety

Proposed benefits of the minimally invasive systems using the lateral approach, compared to an open approach, were limited blood loss, decreased tissue dissection, and shorter recovery times.[19] The safety of the lateral approach has been demonstrated with lower surgical complication rates and lower incidence of nonunion.[22] However, complications do exist and have a reported rate as high as 16.4%.[23] Most complications are minor or self-limited; they can include increased hip, back, and buttock pain and hematoma, although more serious adverse events, such as deep wound infection and nerve root impingement, have been reported.[24] Shamrock et al performed a systematic review of 14 studies.[25] The overall complication rate was reported to be 11.1%, with the most common complication being wound infection (*n* = 17/819, 2%). Nerve root impingement was reported in 1.6% of cases (13/819).

Discussion

LBP is a common condition that is also a great mimicker. The SIJ has been estimated to contribute to pain in as many as 38% of LBP cases.[2–4] SIJ pathology is commonly missed, underdiagnosed, undertreated, and/or misdiagnosed. The diagnostic criteria are not always clear, although some have advocated a clearer pathway for diagnosis and an algorithm for treatment of these patients.[26] Conservative measures are usually employed first, followed by SIJ injection, whether diagnostic or therapeutic. Response to injection aids in patient identification for further treatment, such as surgical fixation. Some insurance carriers may require 50% to 70% pain relief with injections, while others may require two injections prior to fixation.

There are many benefits to the use of surgical fixation. There is a growing need for treatment secondary to increases in proper identification of SIJ pain and pathology, and surgical fixation addresses the actual pathology by immobilizing the joint and eliminating the motion thought to cause inflammation and SIJ pain. Proposed treatment algorithms arrive at consideration of surgical fixation when a patient has persistent moderate to severe pain, has functional impairment, and has failed a minimum of 6 months of conservative care.[26] Surgical or interventional treatments can be performed via lateral or posterior/posterior oblique approaches, with literature supporting both for improving pain and function and maintaining a low adverse event profile. It is clear that most of the literature supports the lateral approach, the most studied approach, with several publications offering Level 1 evidence.

References

1. March L, Smith EUR, Hoy DG, et al. Burden of disability due to musculoskeletal (MSK) disorders. *Best Pract Res Clin Rheumatol.* 2014;28(3):353–366. http://dx.doi.org/10.1016/j.berh.2014.08.002.
2. Yoshihara H. Sacroiliac joint pain after lumbar/lumbosacral fusion: current knowledge. *Eur Spine J.* 2012;21(9):1788–1796.
3. Guentchev M, Preuss C, Rink R, Peter L, Wocker E-L, Tuettenberg J. Technical note: treatment of sacroiliac joint pain with peripheral nerve stimulation. *Neuromodulation Technol Neural Interface.* 2015;18(5):392–396.
4. Cher D, Polly D, Berven S. Sacroiliac joint pain: burden of disease. *Med Devices Evid Res.* 2014;7(1):73–81.
5. Szadek KM, van der Wurff P, van Tulder MW, Zuurmond WW, Perez RS. Diagnostic validity of criteria for sacroiliac joint pain: a systematic review. *J Pain.* 2009;10(4):354–368.
6. Chou LH, Slipman CW, Bhagia SM, et al. Inciting events initiating injection-proven sacroiliac joint syndrome. *Pain Med.* 2004;5(1):26–32.
7. Telli H, Telli S, Topal M. The validity and reliability of provocation tests in the diagnosis of sacroiliac joint dysfunction. *Pain Physician.* 2018; 21:E367–E376.
8. Barros G, McGrath L, Gelfenbeyn M. Sacroiliac Joint Dysfunction in Patients with Low Back Pain. *Fed Pract.* 2019; 36(8):370–375.
9. Diekhoff T, Hermann KG, Greese J, et al. Comparison of MRI with radiography for detecting structural lesions of the sacroiliac joint using CT as standard of reference: results from the SIMACT study. *Ann Rheum Dis.* 2017;76:1502–1508. doi:10.1136/annrheumdis-2016-210640.
10. Guan F, Sun Y, Zhu L. Guan G, Chen M, Chi Z Tian D, Gu J, Yu Z. Risk Factors of Postoperative Sacroiliac Joint Pain for Posterior Lumbar Surgery: ≥2-year follow-up retrospective study. *World Neurosurg.* 2018; 110:e546–e551. doi.10.1016/j.wneu.2017.11.053. Epub 2017 Nov 20.

11. Merskey H, Bogduk N, eds. *Classification of Chronic Pain: Descriptions of Chronic Pain Syndromes and Definitions of Pain Terms.* 2nd ed. Seattle, WA: IASP Press; 1994.
12. Polly DW, Cher DJ, Wine KD, et al; INSITE Study Group. Randomized controlled trial of minimally invasive sacroiliac joint fusion using triangular titanium implants vs nonsurgical management for sacroiliac joint dysfunction: 12-month outcomes. *Neurosurgery.* 2015;77(5):674–690.
13. Polly DW, Swofford J, Whang PG, et al. Two-year outcomes from a randomized controlled trial of minimally invasive sacroiliac joint fusion vs. non-surgical management for sacroiliac joint dysfunction. *Int J Spine Surg.* 2016;10:28.
14. Polly DW Jr. Minimally invasive sacroiliac joint fusion vs. conservative management for chronic sacroiliac joint pain. J Spine Surg. 2019 Sep;5(3):381–383. doi:10.21037/jss.2019.06.10.
15. Dengler J, Kools D, Pflugmacher R, et al. Randomized trial of sacroiliac joint arthrodesis compared with conservative management for chronic low back pain attributed to the sacroiliac joint. *J Bone Joint Surg.* 2019;101(5):400–411.
16. Sturesson B, Kools D, Pflugmacher R, Gasbarrini A, Prestamburgo D, Dengler J. Six-month outcomes from a randomized controlled trial of minimally invasive SI joint fusion with triangular titanium implants vs conservative management. *Eur Spine J.* 2017;26(3):708–719.
17. Dhon BS, Bitan F, Lockstadt H, Kovalsky D, Cher D, Hillen T; SIFI Study Group. Triangular titanium implants for minimally invasive sacroiliac joint fusion: 2-year follow-up from a prospective multicenter trial. *Int J Spine Surg.* 2016;10:13.
18. Sachs D, Capobianco R, Cher D, et al. One-year outcomes after minimally invasive sacroiliac joint fusion with a series of triangular implants: a multicenter, patient-level analysis. *Med Devices (Auckl).* 2014;7:299–304.
19. Lorio MP, Polly DW Jr, Ninkovic I, Ledonio CG, Hallas K, Andersson G. Utilization of Minimally Invasive Surgical Approach for Sacroiliac Joint Fusion in Surgeon Population of ISASS and SMISS Membership. *Open Orthop J.* 2014 Jan 24;8:1–6.
20. *iFuse Surgical Technique.* https://si-bone.com/providers/education/si-joint-ifuse-training.
21. Martin CT, Haase L, Lender PA, Polly DW. Minimally invasive sacroiliac joint fusion: the current evidence. *Int J Spine Surg.* 2020;14:20–29. doi:10.14444/6072.
22. Smith AG, Capobianco R, Cher D, Rudolf L, Sachs D, Gundanna M, Kleiner J, Mody MG, Shamie AN. Open versus minimally invasive sacroiliac joint fusion: a multi-center comparison of perioperative measures and clinical outcomes. Ann Surg Innov Res. 2013 Oct 30;7(1):14.
23. Schoell K, Buser Z, Jakoi A, Pham M, Patel NN, Hseih PC, Liu JC, Wang JC. Postoperative complications in patients undergoing minimally invasive sacroiliac fusion. *Spine J.* 2016 Nov;16(11):1324–1332.
24. Duhon BS, Cher DJ, Wine KD, Lockstadt H, Kovalsky D, Soo CL. Safety and 6-month effectiveness of minimally invasive sacroiliac joint fusion: a prospective study. *Med Devices (Auckl).* 2013 Dec 13;6:219.
25. Shamrock AG, Patel A, Alam M, Shamrock KH, Al Maaieh M. The safety profile of percutaneous minimally invasive sacroiliac joint fusion. *Global Spine J.* 2019;9:874–880. doi:10.1177/2192568218816981.
26. Falowski S, Sayed D, Pope J, et al. A review and algorithm in the diagnosis and treatment of sacroiliac joint pain. *J Pain Res.* 2020;13:3337–3348. doi:10.2147/JPR.S279390. PMID:33335420. PMCID:PMC7737553.

PART 6

Neuromodulation Procedures

18

Percutaneous Spinal Cord Stimulator Trial

Bethany Potere, Nasir Hussain, Timothy Deer, and Alaa Abd-Elsayed

Introduction

Spinal cord stimulation (SCS), a type of neuromodulation, falls under a category of treatments aimed at battling chronic pain caused primarily by neuropathic pain. Fundamentally, the primary mechanism behind SCS applies the gate-control theory, which was first described by Wall and Melzack in 1965.[1–3] The theory proposes that stimulating large A-beta nerve in the substantia gelatinosa of the dorsal horn of the spinal cord inhibits pain signals transmitted by small A-delta and C fibers.[4,5] This further increases the release of inhibitory GABA and decreases release of excitatory glutamate and aspartate, thereby decreasing pain sensation.[1,5] SCS augments this pathway by modulating the dorsal column, which reduces the downstream sensation of pain. In recent years, modulation of the supraspinal pathways has also been realized as an important component of pain and is perhaps also affected by SCS.[3] Ever since the initial application and success of SCS, its use has grown considerably. In addition, the mechanism of action of SCS therapy has been modified with innovations like software that provides potential central mechanisms in the thalamus, combined waveforms that may impact glial cells, and higher frequencies that may work on wide-dynamic-range neurons.[6–8]

Spinal cord stimulator placement is preceded by a percutaneous trial to determine possible candidacy for permanent placement, and extent of pain relief from the trial determines if a patient is a candidate to move forward with long-term placement. This chapter introduces the patient populations and the clinical indications for a percutaneous spinal cord stimulator trial. It also highlights the preoperative optimization of, procedural approach for, and postoperative evaluation of patients undergoing a percutaneous trial.

Indications

SCS is indicated for a variety of conditions in which a patient experiences chronic pain; however, typically it is used for pain in the trunk or limbs, in which conservative therapy has failed.[4] The most common indications include complex regional pain syndrome (CRPS), failed back surgery syndrome (FBSS), or persistent spinal pain syndrome (PSPS), and ischemic lower extremity pain.[9] In patients with back pain who have failed surgery and for whom no further surgical intervention is offered, SCS has increasingly become part of the treatment algorithm.[10,11] Table 18.1 provides the most recent guidelines for the use of spinal cord stimulator trial in three common indications: FBSS, CRPS, and limb ischemia. Other indications include, but are not limited to, neuropathic limb pain, phantom limb pain, visceral abdominal pain, chronic refractory angina, nonsurgical back pain, postthoracotomy pain, intercostal neuralgia, and postherpetic neuralgia;[5,12] however, evidence for these uses is evolving and building. Additional studies are needed to further evaluate the evidence and real-world experience for each indication.

Evidence

Chronic Critical Limb Ischemia

A systematic review of 10 studies with over 440 patients with chronic critical limb ischemia evaluated conservative therapy, which included pharmacologic therapy aimed at vasodilation, anticoagulation, and analgesia, versus conservative therapy plus SCS.[13] The review

TABLE 18.1. Indications and Evidence for Spinal Cord Stimulation (SCS)

	FBSS	CRPS 1	CRPS 2	Limb ischemia	Goal of SCS
NICE[19]	Chronic pain for at least 6 months despite conservative medical management			Only as part of a clinical trial to establish evidence for use	Improve quality of life and functionality
BPS[3]	Evidence supports use of SCS				Relieve pain and improve functionality
IASP[20]	Low back pain with radiculopathy	Not indicated	Indicated	Slowly progressive PVD that is spastic or atherosclerotic in nature	Improvement in pain
ASA[21]	Evidence supports use of spinal cord stimulation				Optimize pain control, improve functional status, improve quality of life

Abbreviations: ASA, American Society of Anesthesiologists; BPS, British Pain Society; Complex Regional Pain Syndrome, Type 1 = CRPS 1, ; Complex Regional Pain Syndrome, Type 2 = CRPS 2, ; EFNS, European Federation of Neurologic Societies; Failed Back Surgery Syndrome = FBBS, ; IASP, Task Force of the European Federation of the International Association for the Study of Pain (IASP); NACC, Neurostimulation Appropriateness Consensus Committee; NEUPSIG, Neuropathic Pain Special Interest Group; NICE, National Institute for Health and Care Excellence; Peripheral vascular disease = PVD.

found that patients with implanted spinal cord stimulators had improved pain relief at 3 and 12 months after SCS implantation. Patients with SCS were also noted to have improved wound healing, improvement in ischemia, and decrease in claudication symptoms.[13] Several recent randomized controlled trials (RCTs) have also suggested long-term pain benefits of SCS in this patient population.

FBSS

In patients with FBSS, numerous RCTs have compared invasive reoperation to SCS, with the majority of the studies suggesting improved pain and analgesic outcomes with SCS.[14] One RCT found that 47% of SCS patients experienced > 50% pain reduction, compared to only 12% of patients who underwent invasive reoperation. The patients with repeat operation also required more opioids.[7,14] Additionally, North et al found that at 6 months, SCS increased the odds of pain control by at least 50% more than in patients who underwent redo spine surgery.[14]

CRPS

Similar improvement in pain and reduction in opioid usage has been seen in SCS for patients with CRPS. Kemler et al demonstrated that in those with CRPS type 1, treatment with SCS plus physical therapy versus physical therapy alone revealed improved pain relief and improved quality of life at 6 months. However, there was no difference in functional status at 6 months.[7,16] Kemler et al extended the study to 24-month follow-up, which revealed continued pain relief in the SCS group.[17]

Patient Selection and Contraindications

A psychological evaluation has become commonplace before SCS consideration, because uncontrolled psychiatric disease has been associated with poor outcomes.[4,7] Pain is a complex biological and psychosomatic process, and a psychological evaluation can help elucidate if mental or emotional factors are driving a patient's pain, in which case SCS may not be warranted until proper treatment or counseling is performed. Finally, active psychosis, severe untreated depression or anxiety, or patients' inability or unwillingness to comply with treatment are all contraindications to SCS.[7]

Other contraindications to spinal cord stimulator trial and permanent placement include patients with thrombocytopenia (platelet count < 50,000) or coagulopathy, or patients who are on antiplatelet or anticoagulants that cannot be safely interrupted.[4,7] Equally as important, potential candidates should be evaluated for both local and systemic infection, and any infection should be thoroughly addressed prior to stimulator implantation.

Perioperative Considerations

Planning for spinal cord stimulator trial should take into consideration both the procedure as well as the patient's existing comorbidities and medications. For diabetic patients, glycemic control to prevent infection is imperative. Patients who smoke should be offered guidance on smoking cessation, again to aid in healing, especially given the sensitive location of the procedure, although in some patients smoking cessation is not achievable. Updated imaging should be considered when possible, ideally with magnetic resonance imaging (MRI) of the spine to evaluate for any anatomic abnormalities, including locations of previous surgical intervention and/or hardware and areas of possible difficulty for lead placement (i.e., due to foraminal stenosis or anatomic variants). Imaging can also guide the clinician–patient conversation on where the generator will be implanted, should the decision be made to proceed with a permanent stimulator.[7] Patient education about wound care and generator care after placement is crucial to promote healing and to prevent infection or malfunction.

Spinal cord stimulator implantation is typically performed using local anesthetic, with or without sedation. However, the physician must be prepared to convert to a general anesthetic if warranted; therefore, an airway examination should be routine in preoperative planning.

General anesthesia is an option based on patient conditions, anxiety status, or positioning difficulty. If general anesthesia is used, intraoperative neuromonitoring should be used to improve the safety of the procedure.

Overall, percutaneous SCS is a minimally invasive, low-risk procedure. In the awake patient or in patients with general anesthesia with intraoperative nerve monitoring (IONM), the risk of nerve injury is small. With regard to bleeding risk, the American Society of Regional Anesthesia and Pain Medicine (ASRA) considers SCS lead placement a high-risk procedure for bleeding and its sequelae.[18] With the population of patients on anticoagulant and antiplatelet therapies increasing, the management of these medications must be a part of routine perioperative management for both trial and permanent stimulator placement. Antiplatelet therapies, such as aspirin, nonsteroidal anti-inflammatory drugs (NSAIDs), and P2Y12 inhibitors, should all be stopped prior to stimulator lead placement. ASRA recommends holding aspirin 4 to 6 days before stimulator placement, depending on if it is prescribed for secondary or primary prevention, respectively. NSAIDs should be stopped for five half-lives prior to the procedure, which corresponds to 1 to 2 days for ibuprofen, diclofenac, ketorolac, and indomethacin and 4 days for meloxicam or naproxen. Direct-acting oral anticoagulants (DOACs) should also be stopped five half-lives before stimulator placement. There are many DOACs in clinical use, and the physician and patient should reference the individual medication label to ensure that the medication is held for an appropriate amount of time. For inpatients who are on a heparin infusion, the heparin should be stopped 6 hours before stimulator lead placement. For patients receiving prophylactic subcutaneous heparin, neuraxial procedures like spinal cord stimulator lead placement are contraindicated in BID or TID dosing. These recommendations, coupled with individual clinician judgment and patient characteristics, aim to reduce the incidence of epidural hematoma and intraspinal bleeding and their subsequent complications. A summary of anticoagulant medication recommendations is given in Table 18.2.

TABLE 18.2. Perioperative Anticoagulant Management[18]

Anticoagulant	Length of Time to Hold before SCS Placement
Aspirin	4–6 days
NSAIDs	5 half-lives
Ibuprofen, diclofenac, ketorolac, indomethacin	1–2 days
Meloxicam, naproxen	4 days
DOACs	5 half-lives*
Heparin infusion	6 hours

Abbreviations: DOACs, direct-acting oral anticoagulants; NSAIDs, nonsteroidal anti-inflammatory drugs.

*Refer to drug-specific instructions for specific times.

Technique

Spinal cord stimulator lead implantation, for both trial and permanent placement, is performed in the operating room on an outpatient basis. The patient is placed in the prone position, and the back is prepped in sterile fashion.[12,14] Often, pillows are placed under the abdomen to improve exposure and curvature of the lumbar spine. Aseptic technique is maintained throughout, and prophylactic antibiotics should be administered. Generally, for trial lead placement, cefazolin alone is sufficient, unless the patient has a penicillin allergy, in which case clindamycin can be used. Subcutaneous local anesthetic is injected prior to insertion of the Tuohy needle. The posterior epidural space is then accessed using the loss-of-resistance technique to air. Care should be taken to avoid entering the anterior epidural space to prevent involvement of motor neurons and potential motor impairment. Under fluoroscopic guidance, the electrodes are then passed into the desired position based upon the indication for stimulator placement.[14] Commonly, the leads terminate in the high to mid-thoracic region for upper extremity pain, in the lower thoracic spine for chronic back pain, and in the low thoracic spine for lower extremity pain due to ischemia.[1,14] Figure 18.1 shows the final location of the lead in the spinal cord. The Tuohy needle is removed with the leads in place using a Seldinger technique, and the leads are secured to the skin using adhesive tape. The electrodes are then connected to an external generator, which is secured to the right or left flank. Large tape is often used to cover the entire setup to protect the hardware from any damage for the duration of the trial.

Postoperative Management and Follow-up

Immediately after device placement, patients should be instructed on how to care for the apparatus during the trial, which is often for 3 to 5 days. The leads and generator cannot get wet for the duration of the trial, which is an important point to emphasize to the patient. Antibiotics are continued throughout the trial period. Following the trial period, pain relief is the main deciding factor for moving forward with more permanent stimulator

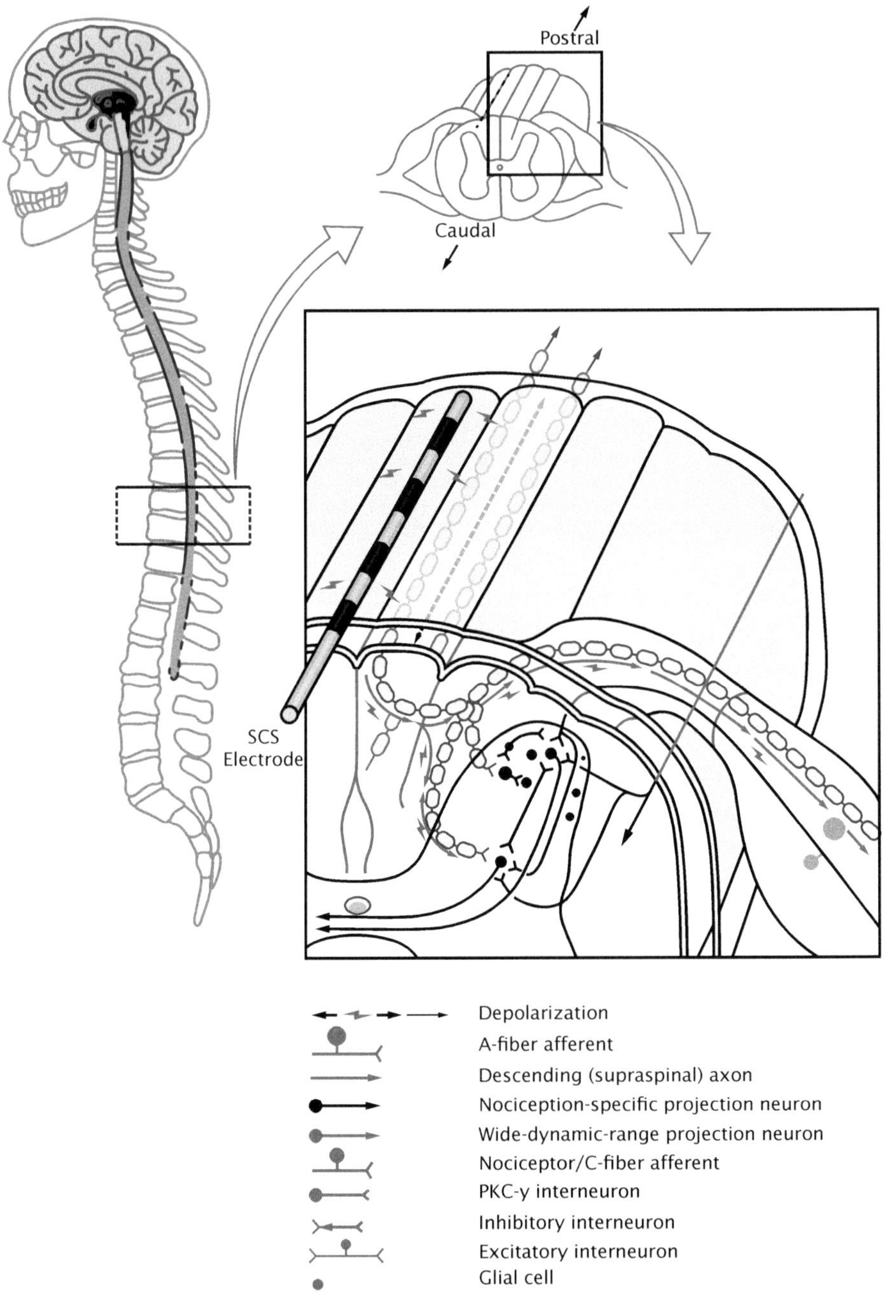

FIGURE 18.1. Final location the SCS lead in the spinal cord.[2]

placement. Patients who receive at least 50% pain reduction are deemed good candidates for permanent lead placement.[7,12,14]

Complications and Management

The most common risks of spinal cord stimulator lead placement are infection, lead migration, and lead breakage.[12] These complications are most common with permanent implants. With a trial placement, the risk for any of these complications is limited and remote. The patient should also be aware of more serious, although less common, risks, such as epidural hematoma, dural puncture, and nerve or spinal cord injury, either directly related to placement or due to lead migration or breakage after successful placement. Lead migration is the most common complication and occurs most often with cervical lead placement, owing to the increased mobility of the cervical spine compared to the thoracic or lumbar spine.[7] Lead migration or fracture is corrected with repair or replacement. Infection is most commonly due to skin flora, such as *Staphylococcus aureus*.[3]

Conclusion

Spinal cord stimulator trial allows both the clinician and the patient to test-drive an intervention, so to speak, before making the commitment to permanent therapy. The test period allows patients who have failed conservative therapies, or even surgery, another avenue for addressing their pain. Spinal cord stimulators are well accepted for a multitude of pain syndromes, and in the era of the opioid crisis, their use has become even more paramount as a part of a multimodal pain strategy. In patients who have satisfactory outcomes from a trial, moving on to a permanent spinal cord stimulator offers a minimally invasive route to pain relief, decreased opioid use, and improvement in quality of life.

References

1. Foreman RD, Linderoth B. Neural mechanisms of spinal cord stimulation. *Int Rev Neurobiol.* 2012;107:87–119. https://onlinelibrary.wiley.com/doi/10.1111/papr.12692.
2. Sdrulla AD, Guan Y, Raja SN. Spinal cord stimulation: clinical efficacy and potential mechanisms. *Pain Pract.* 2018;18(8):1048–1067. https://doi.org/10.1111/papr.12692.
3. British Pain Society. *Spinal Cord Stimulation for the Management of Pain: Recommendations for Best Clinical Practice.* London, England: British Pain Society; 2009. https://www.britishpainsociety.org/static/uploads/resources/files/book_scs_main_1.pdf.
4. Barash PG, Cullen BF, Stoelting RK, Cahalan M, Stock MC. Chronic pain management. In: *Clinical Anesthesia.* 8th ed. Baltimore, MD: Lippincott Williams & Wilkins; 2011:1624–1625.
5. Mendell LM. Constructing and deconstructing the gate theory of pain. *Pain.* 2014;155(2): 210–216. https://doi.org/10.1016/j.pain.2013.12.010.
6. Luecke T, Edgar D, Huse D. 10 kHz spinal cord stimulation for the treatment of chronic back and/or leg pain: summary of clinical studies. *SAGE Open Med.* 2020;8:205031212095136. https://journals.sagepub.com/doi/10.1177/2050312120951369.

7. Deer T, Slavin KV, Amirdelfan K, et al. Success using neuromodulation with BURST (Sunburst) study: results from a prospective, randomized controlled trial using a novel burst waveform. *Neuromodulation.* 2018;21(1):56–66. https://doi.org/10.1111/ner.12698.
8. Fishman M, Cordner H, Justiz R, et al. Randomized Controlled Trial to Study the Effects of DTM-SCS in Treating Intractable Chronic Back Pain. *North American Neuromodulation Society Annual Meeting.* 2020; 25(6, Supplement 2): S1–S9.
9. Christelis N, Simpson B, Russo M, et al. Persistent spinal pain syndrome: A proposal for failed back surgery syndrome and ICD-11. *Pain Med.* 2021;22(4):807–818. https://doi.org/10.1093/pm/pnab015.
10. Stolzenberg D, Ahn JJ, Lendner M, Kurd M. Thoracolumbar spinal cord stimulator trial. *Clin Spine Surg.* 2020; 34(2):51–55. https://doi.org/10.1097/bsd.0000000000000935.
11. Rock A, Truong H, Park YL, Pilitsis JG. Spinal cord stimulation. *Neurosurg Clin North Am.* 2019;30(2):169–194. https://doi.org/10.1016/j.nec.2018.12.003.
12. Butterworth J, Mackey DC, Wasnick J. Chronic pain management. In: *Morgan and Mikhail's Clinical Anesthesiology.* 5th ed. McGraw Hill Professional, New York; 2013:1081–1082.
13. Ubbink D, Vermeulen H. Spinal cord stimulation for non-reconstructable chronic critical leg ischaemia. *Cochrane Database Syst Rev.* 2003;2013(2). https://www.cochranelibrary.com/cdsr/doi/10.1002/14651858.CD004001/full.
14. Lamer TJ, Moeschler SM, Gazelka HM, Hooten WM, Bendel MA, Murad H. The effect of spinal cord stimulation on pain medication reduction in intractable spine and limb pain: a systematic review of randomized controlled trials and meta-analysis. *Mayo Clin Proc.* 2019;94(8), 1475–1487. https://doi.org/10.1016/j.mayocp.2018.12.037.
15. Deer TR, Mekhail N, Provenzano D, et al. The appropriate use of neurostimulation of the spinal cord and peripheral nervous system for the treatment of chronic pain and ischemic diseases: the neuromodulation appropriateness consensus committee. *Neuromodulation.* 2014;17(6):515–550. https://doi.org/10.1111/ner.12208.
16. Kemler MA, Barendse GA, Van Kleef M, et al. Spinal cord stimulation in patients with chronic reflex sympathetic dystrophy. *N Engl J Med.* 2000;343(9):618–624. https://doi.org/10.1056/nejm200008313430904.
17. Kemler MA, De Vet HC, Barendse GA, Van Den Wildenberg FA, Van Kleef M. The effect of spinal cord stimulation in patients with chronic reflex sympathetic dystrophy: two years' follow-up of the randomized controlled trial. *Ann Neurol.* 2003;55(1):13–18. https://onlinelibrary.wiley.com/doi/10.1002/ana.10996.
18. American Society of Regional Anesthesia and Pain Medicine. Regional anesthesia in the patient receiving antithrombotic or thrombolytic therapy. *Reg Anesth Pain Med.* 2018; https://rapm.bmj.com/content/rapm/43/3/263.full.pdf.
19. National Institute for Health and Care Excellence. *Spinal Cord Stimulation for Chronic Pain of Neuropathic or Ischaemic Origin.* NICE; 2008. https://www.nice.org.uk/guidance/ta159.
20. Gybels J, Erdine S, Maeyaert J, et al. Neuromodulation of pain: a consensus statement prepared in Brussels 16–18 January 1998 by the following task force of the European Federation of IASP chapters (EFIC). *Eur J Pain.* 1998;2(3):203–209. https://doi.org/10.1016/s1090–3801(98)90016–7.
21. Rosenquist RW, Benzon HT, Connis RT, et al. Practice guidelines for chronic pain management: an updated report by the American Society of Anesthesiologists Task Force on Chronic Pain Management and the American Society of Regional Anesthesia and Pain Medicine. *Anesthesiology.* 2010;112(4):810–833. https://doi.org/10.1097/ALN.0b013e3181c43103.

19

Percutaneous Spinal Cord Stimulator Implantation (Cervical/Lumbar)

Vinicius Tieppo Francio, Alaa Abd-Elsayed, Timothy Deer, and Benjamin D. Westerhaus

Introduction

The use of electrical stimulation for pain relief has been described since 15 AD, with the earliest documented use in gout treatment by contact with a torpedo fish (electric fish), an approach discovered by the Roman physician Scribonius Largus.[1] Since then, many other scientists and physicians experimented with electrical stimulation and pain relief, but it wasn't until 1967 that Dr. Norman Shealy, the pioneer of contemporary neuromodulation, decided to stimulate large fibers in the dorsal column of the spinal cord,[2] based on the then-new theory of pain mechanisms called the gate-control theory, which had been proposed a few years earlier.[3] In 1968, the first commercially available spinal cord stimulator (SCS) was introduced. Early SCS systems employed platinum leads and large batteries and had a high incidence of lead fractures. Since Shealy's original implant in 1967, spinal cord stimulation has become the most frequently performed surgical procedure for the treatment of chronic pain around the world, and now, in the modern era, spinal cord stimulation is considered one of the most advanced interventional methods and one of the most impressive tools in the treatment for chronic pain syndromes.[4] This chapter discusses the use of the SCS in the treatment of chronic cervical spine and lumbar spine pain syndromes.

Spinal cord stimulation is a particularly important treatment option in chronic spinal pain, which is a highly prevalent condition in the United States, leading to pain, disability, loss of work days, and decline in quality of life (QoL) and function. For instance, chronic neck pain is the fourth leading cause of disability, with an annual prevalence rate exceeding

30%,[5] and chronic low back pain is the leading cause of disability worldwide, with a reported prevalence up to 69%.[6] Chronic spinal pain is a pathological phenomenon that remains poorly understood, incompletely characterized, challenging to treat, and perhaps one of the most important global healthcare problems. The situation has become even more alarming with the onset of the opioid epidemic, the high incidence of drug resistance, and the increase in healthcare costs.[7,8]

The neurophysiologic premise of the therapeutic effects of neuromodulation in chronic spinal pain syndromes is the concept that selective excitation of large afferent fibers activates mechanisms that control pain. This fits the idea that spinal-cord-mediated pain may occur as a result of imbalance between large and small fiber systems that transmit nociceptive information from the site of injury,[9] and that high-caliber fibers exert an inhibitory influence on impulses transmitted in smaller-caliber fibers. This inhibition of sensory impulses has been proposed to occur in the dorsal horn.

Other generalized proposed documented mechanisms of action of spinal cord stimulation include suppression of antidromic active mediators, such as substance P and calcitonin gene-related peptide (CGRP), blockage of transmission to the spinothalamic tract at the dorsal horn, inhibition of collateral or interneurons, upregulation of signaling that provokes wide-dynamic-range (WDR) neuron wind-up, supraspinal feedback loop central inhibition with the thalamocortical system, inactivation of glutamate, and activation of GABA.[8,11]

Over the past decades, ideas about spinal cord stimulation have been rapidly evolving, with new theories, different waveforms, and emerging more solid experimental and clinical high-level studies discussing the role of spinal cord stimulation in chronic refractory low back pain and limited, in chronic cervical spine pain.[12] However, before the mechanisms of action of spinal cord stimulation can be addressed, it is imperative to understand the main components of the stimulator unit and stimulation parameters.

Components of the SCS

The SCS as it is finally implanted has several components.

Leads

The two lead designs in use today are paddle electrodes and cylindrical leads. Paddle electrodes are flat, wide, and rectangular at the distal end, with insulation on one side and the electrodes on the other side, which can number up to 32 electrodes. Originally, the initial lead design meant that leads could only be implanted surgically by laminotomy or laminectomy. More recent designs allow for their implantation under percutaneous technique, and their advantage is more efficient delivery of current. Work by Rosenow in 2006 demonstrated an association between paddle electrodes and complications, infections, and fractures.[13] However, there have not been large, randomized studies comparing cylindrical and paddle leads.[10] Paddle electrodes may be indicated when anatomy, postsurgical changes, or epidural scarring make percutaneous lead implantation technically challenging.

Furthermore, paddle electrodes may be indicated in lead revision due to migration, when better lead stability is required.[14]

Cylindrical leads were designed for percutaneous placement. They have cylindrical polyurethane catheters to insulate the wires as they originate from the stimulator and terminate in platinum-iridium alloy contacts that vary in number, length, and spacing pattern, depending on the make and model. Generally, there are between 8 and 16 contacts per lead. The cylindrical design of the electrodes causes circumferential current flow, which can inadvertently stimulate posterior structures, causing uncomfortable sensations.[10] Leads that have anode and cathode separation of 4 mm have been shown to be mathematically optimal for preferentially stimulating the fibers of the dorsal column rather than dorsal root ganglia.[15] However, anode-to-cathode separation of < 10 mm has been shown to have the most clinical efficacy,[16] because this design confines the stimulation field to along the axis of the lead, which decreases stimulation of extraneous structures, that is, the ligamentum flavum, dorsal root ganglion, etc.[17] The growing trend has been to implant dual, parallel leads over the targeted spinal segment. First, this puts one lead on each side of the physiological midline, allowing better coverage for patients with bilateral pain.[18] Second, having redundancy in the number of leads affords additional flexibility in accounting for slight lead migration in the acute phase after implantation.[19] Finally, it has been suggested that dual leads can create stimulation fields that superimpose and achieve better penetration into the dorsal columns.[20] When accounting for energy efficiency, however, it has been shown that a properly positioned single lead demonstrates the best dorsal column activation with lowest energy utilization.[17]

Implantable Pulse Generator (IPG)

The leads are connected by proprietary connectors to the IPG after proper positioning. Historically, radiofrequency coupling devices were the first pulse generators in the 1970s and 1980s, but they were very inconvenient for the patient, because they required the patient to wear an antenna over the implant during its use, which precluded its use during sleep, swimming, or bathing, in addition to causing possible skin irritation from the taping of the antenna.[17] Current designs employ a primary cell that is either rechargeable or not. The IPG drives the pulse and is programmed based on trial specifications within the parameters defined by the manufacturer and model.[17] Other characteristics of the IPG include MRI compatibility, methods for controlling voltage or current, and ability to interface with the patient and/or programmer.[21] Regarding MRI compatibility, manufacturer guidelines should be followed, because most IPGs are MRI conditional for the head and extremities and some are conditional for whole-body MRI. Over 80% of patients with an implanted SCS require an MRI within 1 year of implantation, so this is an important consideration.[21] Variables for pulse generation are discussed in the next section.

Batteries

The power source for the IPG is a battery that is either part of the IPG (primary cell) or rechargeable. Batteries that are rechargeable are recharged through the patient's skin with external chargers that are held in place by adhesive, belt, or strap. The primary cell battery lasts 4 to 7 years, depending on manufacturer and patient settings, whereas rechargeable batteries can last up to 9 years. Newer IPGs with low-dose burst technology last up to 10 years. When necessary, the IPG is replaced surgically in a manner similar to its implantation.[21]

Parameters for Spinal Cord Stimulation

An understanding of the neurophysiologic and biomedical engineering aspects of spinal cord stimulation and the SCS device and its programming are essential to succeed as an interventional pain physician treating patients with chronic pain. Thorough comprehension of the concepts is very valuable in guiding selection of the proper patient selection and the most appropriate spinal cord stimulation parameters, among all the new technologies. It is outside the scope of this chapter to thoroughly review all the parameters for neurostimulation; however, a direct summary is given below. The concepts were extracted from the studies of Foreman, Miller, Caylor, and Heijmans.[10,22–24]

Pulse, Pulse Width, and Pulse Pair

Pulse is a basic building block of a spinal cord stimulation waveform. It is the length of time that electrical current is delivered through the electrodes. The brief time that current is delivered by the system is called pulse duration and is measured in milliseconds (ms) or microseconds (μs). Pulse width is the length of time that electrical current is "on," whereas the pulse period is the total length of time the current is on and off. The pulse width is also referred to as the duty cycle. Pulse pair is a second pulse delivered in the opposite direction, immediately following the first therapeutic pulse. It is also known as a recovery pulse or a biphasic pulse, and it is used for safety reasons and is not counted in the frequency. In general, increasing the pulse width recruits additional Aβ fibers and broadens the area of paresthesia perception.[23]

Frequency

Frequency is the number of cycles per unit time. Typically, the reference unit of time is 1 second, and therefore frequency is measured in Hertz, or pulses per second. It is calculated inversely from the pulse period, which is the time between when one pulse starts and the next pulse starts. For example, if the time between one pulse and the next is 3 seconds, then frequency is 1/3 Hz; or if the time between pulses is 100 μs, the frequency is 10,000 Hz, which is 10 kHz. It is the number of pulses within 1 second.[10,24]

Amplitude

Amplitude is the relative current of electrical charge delivered to tissues. It is measured in milliamperes (mA), and it affects the number of fibers recruited and the intensity of paresthesia perception.[10]

Current and Impedance

Current is the movement of electrons through a conductive medium. By convention, current—and thereby electrical charges—moves from cathode (the negative terminal) to anode (the positive terminal). Since each pair of pulses passes in opposite directions, when the electrical impulse flows from the device into the body, it is in an anodal direction. When it is flowing in the opposite way (toward the electrodes), it is in a cathodal direction. Impedance is defined as opposition of current flow in any manner that is resistive, conductive, or inductive. A constant current source supplies current to the tissue by adjusting the voltage in response to tissue or lead impedance. In contrast, a constant voltage source adjusts current in response to impedance, maintaining a constant voltage. Changes in impedance can alter the strength of the stimulation during stimulus over time.[25–26] Lead impedance is determined by numerous factors, including the lead/electrode material, lead contact, anatomic target, and anatomic relationships (fibrosis, narrowing, lead migration, lead fracture, spinal hyperflexion, hyperextension, cerebrospinal fluid volume, etc.), which can contribute to chronic elevations of impedance and changes in neurostimulation.[27]

Waveforms

After gaining a basic understanding of the parameters and electrical concepts of neurostimulation, it is essential to comprehend the different waveforms and target sites as they relate to the different proposed mechanisms of action of spinal cord stimulation. A summary of commercially available waveforms is given in Table 19.1.

Tonic Conventional Stimulation

Tonic conventional spinal cord stimulation is governed by three basic elements (frequency, amplitude, and pulse width) and was first introduced by Shealy in 1967, based on the gate-control theory. The perception of paresthesia is determined by the amplitude and pulse width. Generally, higher amplitudes provide stronger paresthesia perceptions, and increasing the pulse width leads to greater fiber recruitment and a broadened paresthesia distribution. Recall, as frequency increases, pulse width must decrease, because they are inversely proportional.[10]

Paresthesia-based tonic stimulation is applied with a frequency ranging from 20 to 120 Hz and a pulse width varying between 200 and 500 μs. This tonic stimulation waveform delivers adjustable amplitudes based on the patient's subjective sensation of paresthesia and induced pain relief. Ideally, the perception of paresthesia should be between perception threshold and the discomfort threshold, also known as the therapeutic window of amplitude stimulation. Pulse width can be adjusted to widen or narrow the electrical field and frequency can be adjusted to alter the perceived sensation.[12,28–30]

The electrical pulses delivered by tonic low-frequency stimulation activate Aβ fibers in the dorsal column of the spinal cord, which, via antidromic transmission (action potential traveling opposite to the physiologic direction), activate inhibitory interneurons in the spinal dorsal horn. The interneurons modulate incoming nociceptive input from Aδ and C fibers and release the inhibitory neurotransmitter γ-aminobutyric acid (GABA) into the extracellular space in the spinal dorsal horn. The release of GABA modulates the inhibitory neurons via nociceptive-specific projections and reduction of multimodal WDR

TABLE 19.1. Summary of Selected Commercially Available Spinal Cord Stimulators

Device	Waveform	Frequency, Amplitude, Pulse Width	Stimulation Setting	Proposed Mechanisms of Action (MOAs)	Features
Abbott	BurstDR (Electrical packets at 40 Hz with five intraburst spikes of 500 Hz) Tonic SCS HF-SCS	200 Hz 0.25–1.6 mA 1,000 μs 40–100 Hz 3.5–8.5 mA 100–400 μs Up to 1,200 Hz	Noncontinuous BurstDR (paresthesia-free, passive recharge) Continuous (paresthesia-based) Continuous (paresthesia-free)	Multiple MOAs proposed, including modulation of lateral and medial pain pathways and the anterior cingulate cortex Dorsal column stimulation WDR inhibition Increase GABAergic neuron and glutamate reduction	Mapping or anatomic placement Rechargeable and nonrechargeable battery options Full-body MRI conditional with leads between T7 and T12
Boston Scientific	Tonic SCS Burst SCS HF-SCS	40–100 Hz 3.5–8.5 mA 100–400 μs 2–1,200 Hz (algorithm base waveform) Up to 1,200 Hz	Continuous (paresthesia-based) Clustered tonic firing burst stimulation (active recharge) Continuous	As previously described Uses two MOAs simultaneously by directing inhibiting WDR neurons and modulating neurons in the dorsal horn without dorsal column stimulation (superception paresthesia-free) and indirectly engages inhibition of dorsal column fibers with tonic stimulation (paresthesia-based)	Mapping placement Rechargeable and nonrechargeable battery options Anodal intensification Full-body MRI conditional (Montage and Alpha)
Medtronic	Tonic SCS HF-SCS DTM (differential targeted multiplex)	40–100 Hz 3.5–8.5 mA 100–400 μs Up to 1,200 Hz 20–1,200 Hz Variable mA 500 μs max	Continuous (paresthesia-based) Continuous (paresthesia-free) Three therapy options with four synchronous signals and six different amplitudes	As previously described As previously described Affects neural-glial interaction and modulates gene expression in the immune and inflammatory processes characteristic of neuropathic chronic pain modulating ion channels and synaptic signaling	Mapping placement Adaptive stimulation Full-body MRI conditional
Nevro	HF10 High-frequency Tonic SCS Low-frequency Pulse dosing Burst	10,000 Hz 1–5 mA 30 μs 2–1,200 Hz 2–8 mA 100–500 μs	Continuous stimulation Same as above Intermittent HF10 (25% on and 75% off) Noncontinuous stimulation	Direct dorsal horn inhibition, WDR neuron inhibition, and small fiber recruitment, paresthesia-free Dorsal column stimulation WDR inhibition Increase GABAergic neuron and glutamate reduction	Anatomic placement Rechargeable battery Full-body MRI conditional

	(five impulses with an intraburst frequency of 500 Hz) Burst 10k (Burst stimulation with HF10 during interburst time periods) Frequency pairing (Tonic SCS with HF10 stimulation between electrical impulses)	Same as above Burst packets repeated at frequency of 40 Hz 1,000 μs and 2–8 mA 10,000 Hz 1,000 μs and 2–8 mA 10,000 Hz 1,000 μs and 2–8 mA	Continuous Continuous	Direct dorsal horn and WDR neuron inhibition Dorsal column stimulation with WDR neuron inhibition and GABAergic action Same as above A combination of both mechanisms described previously with direct neural inhibition in the dorsal horn and dorsal column stimulation with paired waveforms	
Nalu	Tonic SCS with a pulsed stimulation pattern (PSP), layered pattern waveform	2–1,500 Hz Up to 10.2 mA 12–1,000 μs	PSP (paresthesia-free) with narrow pulses, high-rate train, long train, and low-rate train	Narrow pulse stimulation includes modulation of low-threshold fiber, dorsal horn, dorsal root, and glial cells. High-rate train (onset/offset) increases fiber recruitment, while long train (charge delivery) modulates high-threshold fibers, dorsal column, lateral and medial pathways, and low-rate train (onset/offset) accommodation, medial and lateral pathway.	Anatomic placement Wireless external charging therapy disc IPG free Full-body MRI conditional
Saluda	Evoked compound action potential (ECAP) closed-loop	Variable based on ECAP closed-loop feedback	Closed-loop stimulation	ECAP closed-loop stimulation measures the spinal cord nerve fibers' response to stimulation via ECAP and automatically adjusts stimulation within the therapeutic window to maintain ECAP at a consistent level. ECAP activation of the dorsal column fibers with antidromic and orthodromic inhibitory effects.	Mapping placement Measures response to stimulation and adjusts amplitude to maintain ECAP Unknown MRI compatibility

neurons' spontaneous firing. WDR neurons differ from most other neurons in that they experience the wind-up phenomenon, which allows for the intensity of their response to increase with an increased frequency of stimulus, and vice versa. WDR neurons are integrated into the lateral discriminatory pathway and are activated in tonic stimulation, disrupting the ascending pain pathway. Recall that the lateral discriminatory pathway provides input on the location, quality, and intensity of pain. This is in contrast to the medial affective ascending pathway, which drives attention or perception to pain via nociceptive-specific neurons, which are activated in passive-recharge burst stimulation, described later in this chapter.[8,11,24,28,31–32]

Tonic stimulation frequencies of 30 to 100 Hz maximally inhibited WDR neurons, while frequencies under 30 Hz and over 100 Hz excite WDR neurons.[33] Adding to the spinal segmental effects, tonic stimulation also modulates pain through supraspinal feedback loops by modulating nociceptive transmission in the dorsal horn via descending serotonergic and noradrenergic projections.[11,24,32]

Glial cell modulation is another proposed mechanism of action described in animal and preclinical studies for both conventional and differential target multiplexed (DTM) stimulation. The release of glutamate by glial cells is associated with abolishment of spinothalamic pathways, and it is well known that glial cells, particularly microglia and astrocytes, play an important role in the development and maintenance of chronic neuropathic states, moderated by glial-mediated sensitization. It has been shown that the number of glial cells in the posterior aspect of the spinal cord between T8 and T11, where stimulation is usually applied, outweighs the number of neurons, with a measured ratio of 20:1.[34] Hence, spinal cord stimulation, particularly with 60 Hz and 4 Hz, modulates glial cells by the release of GABA, inhibiting microglia and astrocytes, suggesting reduction of central excitability. Glial cell activation has been implicated in the development and maintenance of persistent neuropathic pain, and glial inhibition improves mechanical allodynia in animal models.[34–35] Tonic spinal cord stimulation showed decreased glial cell activation with improved withdrawal responses and decreased immunostaining of microglial markers in the dorsal horn lamina and dorsal root ganglion (DRG).[29,33–36]

There are different modes of tonic stimulation. Tonic stimulation with clustered firing is called clustered tonic firing burst stimulation and is based on the Boston Scientific burst tonic stimulation waveform. With this waveform, there is a cycling burst mode delivering 4 to 5 spikes, each being individually active biphasic spikes.[23,29,37] This burst waveform uses active recharge to repeatedly balance the charge after every spike and does not exhibit a charge summation. Therefore, it has been suggested to be termed clustered tonic firing stimulation to differ from the BurstDR stimulation waveform by mimicking a cluster tonic firing model and a linear build-up of cellular calcium, in addition to pain-modulatory effects via GABAergic mechanisms and lateral thalamic pathway modulation. The BurstDR stimulation modulates lateral and medial pain pathways without interspinal GABAergic action; however, both waveforms are directed at the levels of the dorsal columns. Electrophysiological monitoring studies of clustered tonic firing showed typical biphasic spikes, each individually followed by electromyography spikes, a response that mirrors typical tonic stimulation but differs from BurstDR. Therefore, the mechanisms of action of clustered tonic burst firing differ from the mechanisms of action of BurstDR at cellular, neurochemical, anatomic, and electrophysiological levels.[8,37–38]

BurstDR Stimulation

The BurstDR waveform (Abbott, Austin, TX) was introduced in 2010 by Dirk DeRidder (thus the DR suffix after the name of the waveform).[39] The main difference between tonic burst stimulation and BurstDR stimulation is the actively charge-balanced stimulation in clustered tonic stimulation versus the passively charge-balanced stimulation in BurstDR.[40] There are fundamental differences between the two waveforms. The BurstDR waveform is a 5-pulse train waveform with a passive quiescent phase, running with a pulse width frequency of 40 Hz and intraburst frequency of 500 Hz, with an advanced mode of programmed pulse stimulation that mirrors the dual-firing qualities of the thalamus. This is different from the clustered tonic firing burst stimulation already described.[23,29,37,39]

BurstDR tries to mimic physiologic burst firing, which involves closely spaced high-frequency sodium spikes nested on a nonlinear build-up of calcium in a cellular and electrophysiological level.[40] This leads to a summated electromyographic (EMG) response when measured intraoperatively, whereas each spike in tonic burst stimulation results in one small EMG spike, demonstrating a clear difference in the stimulation designs. This response makes sense because passive charge balancing will have outstanding or "lost" current for a time, which then produces a summative action, whereas active charge balancing would not have outstanding current and its EMG spikes are then discrete. Additionally, the amplitude needed to achieve an EMG response is different, with a much lower amplitude for BurstDR than for clustered tonic stimulation. Last, upon cessation of BurstDR stimulation, the subsequent threshold of EMG is much lower for multiple minutes, suggesting short-term neuroplastic changes not present with any other stimulation waveform. This is consistent with the understanding of the electrophysiologic responses of the neuromuscular junction with repetitive-stimulation nerve conduction testing at supraphysiologic frequencies. Some studies suggest that BurstDR activates spinal GABAergic neurons, and other studies suggest that only tonic burst stimulation stimulates GABAergic neurons, but both modulate descending inhibitory pain pathways, with BurstDR activating the medial pain pathway and also affecting the anterior cingulate cortex of the brain. It is postulated that the medial (affective) pain system is triggered by nociceptive neurons in lamina I of the dorsal horn and that this is achieved by BurstDR, and not by tonic burst stimulation.[29,37,39–44]

High-Frequency Stimulation

High-frequency stimulation (HF-SCS) , 10-kHz stimulation, involves a paresthesia-free paradigm because stimulation occurs below the sensory threshold.[24] A focus on charge delivery or dosing, in contrast to amplitude and pulse delivery, may be of greater importance in pain modulation.[23] HF-SCS delivers tonic pulses to the dorsal column at higher frequencies than traditional spinal cord stimulation, typically at 10 kHz. There is no general consensus on the mechanisms of action of HF-SCS, but it has been proposed that HF-SCS works by selectively activating inhibitory interneurons in the dorsal horn or the dorsal root entry zone, without activating dorsal column fibers, thus recruiting small and medium fibers while blocking large axons, leading to suppression of interneurons without paresthesia.[45–47]

HF-SCS employs a paresthesia-free mechanism, delivering high-frequency and low-amplitude pulses to maximize total charge delivery without generating a paresthesia by using direct neural inhibition targeting the dorsal horn cells while avoiding activation of Aβ axons in the dorsal horn. Furthermore, only with the use of 10-kHz modulation were pain neurons and the wind-up response of WDR inhibited without acting in the dorsal column.[24,46,48] Several working hypotheses for the mechanisms of pain relief with HF-SCS have been proposed, including a reversible depolarization blockade (limiting the propagation of nociceptive signals). Other working hypotheses include desynchronization of neural signals, which can result in pseudospontaneous or stochastic neuronal activity in the spinal gate, membrane integration, glial–neuronal interaction, and induced temporal summation, which attenuates the WDR wind-up phenomenon, representing suppression of hyperexcitability in spinal cord neurons.[23,29,32,49–51] HF-SCS with 10 kHz has been shown to selectively activate inhibitory interneurons in the superficial dorsal horn without meaningfully activating dorsal column fibers and excitatory interneurons. Direct neural inhibition by directly targeting the dorsal horn has been shown with frequencies above 5 kHz, in contrast to dorsal column fibers inhibition at lower frequencies (500 Hz) with different waveforms (traditional tonic or burst). Studies have shown that HF-SCS increases dorsal horn expression of c-Fos, an indirect marker of neuronal activation produced during noxious stimulation. An increase of c-Fos immunoreactive cells in the dorsal horn after spinal cord stimulation suggests early cellular activation, further supporting dorsal horn neural circuit modulation.[52] HF-SCS has been postulated to result in significant local heat by modulating neuroinflammatory changes in the 72-kDa heat shock protein, known to inhibit activation of proinflammatory transcription factors on the dorsal structures in the spinal cord.[53]

At present, not much is known about the physiological mechanisms of HF-SCS compared to tonic conventional spinal cord stimulation and how one stimulation produces paresthesia and the other does not. The literature is in its infancy and is controversial. New insights have been described about how the mechanism of action differs between the two, but one working hypothesis suggests that HF-SCS neither activates nor changes the conduction properties of dorsal column fibers. HF-SCS may induce depolarization blockade of lower-threshold large-diameter fibers in the dorsal column, which carry mostly vibration and pressure, and therefore avoid paresthesia. The same stimulation activated medium- and small-diameter fibers, which leads to spinal pain inhibition, with neural inhibition at the level of the dorsal horns. The lack of dorsal column activation, weak inhibition of WDR neurons, and slow onset of pain inhibition suggest that HF-SCS may act through different mechanisms than apply in conventional tonic paresthesia-based stimulation.[8,32,54–55]

DTM Stimulation

DTM programming (Medtronic, Minneapolis, MN) is a stimulation approach in which electrical signals are synchronously delivered to the dorsal aspect of the spinal cord to target multiple cells, including microglia and astrocytes.[56] DTM stimulation delivers three therapy options, with each option delivering four stimulation signals, targeting six different anatomic targets with six different amplitudes. This algorithm involves multiple pulsed signals combined spatially and temporally. Each DTM therapy option is multiplexed, which means that it involves the coordination of four synchronous signals: one base and three prime signals with different frequencies and pulse widths, meaning that each therapy option differentially aims to six anatomic targets collectively.[34,57]

The role of glial cells in the chronic pain state has been described previously, as both microglia and astrocytes play an important role in the development and maintenance of chronic neuropathic states, moderated by glial-mediated sensitization. DTM has been studied in animal models to target and modulate the expression of cell-specific genes in the direction of the healthy state, thus regulating neuronal–glial interaction processes in chronic pain. In addition, preclinical studies in animal models suggested that the DTM waveform has a greater impact in the neural–glial interaction than other frequencies by more effectively modulating genes associated with pain-related processes and returning their expression toward the healthy nonpain state. DTM provides an effective way of modulating immune-related processes, synaptic neurotransmission, signaling, and biological processes that are key to neuroglial interactions in the healthy and chronic pain state.[34,56]

Evoked Compound Action Potential (ECAP) Closed-Loop Stimulation

Available SCS systems, regardless of the stimulation parameters, are open-loop systems, in that they are simply providing stimulation without the ability of sensation of spinal cord activation and active adjustment of waveforms. This is in contrast to the newly described closed-loop stimulation system with ECAP monitoring. An ECAP is a measurement of the response of dorsal column fibers to electrical stimulation in the spinal cord. The ECAP can be controlled in real time with closed-loop stimulation to keep a stable electrical activation within the spinal cord. In lay terms, the advantage of ECAP is that it provides real-time recording of how much stimulation is reaching the target of the spinal cord, and by using objective neurophysiologic measurements, one can keep a stable activation within the spinal cord by maintaining a stable ECAP.[58–60] The feedback occurs at one electrode pair on the SCS lead that sits in the distal epidural space. After receiving the information, the IPG will modify the amplitude of the next electrical signal to the spinal cord, thus maintaining the programmed ECAP to remain within the therapeutic window at a higher rate than in open-loop systems.[59,61]

ECAPs are the sum of multiple action potentials that result from activation of multiple nerve fibers by an electrical stimulus, and in spinal cord stimulation they are equal to a direct measure of spinal cord fiber activation. In closed-loop spinal cord stimulation, the difference between the measured ECAP and the target ECAP amplitude is minimized by automatically adjusting the stimulation current to maintain consistent spinal cord activation.[59–60,62] Perhaps the greatest importance of ECAP stimulation is the monitoring feedback to address variants, such as position, distance, physiological, and anatomic variants. This is important because when using open-loop stimulation, the electrical field strength reaching the spinal cord varies with changes in distance between the electrodes and spinal cord during changes in positioning, breathing, movement, or normal activity, which may result in over- or underactivation of the spinal cord fibers. Yet, the ECAP-controlled closed-loop spinal cord stimulation reduces this variation with posture by adjusting its amplitude automatically.[58,60–62]

Pulsed Stimulation Pattern

Pulsed stimulation pattern (PSP; Nalu Medical, Carlsbad, CA) is a novel mode of electrical delivery that incorporates multiple elements or layers within the waveform, which can implicate different mechanisms of action. PSP involves narrow pulses, high-rate train, long train, and low-rate train. The theoretical mechanisms of action of narrow pulse stimulation include modulation of low-threshold fibers, dorsal horn, dorsal root, and glial cells. High-rate train (onset/offset) increases fiber recruitment, while long train (charge delivery) modulates high-threshold fibers, dorsal column, lateral and medial pathways, and low-rate train (onset/offset) accommodation modulates medial and lateral pathways. These varying stimulation patterns may evoke a wide range of underlying analgesic mechanisms of action similar to other stimulation patterns (i.e., HF-SCS, burst, and traditional stimulation). Early ongoing research suggests that PSP blends multiple mechanisms of action based upon varying temporal response, neurophysiologic modulation, epigenetic (channel and protein up/down regulation), priming glial–neural interaction, and higher-order neuronal modulation.[63]

Indications and Contraindications

In the United States, the utilization of spinal cord stimulation may differ from its use in Europe or other locations across the globe; however, in general, SCS therapy should be considered for patients suffering from intractable chronic pain of the spine or limb who have failed conservative measurements, which is an indication approved by the U.S. Food and Drug Administration.[21] Historically, spinal cord stimulation was used as a last-resort treatment in chronic pain syndrome of the spine and limbs after failure in multiple trials of standard medical care. However, in the new algorithm for the treatment of pain, spinal cord stimulation is moving to earlier use, as the body of evidence continues to grow showing better pain control, decreased opioid utilization, improved long-term functional outcomes with newer technology, and better understanding of neuromodulation therapy. At the time of this writing, the Centers for Medicare & Medicaid Services National Coverage Determination still required this technology be used as a "late resort (if not a last resort) for patients with chronic intractable pain," despite the last revision of this policy being more than 25 years old.[64]

In brief, thoracolumbar spinal cord stimulation is recommended for failed back surgery syndrome (FBSS), neuropathic pain in postlaminectomy, complex regional pain syndrome (CRPS), and as a last-resort treatment of moderate to severe chronic neuropathic pain of the spine and/or extremities that is refractory to standard conservative care. Pain must be neuropathic in nature, and not nociceptive, including chronic postlaminectomy neuropathic pain, chronic radiculopathy, plexopathy, and other chronic pain syndromes.

Note that for cervical or thoracolumbar permanent SCS implantation, SCS trials must demonstrate at least 50% pain relief, and very specific patient criteria must be met, which are described in detail later in this chapter.[4,8,21,64–70]

Recommendations for cervical spinal cord stimulation are controversial, with perhaps the its use for CRPS being the only unanimous position among clinical policies.[67–68] Conditional recommendations on a case-by-case basis, particularly for cervical spinal cord stimulation, include failed neck surgery syndrome, chronic cervical radiculopathy, brachial plexopathy, and chronic pain syndromes of the head, face, neck, and upper extremities that have not responded to traditional conservative care. However, these have not been as extensively studied as thoracolumbar spinal cord stimulation, and literature to support cervical spinal cord stimulation is limited but promising.[21,65,71–72] Studies describing the use of cervical spinal cord stimulation in CRPS, plexopathy, chronic cervical radiculopathy, failed neck surgery syndrome, intractable chronic neck and upper limb pain, intractable migraines, and others have been published,[72–83] and the literature continues to grow with the simultaneous improvement in neuromodulation devices, techniques, understanding of mechanisms of action, patient criteria, and scientific evidence, as described in detail in this chapter. Table 19.2 summarizes the indications for spinal cord stimulation.

The contraindications to SCS implants are quite similar to the general contraindications to other minimally invasive spinal procedures. There are a few more direct considerations and contraindications to SCS implantation, including anatomic, medical, and psychosocial reasons. Anatomic contraindications include critical canal stenosis, serious neurological deficit, spinal instability with surgically correctable pathology, spinal instability at risk for progression, and pregnancy. There are numerous medical considerations regarding SCS implantation, particularly active infection, coagulopathy, thrombocytopenia, immunosuppression, conditions that greatly increase surgical risk, and depending on the device used, the need for MRI in the future. It is also fundamental to consider psychosocial factors, such as cognitive impairment, active substance abuse, a hazardous living environment, severe depression, anxiety, bipolar disorder, other psychosomatic disorders, and unrealistic patient expectations.[84–85]

TABLE 19.2. Summary of SCS Indications

Recommendations (sources)	Indications for Thoracolumbar SCS	Indications for Cervical SCS
Clinical guidelines, society consensus, insurance clinical policies	Failed back surgery syndrome Chronic neuropathic pain postlaminectomy Complex regional pain syndrome	Complex regional pain syndrome
Guidelines and high-level research studies	Chronic lumbar radiculopathy and/or plexopathy Painful peripheral vascular disease Intractable angina	Failed neck surgery syndrome Chronic cervical radiculopathy and/or plexopathy
Limited studies and anecdotal evidence	Visceral and pelvic pain Other chronic pain	Chronic pain of the head, face and upper limb Intractable chronic migraine

Evidence

There are numerous high-quality studies with strong evidence supporting the use of spinal cord stimulation. Studies have demonstrated pain relief and functional outcomes with spinal cord stimulation that are superior to what is achieved with comprehensive medical management, as well as opioid utilization reduction.[4,8,70,86–92] The sentinel evidence supportive of spinal cord stimulation has been documented using tonic stimulation; however, more recently, burst, HF-SCS, DTM, and ECAP stimulation waveforms have demonstrated favorable outcomes.[8,70] A 2019 meta-analysis of approximately 1,000 patients with intractable spine and limb pain of various etiologies, including postlaminectomy syndrome, chronic back or leg pain, diabetic neuropathy, peripheral vascular disease, and CRPS, found that spinal cord stimulation had better pain outcomes than medical treatment, with increased odds of > 50% pain reduction.[70]

Thoracolumbar Spinal Cord Stimulation

FBSS

Spinal cord stimulation is a recommended treatment option for patients who meet the selection criteria and who have FBSS with persistent leg pain that is determined to be related to nerve damage from the initial pathology and/or surgery, as confirmed by diagnostic imaging and/or electrodiagnostic study.[21,65–66] The body of evidence regarding spinal cord stimulation for FBSS, chronic pain, and neuropathic pain continues to grow, as the technology for spinal neuromodulation evolves. There is moderate-quality evidence supporting the use of spinal cord stimulation in patients with persistent radicular pain due to FBSS.[21] The earliest studies that demonstrated statistically significant improvements in pain control with SCS implant in contrast to repeat lumbar surgery and comprehensive medical management were first described in 2005 and 2007 by North et al,[89] and Kumar et al,[93] respectively. In particular, the crossover randomized controlled trial (RCT) by North described that 47% of patients with SCS implantation and 12% with lumbar reoperation achieved at least 50% pain relief of low back pain due to FBSS.[89] The international multicenter RCT with 6-month follow-up published by Kumar et al compared spinal cord stimulation to conventional medical management in treating postsurgical low back pain and radiculopathy, and found that 48% of patients in the SCS group achieved at least 50% pain relief, in contrast to only 9% in the medical group.[93]

Subsequently, the crossover study by Manca et al compared spinal cord stimulation and active medical management with NSAIDs, antidepressants, anticonvulsants, opioids, epidural corticosteroids, nerve blocks, rehab therapy, and chiropractic with 6-month and 12-month long-term follow-up. At 6 months, 9% of the patients in the medical management group and 48% of the patients in the SCS group had at least 50% pain relief. By 12 months, 34% of patients in the SCS group and 7% of patients in the medical group achieved at least 50% pain relief; the conclusion was that in comparison to conventional medical management, spinal cord stimulation generates important improvements in pain relief and patients' QoL outcomes.[94] Frey et al conducted a systematic review of level II-1 and II-2 evidence regarding the use of spinal cord stimulation in FBSS and concluded that 60% of selected patients could expect at least a 50% reduction in chronic pain on a long-term basis.[95] According to the summary review by Rock et al, spinal cord stimulation is recommended by the National Institute for Health and Care Excellence, the British Pain Society, the Neurostimulation Appropriateness Consensus Committee (NACC), and other societies when the patient selection criteria described on this chapter are met,[92] and particularly the British Pain Society guidelines conclude that multiple high-level studies of SCS use in FBSS have demonstrated improved pain relief, reduction in medication use, improved QoL, and greater patient satisfaction.[95–96]

With advancements in SCS technology, new studies were published discussing the efficacy of spinal cord stimulation in FBSS using different waveforms. Sweet et al published a level II randomized crossover trial comparing conventional spinal cord stimulation and subthreshold high-density spinal cord stimulation with sham stimulation and found that subthreshold spinal cord stimulation yielded significantly greater improvement in pain relief (primary outcome 50%) than was achieved with conventional spinal cord stimulation.[97] In a double-blind crossover RCT published in 2014, Schu et al found that patients receiving burst stimulation had significantly lower pain scores than patients receiving tonic and placebo stimulation and concluded that burst was superior to tonic stimulation in short-term pain relief.[98] Kapural et al published a multicenter RCT of patients with heterogeneous diagnoses and compared HF-SCS with traditional spinal cord stimulation.[88] Data suggested that at 24 months the HF-SCS group had a greater response rate than the tonic stimulation group as well as greater pain reduction in both back and leg.[88] A year later, De Andres et al published a non–industry-sponsored RCT that compared conventional spinal cord stimulation to HF-SCS in patients with FBSS.[99] Results showed no difference in pain or functional scores between the two groups at 12 months, and both tonic stimulation and HF-SCS caused significant pain reduction relative to baseline.[99] Bolash et al compared tonic stimulation and HF-SCS and concluded that HF-SCS waveform was noninferior to the low-frequency waveforms in regard to back and leg pain at multiple endpoints in the first 6 months,[100] while the studies by Kinfe et al and Muhammad et al concluded that burst stimulation and HF-SCS were both equally safe and effective in decreasing back and leg pain, although burst was slightly better at decreasing leg pain.[101–102] De Voss et al conducted a prospective crossover study comparing tonic and burst stimulation for FBSS and found that burst stimulation provided additional pain benefit (approximately 30%) compared to tonic stimulation, with a patient preference for tonic stimulation.[103] Courtney et al, in a prospective study comparing tonic and burst stimulation for FBSS, concluded that overall pain scores reduced 46% from tonic to burst stimulation, and almost all patients had a preference for burst stimulation over tonic, findings comparable to those in the study by De Ridder in 2015.[104] The study by De Ridder et al was a prospective crossover study comparing tonic and burst stimulation for FBSS and found that burst stimulation was superior to both tonic and placebo stimulation; furthermore, when patients from the tonic stimulation group crossed over to the burst stimulation group, meaningful benefit in pain reduction was achieved, with a subjective patient preference for burst stimulation.[105]

To summarize, over the past two decades, studies have demonstrated the clinical and statistical efficacy of spinal cord stimulation in patients with chronic refractory low back pain caused by neuropathic pain and postlaminectomy syndrome. Some of the studies reviewed appear to have shown a small favorability of HF-SCS over tonic stimulation and a small superiority of burst stimulation over tonic stimulation. However, due to limited data, superiority cannot be clearly established. Evidence comparing HF-SCS and burst stimulation is limited, but small studies have suggested equal effectiveness for improving back pain, with a slight superiority of burst stimulation for decreasing leg pain. Spinal cord stimulation should be used as recommended by clinical guidelines, and a case-by-case patient-selection, device-selection, and waveform-selection approach remains the best method for achieving a successful treatment plan.

CRPS

Spinal cord stimulation in patients with CRPS selected per the criteria described in this chapter can provide substantial pain reduction and improvement in health-related QoL.[106–109] Spinal cord stimulation can be an adjunct therapy for CRPS refractory to conventional therapy, particularly in patients with disease limited to one extremity.[21] In one series of studies, spinal cord stimulation in CRPS was shown to decrease pain scores more significantly than physical therapy alone at 6-month follow-up, to 24 months. At 6 months and 2 years, the SCS group had reduced severe burning pain, but no change was found in allodynia, hypesthesia, or function. The authors concluded that SCS implant plus physical therapy reduced pain and improved health-related QoL more than physical therapy alone for up to 2 years but did not improve functional outcome measures, and they noted that despite the diminished effectiveness over time, 95% of patients would proceed with SCS implant again for their CRPS.[106–108] Harke et al conducted a prospective trial that evaluated the use of spinal cord stimulation in CRPS and found that SCS implant was considered effective, with substantial pain relief up to 35 months' follow-up.[110] Along the same line, Van Eijs et al, in a small prospective study using tonic spinal cord stimulation in CRPS, concluded that tonic stimulation reduced pain by 35% up to 12 months and suggested that the feasibility of early use for SCS in CRPS was low.[111] Sears et al, in a retrospective cohort study, found that patients with SCS had a high degree of satisfaction, but their pain relief rate was lower[112] than in other studies, such as that by Geurts et al, who found sustained pain relief with SCS in patients with CRPS with 11 years of long-term follow up.[113] Gopal et al, in a retrospective review of 80 cases of SCS for patients with a diagnosis of FBSS and CRPS who had undergone prior comprehensive medical management and interventional treatment with no sustained benefit, found that SCS implantation was the most effective treatment for FBSS and CRPS that has proven resistant to medical management.[114] A comprehensive review reported that SCS is a favorable and effective modality for treating CRPS, with high-level evidence (IB+) supporting its role in improving patients' perceived pain relief, pain score, and QoL.[115]

With advancements in SCS technology, new studies were published discussing the efficacy of spinal cord stimulation in CRPS using different waveforms. Kriek et al concluded that standard tonic stimulation frequency is an effective therapy for patients with CRPS.

However, they also demonstrated that patients can often gain better pain reduction with nonstandard frequencies of stimulation. Significant pain reduction and patient satisfaction were achieved at four different settings. Standard stimulation was preferred by 48% of the patients, while 52% preferred nonstandard stimulation.[116] Stimulation settings at 40, 500, and 1,200 Hz and burst were equally effective in relieving neuropathic pain related to CRPS and were significantly better than placebo.[116] A review published in 2019 by Hoydonckx et al identified 13 studies discussing new waveforms for stimulation in CRPS, including burst, HF-10, and high-density, and concluded that novel SCS models have the potential to provide analgesia in patients with CRPS, with patients reporting 30% to 100% pain reduction, as well as significant improvement in QoL.[117] To summarize, the National Institute for Health and Care Excellence, the British Pain Society, the NACC, and other societies recommend the use of SCS for adults with CRPS 1 and CRPS 2 who continue to experience chronic pain despite medical management, and these recommendations are based on clinical evidence, level IIa-III data, with degree recommendation A based on available data.[92]

Other Chronic Pain

Although the relevant literature is less robust than the literature on the other major indications, there are multiple painful syndromes that might be successfully treated with spinal cord stimulation. Chronic neuropathic pain, painful diabetic neuropathy, postherpetic neuralgia, intercostal neuralgia, postthoracotomy neuralgia, and phantom limb pain after spinal cord injury have been described in the literature to have been successfully treated with SCS implant.[4,92,118–120] Level I evidence already exists for the efficacy of SCS in treating CBLP, and it is supported by real-world clinical experience.[121]

Numerous studies have evaluated the use of SCS implantation in chronic back pain "maiden back" ineligible for spinal surgery or surgery-naive. Van Buyten et al studied the use of SCS for the treatment of chronic back pain in patients with or without leg pain and with no history of surgery, and the authors found that 60% of patients reported long-term pain reduction of more than 50% from baseline at 24 months, and 71% of subjects reported leg pain reduction of more than 50% at 24-month follow-up.[122] De Ridder et al, in a prospective crossover double-blind RCT, described the use of spinal cord stimulation for limb and back pain in SCS-naive patients. They compared tonic and burst stimulation versus placebo and found that burst stimulation was noninferior and superior to tonic stimulation in the treatment of chronic neuropathic limb and back pain, with patients preferring burst stimulation.[43] These findings are in agreement with the study by Deer et al in SCS-naive patients with chronic pain of the back and limbs; the authors concluded that patients had improvement in pain and significantly preferred burst stimulation over tonic.[86] In a series of studies from 2017 to 2020, Al-Kaisy confirmed with long-term follow-up data the benefits of SCS for chronic neuropathic pain in patients without surgical history.[123–125] The 2017 study concluded that there was an average reduction of VAS score of 4.7 points at 6 months and a reduction of 5.6 points at 12 months.[123] The authors recommended the use of 10-kHz SCS instead of surgery in patients with clear and unequivocal correlation between clinical symptoms and radiological findings. Subsequently, in a 36-month follow-up prospective open-label study examining the use of 10-kHz SCS for treatment of low back pain in patients with no history of spinal surgery, 17 of 20 patients reached the 36-month endpoint, and the authors indicated that SCS can be used when surgery is not appropriate; however, further data are needed.[123–124] Furthermore, several studies have discussed real-world data regarding the benefits of SCS, particularly HF-SCS, in patients with nonsurgical refractory back pain, with the studies reporting on a small sample of patients with statistically and clinically significant improvements in numerous outcomes, including pain relief, function, disability, QoL, global health perception, and opioid utilization reduction, with benefits noted at 12 months postimplantation and clinical benefits sustained after 3 years of stimulation.[121,124,126–127] Data have shown that 10-kHz HF-SCS is a promising therapy for nonsurgical refractory back pain, with average back pain decreased by 70% at 3-month follow-up. The results was sustained at 12 months, with a 73% back pain and leg pain responder rate and a 68% remission rate. At 12 months, the combined cohort of two large studies had an average decrease in disability scores of 15.7% points from baseline, and opioid use decreased more than 50%. The authors conducted subanalysis of prospectively collected clinical outcome data from the independent cohorts of two previous studies (SENZA-RCT and SENZA-EU) and concluded that 10-kHz SCS reduced pain, disability, and opioid consumption for patients with nonsurgical refractory back pain, suggesting that application of 10-kHz SCS may improve care for nonsurgical refractory back pain.[128]

Among other painful syndromes in which SCS has been studied, painful diabetic neuropathy has been the subject of clinical and research interest. The study by De Voss et al randomized patients with diabetic neuropathy into two groups, one group with conventional medical management plus SCS, and the second (control) group with medical management but no additional SCS therapy. After 6 months of treatment, the average pain score was significantly reduced, from 73 to 31, in the SCS group ($P < .001$), but it remained 67 ($P = .97$) in the control group. QoL questionnaires also showed that patients in the SCS group, unlike those in the control group, experienced reduced pain and improved health and QoL after 6 months of treatment. The authors concluded that in patients with refractory painful diabetic neuropathy, SCS therapy significantly reduced pain and improved QoL.[129] Slangen et al also demonstrated durable pain relief for painful diabetic neuropathy with SCS treatment, with sustained benefits up to 6 months.[130] Numerous other studies have also been published discussing the use of SCS in painful diabetic neuropathy. For example, multicenter studies by Petersen et al and Galan et al reported the outcomes for painful diabetic neuropathy treated with HF-SCS and found that pain relief was sustained at 12 months by 74% of patients, and a total of 86% of patients were responders at 12 months, with up to 71% reporting improvement in peripheral sensory neuropathy and reflexes. Patients showed improvement in pain scores, disability index scores, global function, and sleep scores, with 85% reporting they felt moderately better, better, or significantly better at 12-month follow up.[131–132]

Intractable Angina

It is outside the scope of this chapter to discuss spinal cord stimulation use in non-spine-related pathologies. However, it is important to note that SCS implantation has been widely studied for the treatment of intractable refractory angina providing anti-ischemic effects that has been known to improve QoL and the New York Heart Association (NYHA) functional class, and it is recommended by multiple sites and clinical guidelines as a treatment option.[21] Note that, in contrast to the traditional thoracolumbar SCS implant, the SCS implant for angina treatment is at the T1–T2 level. The largest trial of SCS implants for intractable refractory angina concluded that SCS reduced angina and nitrate use as much as coronary artery bypass graft surgery (CABG) did and was associated with lower 6-month mortality and stroke event rates than CABG. However, SCS had no effect on ischemic ST changes; therefore, the SCS-related reduction in anginal symptoms suggested mainly an analgesic effect. Consequently, it is suggested that SCS should be reserved for a few carefully selected patients who cannot undergo CABG.[133–134]

Painful Peripheral Vascular Disease

In contrast to the United States, where SCS implantation is most commonly used for chronic back pain with neuropathic features, in Europe, the most common indication for SCS implant is painful inoperable peripheral vascular disease.[21] However, because it is outside the scope of this chapter to discuss SCS use for other than spine-related pathologies, the topic of peripheral vascular disease is only briefly considered here. To note, a few studies have shown that SCS implant was effective for limb analgesia, delay of amputation, and improved limb survival, and a systematic review in 2013 concluded that the risk of limb loss after 12 months was significantly lower in the spinal cord stimulation group, while there were no significant differences in ulcer healing. The authors concluded that there was evidence favoring SCS use over standard conservative treatment alone to improve limb salvage, but the benefits of SCS must be considered in non-vascular surgical candidates.[135] In 2020, Saini et al concluded that the literature supports the use of SCS implants for intractable peripheral vascular disease and intractable angina, and patients with SCS showed improvement in cerebral blood flow, increased capillary recruitment, better QoL, increased exercise capacity, and significant reductions in both narcotic drug use and daily attacks.[136]

Cervical Spinal Cord Stimulation

The applications of cervical spinal cord stimulation are based on the obvious similarities to thoracolumbar SCS applications and on anecdotal experience. Yet, cervical spinal cord stimulation is an area where many evidence gaps still exist, guidelines are not clear, and recommendations differ.[137] Perhaps the only unanimous indication for the use of cervical SCS is in CRPS. However, as more studies have been published discussing SCS for cervical pathologies, and with new technological advancements in waveforms, the use of cervical SCS for intractable cervical axial and radicular pain will continue to grow and show value, particularly with paresthesia-free waveforms. Presently, literature to support cervical SCS for failed cervical spine surgery, cervical axial spine pain, and radicular pain is limited to case series, retrospective studies, and prospective studies with level II evidence. Cervical SCS is an important treatment option in the management of chronic refractory neck pain, radicular pain, failed neck surgery, CRPS, pain of the head, face, and jaw, intractable headache, and occipital neuralgia, among other conditions.[21,65,72–83]

In 2014, one of the first cervical SCS studies, a prospective study, evaluated the benefits of cervical SCS in patients with heterogeneous cervical spine diagnoses and not necessarily failed cervical surgery. The patients treated with cervical SCS reported pain relief of 54.2% at 3 months, 60.2% at 6 months, and 66.8% at 12 months.[65] In the same year, a case series report on cervical SCS for indications including failed cervical spine surgery reported pain reduction averaged at least 50% (28.6%–70%) across all groups, with pain relief lasting a mean of 3.5 years (0.5–13 years) for all diagnostic categories and a mean of 2.4 years for failed neck surgery syndrome.[79] Haider et al demonstrated that both percutaneous and paddle implant cervical SCS can improve pain and function in patients with failed neck surgery syndrome, CRPS, and neuropathic pain (cervical radiculopathy), with sustained relief at 6-month and 12-month follow-up.[76] The authors discussed the comparable efficacy, safety, and long-term patient satisfaction with cervical SCS and thoracolumbar SCS. Additionally, the authors discussed the use of paddle versus percutaneous electrodes and concluded that if percutaneous trial was effective in covering the pain, the recommendation was to proceed with percutaneous electrodes. Placement of cervical leads is particularly challenging, being more risky and more difficult. Displacement of cervical leads is twice as likely, due to enhanced cervical spine mobility, and is more likely to require surgical revision. Overall, due to the size and shape of paddle leads and the narrowed cervical spinal canal, percutaneous leads may be favored.[71,76]

The study by Hunter et al concluded that the application of cervical SCS for failed cervical spine surgery is effective in reducing pain, in improving QoL, and in increasing patient satisfaction, but further studies are needed. In the study, 65.2% pain relief was observed at 3 months, 62.4% at 6 months, and 71.9% at 12 months after cervical SCS implantation. Statistical analysis also concluded that pain, disability, and QoL scores were statistically and clinically significantly improved up to 12-month follow-up.[138] These data are congruent with previously published data that evaluated tonic cervical SCS and demonstrated pain relief at 6 months and 1 year.[51,72,75,79,139]

The introduction of new waveform technology triggered a new direction in the clinical research use of cervical SCS, particularly after the SENZA study utilizing HF-SCS and the SunBURST study utilizing burst stimulation.[86,88] These studies suggested statistical superiority with pain relief (both SENZA and SunBURST) and clinical superiority (SENZA) compared to tonic SCS. The clinical efficacy of tonic low-frequency SCS in the cervical spine is challenged in clinical practice by the difficulty of obtaining sensory paresthesia in the axial neck region, with high variability of the paresthesia secondary to the inherent, dynamic neck and upper limb movements. The variability may result in excess, not enough, or discomfort that leads to suboptimal outcomes. Therefore, the use of new waveforms, such as burst and 10-kHz HF-SCS, is particularly interesting in the cervical spine. The study by Grider et al evaluated the use of a monophasic burst waveform cervical SCS in patients with chronic cervical axial pain with and without radicular pain and concluded that the use of burst cervical SCS improved function, QoL, and pain in these patients and patients with cervicogenic headache.[83] Patients were followed up to 1 year postoperatively and outcome measurements suggested statistically and clinically significant improvements in Oswestry Disability Index (ODI), global pain scale score, and opioid utilization reduction (93% reduction). The retrospective open-label study by El-Majdoub et al evaluated the efficacy of 10-kHz HF-SCS in chronic neck and upper limb pain, and the authors concluded that HF-SCS of the cervical spine was effective in reducing pain and in improving functional capacity.[82] Pain relief for axial neck pain at 3 months was reported at 71.6%, 70.9% at 6 months, and 74.1% at 12 months. Pain relief for upper limb pain at 3 months was 72%, 72.2% at 6 months, and 76.7% at 12 months. ODI score measured a 35.5% decrease by 3 months and remained stable at 6 and 12 months. Decrease of total morphine equivalents was also documented at 55.9% at 12 months, and the total dose of anti-inflammatory steroidal drug use decreased by 78.9% after 12 months.[82] These findings were corroborated by the studies of Deer et al 2014 and Chivukala et al 2014.

The study by Amirdelfan et al in 2020 excluded patients with previous cervical spine surgery and evaluated the use of cervical SCS in chronic axial neck pain with and without radiculopathy. The authors concluded that 10-kHz HF-SCS provided long, durable pain relief and improvement in QoL. The primary endpoint was > 50% pain relief at 3 months and was achieved by 86.7% of patients. At 12 months, 89.2% of patients with neck pain and 95% of patients with upper limb pain had > 50% pain relief from baseline. Additionally, 95% of patients reported to be satisfied or very satisfied with the intervention, and 30% either eliminated or reduced their opioid intake. 10-kHz HF-SCS cervical treatment resulted in a nearly 25-point reduction in pain disability index, nearly 2.5-fold greater than the value needed for statistically meaningful clinical difference, which is higher than previous data from low-frequency tonic SCS.[81] Foremost, the studies by Sayed et al and Burgher et al evaluated real-world outcomes of 10 kHz HF-SCS in patients with upper limb and neck pain.[121,140] The primary outcome was > 50% pain relief at the end of the trial, and all patients reported a successful response. More than 75% of patients reported continued improvement at last follow-up, while 72% of patients reported improvement in function, 53% of the patients reported improvement in sleep, and 36% of patients reported reducing their medication at the last follow-up period.[121] The study by Burgher et al added to the growing body of literature supporting the recent findings by Amirdelfan et al and Sayed et al, adding that HF-SCS, particularly at 10 kHz, is effective for chronic upper extremity and neck pain, with a great safety profile and patient satisfaction level, with 84.4% of patients at 12-month follow-up satisfied or very satisfied with their treatment, along with 78.1% upper limb pain relief, 85.2% shoulder pain relief, and 75% neck pain relief at 12-month follow-up.[140]

As the field of neuromodulation continues to evolve with new devices, waveforms, understanding of mechanisms of actions, and surgical techniques, pain physicians will become more comfortable in adding cervical spinal cord stimulation to their clinical practice, concomitantly as new evidence grows through continued research on use of cervical spinal cord stimulation.

Other Notable Evidence

Salvage Therapy

Initiating use of a newer form of SCS after failure of a conventional unit is considered investigational[65]; however, several studies have demonstrated statistical and clinical significance of results when newer waveform technologies are used in previously failed SCS therapy.[141] The review by Reddy et al in 2020 examined a total of eight studies and four abstracts on salvage therapy and concluded that, from data currently available, the conversion from conventional tonic stimulation to new waveforms (burst, HF, multiple waves) may be appropriate in selected patients.[142] The study by Ghosh et al corroborated these findings: patients who had experienced failed tonic stimulation primarily from poor paresthesia coverage underwent a trial and implantation with 10-kHz HF-SCS and reported great response, findings suggesting that, in a significant proportion of patients with previously failed tonic stimulation, HF-SCS may achieve clinically meaningful and durable pain relief up to 8 months.[143] Kapural et al conducted a retrospective data review of 120 patients across two clinical sites and found that, of cases with previous failed low-frequency SCS, 81% reported at least 50% pain relief upon utilization of 10-kHz HF-SCS and a significant decrease of opioid utilization at 12 months after salvage therapy. The authors concluded that HF-SCS should be considered an appropriate option to rescue failed low-frequency SCS.[144]

Adjunctive Treatment to Decrease Opioid Use

There is high-quality evidence from RCTs, systematic reviews, and meta-analyses discussing the role of SCS as an adjunctive treatment to decrease opioid utilization; however, society recommendations and clinical guidelines still debate the effect of spinal cord stimulation on the likelihood of opioid use. Considering the ongoing opioid epidemic in the United States, where more than 47,000 Americans died of opioid overdose in 2017 and more than 153,260,450 prescriptions for opioids were written in 2019, it is common sense to consider nonpharmacological interventions, such a SCS, as an adjunct to help decrease opioid utilization. Recent data are clear that SCS use helps decrease opioid utilization. For example, the systematic review of RCTs and meta-analysis conducted by Pollard et al in 2019 concluded that, in patients with intractable spine and limb pain, SCS use was significantly associated with reduced opioid consumption. The study reviewed data from five trials, with a total of 489 patients, and examined the odds of reduced opioid consumption with SCS in comparison to medical treatment. The authors concluded that the odds of reducing opioid consumption were significantly increased in the SCS group compared to the medically treated group.[145]

It is important to note that a study by North et al in 2005 found that patients taking high-dose opioid analgesics were more likely to fail SCS treatment[89] and a study by Kapural et al in 2015 reported that 35.5% of HF-SCS patients decreased or eliminated opioid utilization.[88] On the other hand, the observational study by Dougherty et al reviewed 145 charts and the trend of opioid utilization after SCS implantation.[146] They found that the daily morphine equivalent dose of 65 was the most statistically meaningful preoperative dose threshold, and approximately 50% of patients decreased opioid use by > 20% after SCS implantation. The authors concluded that, although there was statistically significant opioid reduction after SCS implant, not all patients saw benefit from SCS, and there is still much room for further research regarding the opioid-sparing effects of SCS.[146] Al-Kaisy et al reviewed multiple prospective and retrospective studies of patients with intractable pain who received HF-SCS; the authors demonstrated that in patients treated with HF-SCS, the mean daily dose of opioids was reduced after SCS treatment, and on average over 60% patients either reduced or eliminated opioids at the last follow-up.[147] Studies have documented that higher use of opioids before and during SCS implant use has been shown to be associated with higher rates of explant, and patients who eliminate opioid use completely have been reported to have clinical outcomes in pain scores and disability that are superior to outcomes for patients who remain on opioids. High-dose opioid use is known to be associated with an increased odds ratio of treatment failure.[89,148] Overall, studies have shown that elimination of opioid dependence after SCS implant has been found to be highly dependent on pre-implant dose, with patients on a morphine equivalent dose ≤ 30 mg/day being most likely to wean completely after spinal cord stimulation.[149]

Spinal neuromodulation can help stabilize or decrease opioid use; therefore, it is plausible to consider, on a case-by-case basis, earlier SCS intervention in pain treatment, before escalating opioid use, as it has been documented that spinal cord stimulation has the potential to decrease/eliminate opioid use and to improve pain, function, and QoL outcomes in complex chronic pain patients. As has been described by Lad et al, healthcare resource utilization increases with longer pain-to-SCS time, suggesting that considering spinal cord stimulation earlier in the care continuum for chronic pain improves patient outcomes, with reductions in hospitalizations, clinic visits, and opioid usage.[150]

Spasticity

Research into chronic and intractable spasticity as another potential indication for SCS implantation had initial traction with the burgeoning of the technology in the 1980's.[151–154] However, momentum waned because complications remained relatively high and efficacy was questioned in a small retrospective study of just 17 patients in 1998 that became widely cited.[155] Thankfully, technology has advanced, complications have dramatically decreased, and recently there has been renewed research into this indication.[156–159] Spasticity as an indication for SCS implant remains less researched and incompletely understood, but it illustrates the exciting point that patients with formerly intractable painful conditions may take renewed hope from expanding SCS technology.

Patient Selection and Criteria

Perhaps the most important factor for the overall success of SCS treatment in chronic pain is proper patient selection. Failure in proper selection can lead to poor patient outcomes, increased healthcare costs, higher demand for medications, elevated psychological and emotional burden, increased risk of litigation, and disease progression. (Of course, in addition to proper patient selection, proper SCS device selection is an integral factor for success, especially considering the continuous technological evolution of devices, waveforms, and

SCS programming, but it is outside the scope of this chapter to discuss the specifics of device and waveform selection.)

Appropriate patient selection for spinal cord stimulation must meet the following criteria as defined by current literature and commercial insurance providers: [4,21,65,67–69,92]

- The patient must have a documented medical diagnosis amenable to SCS treatment (e.g., FBSS, CRPS, intractable chronic neuropathic pain), as described in the indications section of this chapter
- The pain source addressed must be neuropathic, as confirmed by physical exam, diagnostic imaging, and electrodiagnostic findings when appropriate
- The patient must have had suboptimal response to, must have failed, or must be judged unsuitable for, conservative therapy (e.g., pharmacological therapy, psychotherapy, physical therapy, spinal injections)
- There is a high correlation between favorable response to SCS and complex psychological testing as part of preoperative evaluation and proper patient selection. The goal is to maximize the probability of improvement in functional outcomes and pain while establishing functional goals to reinforce that improvement in pain is not the primary endpoint, but rather the return to functional activity.
- The patient must have demonstrated at least 50% pain relief with SCS trial
    - The delay between trial and implant is important; the longer the period between the end of the trial and the actual implant is, the lower the effectiveness of SCS is.

Exclusion criteria for SCS vary widely; however, some common exclusion criteria reported in multiple studies are spinal instability, spinal malignancy, pregnancy, thrombocytopenia, coagulopathy, active malignancy, spinal infections, and contraindications to device implantation or the surgical procedure.

Predictability of a successful SCS implant is directly proportional to SCS trial response. However, mounting evidence has suggested that increased BMI, smoking, substance abuse, and psychiatric illness (untreated depression and anxiety) tend to correlate with less favorable outcomes. Other risk factors associated with failure include somatization disorder, substance-use disorder, lack of social support, and high-dose opioid therapy(≥ 90 mg of daily morphine equivalents prior to implant).[65]

Perioperative Management

Planning for, and perioperative management of, spinal cord stimulator implantation are of heightened importance to the interventional pain physician, because this procedure is one of the most technically challenging in the field today. Foremost, proper patient selection is critical to successful outcomes. Preoperative preparation includes medical optimization of the patient, identification of contraindications, evaluation of psychological factors, and recognition of potential complications. And, of course, implantation of the SCS presupposes a successful trial phase of SCS implant (discussed at length in Chapter 18).

Preoperative Testing

The extent of preoperative testing is dictated by several factors, including the decision about general anesthesia or sedation, the comorbidities present, and the use of other bioelectrical devices (e.g., pacemaker, implantable cardiac defibrillator, peripheral nerve stimulator, deep brain stimulator, intrathecal pump, etc.). If the decision is to use general anesthesia, then preanesthesia evaluation should include a specific history and physical exam, airway assessment, and appropriate laboratory tests.

Laboratory evaluation is dictated by medical history, comorbidities, and demographics. It is appropriate to have female patients of child-bearing age get a pregnancy test, because SCS implants are not done in pregnant patients. It is prudent practice to get a preoperative complete laboratory evaluation, including CBC, PT, PTT, INR, bleeding time, and blood type and cross. If the patient has a history of easy bruising or potential for infection, a CBC is reasonable to rule out thrombocytopenia and leukocytosis, respectively. PT/INR can be helpful in identifying coagulopathies. Uncontrolled coagulopathy and severe thrombocytopenia (< 50k platelets) are absolute contraindications to SCS implantation.[160] As is discussed under "Anticoagulation Guidelines," anticoagulants, including warfarin, clopidogrel, aspirin, nonsteroidal anti-inflammatories, and others, should be discontinued before surgical interventions, usually within 7 days of the procedure, although often patients can continue to use acetaminophen. Also, as the standard of care for surgical interventions, the preoperative workup should include urinalysis, chest x-ray, electrocardiogram, and a metabolic panel.

One important consideration is addressing patients with bioelectrical devices, especially cardiac devices: device compatibility should be researched and established prior to implantation of the SCS. For patients with cardiac devices, it is advisable to consult with the patient's cardiologist prior to SCS implantation and to obtain all cardiac laboratories indicated. An implantable cardiac defibrillator requires elevated attention to ensure that the SCS does not discharge the defibrillator, and it is paramount to check with the SCS device manufacturer to ensure compatibility.[160]

Preoperative patient education and counseling ares fundamental for successful outcomes and minimization of complications. Patients should be counseled about medications to hold temporarily prior to the procedure, about tight glucose control, about reduction of BMI, and against tobacco use, especially because nonsmokers and healthy-weight patients have lower risk of postoperative infection and wound dehiscence.[161]

Advanced imaging is routinely obtained prior to SCS implantation. An MRI within the past 6 months, and assuming there have been no interval surgeries, should suffice in providing proper preoperative planning in anticipation of potential technical difficulties and optimal lead placement. If it is not possible to complete an MRI, a CT scan of the thoracolumbar spine is an alternative, and it may or may not include a myelogram. Assessment of the most patent interspinous spacing for lead placement may be achieved with MRI or CT scan.[160] Critical central canal stenosis and anatomic spinal instability at risk for progression are both contraindications to the procedure, as are serious neurologic deficits or significant dynamic spine instability with surgically correctable pathology.[85,162] Other anatomic factors evaluated by advanced imaging include severe scoliosis, kyphosis, severe degenerative changes with facet hypertrophy and osteophytes, and previous spine surgeries, including fusion and hardware placement. These conditions can make fluoroscopic visualization of landmarks more difficult.[162]

Biopsychosocial Screening

Biopsychosocial screening is uniquely important to the SCS implant procedure. It is typically performed prior to SCS trial; the reader is referred to the discussion of this topic in Chapter 18 on the SCS trial. Recall that it is known that there is a high correlation between complex psychological testing and favorable response to SCS, meaning a biopsychosocial screening prior to SCS trial leads to better outcomes. The aim is to maximize the probability of improvement in functional outcomes and in pain relief and to establish function goals, in order to reinforce to the patient that the primary endpoint is not improvement in pain, but the return to functional activity.

Briefly, biopsychosocial screening is the most comprehensive and heuristic approach to evaluating the complex interactions of medical disorders.[163] It is good practice to consult a psychiatrist or trained psychologist early in the patient's chronic pain treatment journey to evaluate the patient's mental and emotional stability, particularly before the patient undergoes the SCS implantation procedure. The evaluation typically uses a combination of assessment tools, including the Oswestry Disability Questionnaire, Beck Depression Inventory, Pain Medication Questionnaire, MMPI, SF-36, and Coping Strategy Questionnaire. It is important to gather the patient's pain symptoms, demographic information (including marital status, employment status, education level), date of onset of pain, details of the pain condition, prior treatments or surgeries attempted, disability payment status, workers' compensation or personal injury litigation involvement, healthcare utilization, and other comorbid chronic health problems.[164] Psychosocial risk factors include occupational strife, physical or emotional abuse, lack of spousal support, substance abuse, anger, depression, and anxiety. Medical risk factors include pain lasting more than 2 years, prior surgery, nonorganic signs, abnormal pain drawing, smoking status, and obesity.[165–167]

Biopsychosocial contraindications include severe cognitive impairment, active substance abuse, living environment that could be potentially hazardous, inability to provide informed consent, or unrealistic patient expectations.[84–85] Relative contraindications include poor social support, lack of reliable means for follow-up, or untreated psychological disorder. Psychosocial conditions that should be optimized prior to deciding to proceed with SCS implantation include personality disorders, unstable or unsupportive family environment, suicidal ideation, severe depression, severe sleep disturbances, somatization/somatoform disorder, active alcohol or drug use, and marked cognitive impairment.[162]

Antibiotics

In 2017, the NACC for Infection Prevention and Management published a comprehensive set of guidelines, and the reader is referred to the NACC's publication for exhaustive discussion of this important topic.[167] The NACC recommendations for infection management practices, which provide the basis for the discussion here, are listed in Table 19.3.

TABLE 19.3. The Neurostimulation Appropriateness Consensus Committee (NACC) Recommendations for Infection Management Practices, with Origin of Practice[a]

NACC Recommended Practices	Evidence Level	Recommendation Strength	Consensus Strength
Preoperative practices			
Identify and treat all remote infections	II-2	B	Strong
Optimize glucose control	II-2	B	Strong
Discontinue tobacco use	II-2	B	Strong
Decolonize MSSA and MRSA carriers through the application of mupirocin nasal ointment and chlorohexidine baths	I	A	Strong
Utilize preoperative antibiotics	I	A	Strong
Utilize preoperative weight-based antibiotic dosing	I	A	Strong
Use appropriate preoperative timing (within 1 hour before surgical incision, excluding vancomycin) for prophylactic antimicrobial administration	I	A	Strong
Remove hair (when required) with electric clippers immediately prior	I	A	Strong
Perform preoperative surgical scrub for a minimum of 2 to 5 minutes with an appropriate antiseptic	II-2	B	Strong
Keep nails short and do not wear artificial nails	II-3	B	Strong
Do not wear hand or arm jewelry	III	B	Strong
Intraoperative practices			
Wear a surgical mask	II-3	B	Strong
Wear a surgical cap or hood to fully cover hair	II-3	B	Strong
Use sterile gown and gloves	II-3	B	Strong
Double glove	II-1	B	Strong
Utilize chlorhexidine gluconate for preoperative skin antiseptic	I	A	Strong
If an incise drape is used, then iodophor-impregnated drape is recommended	I	A	Strong
Use laminar flow and HEPA filters in the OR	I	A	Strong
Limit procedure room traffic	I	A	Strong
Keep procedure room doors closed	II-3	B	Strong
Limit tissue trauma, maintain hemostasis, eradicate dead space, and avoid electrocautery at tissue surface	III	B	Strong
Irrigate with saline through a bulb syringe prior to closure of surgical wound	I	B	Strong
Employ implant strategies to limit operative time	II-2	B	Strong
Postoperative practices			
Apply an occlusive dressing for 24 to 48 hours	II-2	B	Strong
Do not routinely use topical antimicrobial agents for surgical wounds that are healing by primary intention	II-2	B	Strong

(continued)

TABLE 19.3. Continued

NACC Recommended Practices	Evidence Level	Recommendation Strength	Consensus Strength
Understand maximum time criterion for defining a deep SSI of an implantable device (1 year postimplant)	III	B	Strong
Do not continue antibiotics into the postoperative period beyond 24 hours	I	A	Strong
Educate patient and family on proper incision care, symptoms of SSI, and importance of reporting symptoms	III	B	Strong
Wash hands before and after dressing changes	III	B	Strong
Use sterile technique for dressing changes	III	B	Moderate
For suspected SSI, prescribe antibiotic therapy that covers the likely causative organisms, and consider local resistance patterns and culture results/ sensitivities in choosing an antibiotic	III	B	Strong

[a] Adapted from Deer et al.[167]

The NACC recommendations are divided into preoperative, intraoperative, and postoperative practices.

Preoperatively, optimizing glucose control and discontinuing tobacco use are level B recommendations. Level A recommendations include decolonizing MSSA and MRSA through application of mupirocin nasal ointment (three times a day for 3–5 days before implantation) and chlorhexidine baths (twice daily for 3–5 days prior to implantation), weight-based dosing of preoperative antibiotic for trials and implants, appropriate preoperative timing of prophylactic antibiotics (30–60 minutes prior to incision for cephalosporins, clindamycin, sulfonamides, and aminoglycosides, or within 120 min of incision for vancomycin), and removing hair with electric clippers immediately prior to the procedure, when required. These recommendations have the strongest evidence of postoperative infection prevention. Last, for medical personnel it is recommended that preoperative surgical scrub be performed for 2 to 5 minutes with appropriate antiseptic, that nails be kept short, that artificial nails not be applied, and hand or arm jewelry not be worn for the surgical procedure. Antibiotic selection should be effective against most common pathogens (*Staphylococcus aureus* and *S. epidermidis*). Consulting with a pharmacist about your community's antibiogram is advised. For SCS implantation, the antibiotic coverage recommended is a single dose of a cephalosporin (e.g., cefazolin 1–2 g). If the patient has beta-lactam allergy, clindamycin or vancomycin may be utilized.[167] Table 19.4 details antibiotic selection and weight-based dosing.

Intraoperative infection control practices should include wearing a surgical mask, cap, and sterile gown, as well as double gloving, which are level B recommendations. Level A recommendations include utilizing chlorhexidine gluconate for preoperative skin antiseptic, using iodophor-impregnated drapes, using laminar flow and HEPA filters in the operating

TABLE 19.4. Prophylactic Antibiotic Recommendations[a]

Antibiotic	Standard IV Dosing	Timing before Incision	Redosing Interval (Hours)	Indications
Cefazolin	1 g for ≤ 80 kg	Within 30–60 min	3–4 (CrCl > 50 mL/min)	First-line
	2 g for > 80 kg		8 (CrCl 20–50 mL/min)	
	3 g for > 120 kg		16 (CrCl < 20 mL/min)	
Clindamycin	1 g for ≤ 80 kg	Within 30–60 min	6 (CrCl > 50 mL/min)	Beta-lactam allergy
	2 g for > 80 kg		6 (CrCl 20–50 mL/min)	
	3 g for > 120 kg		6 (CrCl < 20 mL/min)	
Vancomycin	1 g for ≤ 80 kg	Within 120 min	8 (CrCl > 50 mL/min)	Beta-lactam allergy
	2 g for > 80 kg 3 g for > 120 kg		16 (CrCl 20–50 mL/min) None (CrCl < 20 mL/min)	Known MRSA colonization or endemic presence of MRSA in community
				Procedure performed in a facility with a recent MRSA outbreak
				Patients with recent, prolonged hospitalization or institutionalized

[a] Adapted from Deer et al.[167]

room (OR), and limiting OR traffic. Other level B recommendations include keeping the OR doors closed, limiting tissue trauma, maintaining hemostasis, eradicating dead space, avoiding electrocautery at the tissue surface, irrigating with normal saline—and at times with bacitracin irrigation using a bulb syringe prior to closure of the surgical wound (sometimes with vancomycin powder)—and employing implant strategies to limit operative time. These practices are summarized in Table 19.3.

Postoperative guidelines for infection control include one level A recommendation not to continue antibiotics into the postoperative period beyond 24 hours. The level B recommendations are: applying occlusive dressing for 24 to 48 hours after implantation; not routinely using topical antimicrobial agents for surgical wounds that are healing by primary intention; understanding maximum time criteria for defining deep surgical site infection (SSI) of an implantable device (up to 1 year postoperatively); educating the patient and family on proper incision care, symptoms of SSI, and importance of reporting symptoms; washing hands and using sterile technique before and after dressing changes;

and, when SSI is suspected, prescribing a course of antibiotics that covers the likely causative organisms.

Anticoagulation

Because of the invasiveness of SCS implant procedure, coupled with its proximity to the spinal cord across many segments, there is a heightened risk of spinal epidural hematoma, which would result in neurologic impairment, and SCS implantation is considered a high-risk procedure. Fortunately, bleeding during SCS procedures is relatively rare, occurring in 0.3% to 0.7% of cases.[168] The heightened risk for epidural hematoma is attributable to the extensive, thin-walled, valveless venous plexus, which is vulnerable to damage during approach of the epidural needle as well as advancement of the SCS leads, and fagility of the vessels increases with age. The plexuses localize primarily in the lateral and anterior aspects of the epidural space.[169–171]

Regarding anticoagulation, the Joint Guidelines for Interventional Spine and Pain Procedures in Patients on Antiplatelet and Anticoagulant Medications were ratified by multiple pain societies in 2018.[168] The timing of when to hold anticoagulation medication is dependent on its pharmacokinetics and pharmacodynamics. In general, the guidelines recommend that the paradigm of 5 half-lives be used to approximate the hold duration for anticoagulants. Given the high-risk nature of the SCS implant procedure, the most conservative interval for cessation of anticoagulant is recommended. NACC/ASRA guidelines recommend discontinuing anticoagulation between 1 and 7 days before the procedure, depending on the medication, and if needed, monitoring of INR. The time to restart anticoagulation is also specific to the anticoagulant in question, but it is usually within 12 to 24 hours postoperatively. The recommendations are detailed by specific anticoagulation drugs in Table 19.5. For nuanced discussion of this important subject, the reader is directed to the latest guidelines.

Anesthesia

The selection of general anesthesia (GA), monitored anesthesia care (MAC), spinal anesthesia, or local anesthetic with or without sedation should be discussed by the interventional pain physician and the patient, with the decision involving the anesthesiologist as indicated. Some patients prefer GA for a procedure of this level of invasiveness, and others may prefer no systemic anesthetic medications, while for others, their comorbidities may dictate the decision. Typically, the patient's anxiety level, the ability to lie prone for the duration of the procedure, and airway management, in addition to the surgeon's preference, dictate the choice of anesthetic. Although implantations for trials are generally performed under local anesthesia and conscious sedation, permanent implants may be performed with the patient asleep (under GA) versus awake and with or without intraoperative monitoring, with some reports suggesting similar or superior outcomes with the use of GA.[82] Certainly, for paresthesia-based lead placement, which requires the active feedback of the patient, implantation is usually performed with local anesthetic, moderate conscious sedation, and MAC.[160]

Generally, the use of MAC is preferred because it allows the patient to report pain and sensation that could indicate nerve trauma; however, for patients who require GA,

TABLE 19.5. Management of Anticoagulants and Antiplatelet Medications for SCS Implantation[a]

Drug	When to Stop	When to Restart
Aspirin (ASA) and ASA combinations	Primary prophylaxis: 6 days Secondary prophylaxis: shared assessment and risk stratification	24 hours
NSAIDs	5 half-lives	24 hours
▪ Diclofenac	1 day	
▪ Ketorolac	1 day	
▪ Ibuprofen	1 day	
▪ Etodolac	2 days	
▪ Indomethacin	2 days	
▪ Naproxen	4 days	
▪ Meloxicam	4 days	
▪ Nabumetone	6 days	
▪ Oxaprozin	10 days	
▪ Piroxicam	10 days	
Phosphodiesterase inhibitors		24 hours
▪ Cilostazol	2 days	
▪ Dipyridamole	2 days	
ASA combinations	Follow ASA guidelines	
Anticoagulants		
▪ Coumadin	5 days, normal INR	6 hours
▪ Acenocoumarol	3 days, normal INR	24 hours
▪ IV heparin	6 hours	2 hours
▪ Subcutaneous heparin	24 hours	6–8 hours
▪ LMWH		
▪ Enoxaparin (ppx)	12 hours	12–24 hours
▪ Enoxaparin (tx)	24 hours	12–24 hours
▪ Dalteparin	24 hours	12–24 hours
Fibrinolytic agents	48 hours	N/A
Fondaparinux	4 days	24 hours
P2Y12 inhibitors		
▪ Clopidogrel	7 days	12–24 hours
▪ Prasugrel	7–10 days	24 hours
▪ Ticagrelor	5 days	24 hours
▪ Cangrelor	3 hours	24 hours
Direct-acting oral anticoagulants		
▪ Dabigatran	4 days	24 hours
▪ Rivaroxaban	3 days	24 hours
▪ Apixaban	3 d	24 hours
▪ Edoxaban	3 d	24 hours

(continued)

TABLE 19.5. Continued

Drug	When to Stop	When to Restart
GP IIb/IIIa inhibitors		
▪ Abciximab	2–5 days	8–12 hours
▪ Epifibatide	8–24 hours	8–12 hours
▪ Tirofiban	8–24 hours	8–12 hours
Antidepressants and SRIs	routine discontinuation not recommended	

[a] Adapted from Narouze et al.[168]

neuromonitoring is used during the procedure. MAC use during SCS implant is with sedation and local anesthetic infiltration, with the level of sedation increased as needed after paresthesia converge testing. While sedation is titrated, the patient is carefully monitored and ventilation and airway patency are assessed. MAC medications and doses should be individualized based on the patient and intervention, and most often include intravenous (IV) low-dose, titrated propofol infusion (0.5–1 mg/kg IV), dexmedetomidine, and other rapid-onset, short-duration medication combinations. One common example is midazolam (1–2 mg IV) and fentanyl (50–100 μg IV), which can be followed by small titrated supplemental doses of midazolam (0.5–1 mg IV) and fentanyl (25 μg IV).

Neuromonitoring

Neuromonitoring is increasingly used in SCS implantation, and it is particularly useful with lead placement under GA to assess for motor response, nerve damage, and dermatomal coverage; with anatomically placed leads for paresthesia-free percutaneous SCS under GA; and with cervical SCS implantation.[160] There are two primary methods for placing leads under GA with neuromonitoring, including electromyography (EMG) compound muscle action potentials (CMAPs) and collisions between somatosensory evoked potentials (SSEP).[172–173] The data obtained with these methods indicate that the yield is better with the EMG technique than with the SSEP collision technique. An increase in the latency between stimulus and CMAP and/or a reduction in the amplitude of the CMAP may indicate nerve injury. Muscle coverage for EMG responses is the primary concern in utilizing neuromonitoring for the placement of SCS electrodes under GA. In addition, neuromonitoring allows monitoring of the spinal cord in case of injury during placement of an electrode. Sterile, 1.3-cm, 27-gauge subdermal needle electrodes are placed in pairs for bilateral coverage. Symmetrical placement of the monitoring leads is imperative given that the basis for the neurophysiologic mapping is response amplitude comparisons. EMG responses are determined with the addition of the surgeon's interpretation of the placement of the electrode, as well as fluoroscopy for confirmation. This interpretation is then utilized to determine the physiological midline, laterality, and orientation of the electrode, as well as myotomal coverage as a marker for anticipated dermatomal paresthesia. One recommended typical muscle set-up depends on the area and the patient's pain region but may include EMG response from bilateral upper-lower rectus abdominis, iliopsoas, adductor, quadriceps, tibialis anterior, medial gastrocnemius, and abductor hallucis extensor and hallucis brevis for thoracolumbar SCS placement, and middle trapezius, deltoid, biceps, triceps, abductor pollicis brevis, and abductor digiti minimi for cervical SCS.

Technique

SCS implantation is performed under fluoroscopic guidance as an outpatient procedure ina fully equipped operating room (OR) with C-arm fluoroscopy, a resuscitation cart, and full surgical staff (circulating nurse, anesthesiologist, surgical technician, and surgeon).[174] The SCS implantation is performed under sterile technique with antibiotic prophylaxis, skin preparation and draping, and the equipment described here.

Surgical Equipment

For C-arm fluoroscopy, equipment includes protective lead aprons and thyroid guards, lead glasses/eyewear, and head cap. Full surgical attire is used, including gowns and sterile gloves (double-gloving is recommended). Other supplies include surgical drapes (lap drapes, half drapes, sterile drapes), sponges, towels, and suction equipment. Sterile skin preparation is done with chlorhexidine scrub and ChloraPrep solution. Mayo stand, suture scissors, retractors of preference, forceps, clamps, tunneling tool, needle drivers, holders, surgical needles, adhesive and sutures (absorbable Vicryl and Monocryl and non-absorbable Ethibond). Scalpel blades No. 11 and No. 15, bipolar electrosurgery unit and grounding pad, loss-of-resistance (LOR) pulsator syringe, percutaneous leads, IPG, 14-gauge Tuohy needle, and other needles of choice (18-gauge 1½ inch, 22-gauge 1½ inch, 25-gauge 1½ inch). Medications used include 1% lidocaine with epinephrine, NaCl irrigation with bacitracin, tissue adhesive (such as Dermabon or Indermil), antibiotics (cefazolin, clindamycin, or vancomycin), and sedation/anesthesia medications (fentanyl, midazolam, propofol), as previously described.[174]

Patient Positioning

Patient positioning is important step in optimizing lead placement and a successful SCS implant. The patient is positioned prone on a radiolucent table, with pillows under the thorax and/or abdomen to help bring the spine into flexion and open the interlaminar space. Cushions are placed under any hard or bony pressure points of the patient's body to prevent direct bony contact and pressure sore formation.[174] If a patient is under GA, additional positioning factors may be employed per athe nesthesiologist. Likewise, if neuromonitoring is utilized, additional positioning or securing of devices may be needed. If electrocautery is to be used, ensure that the grounding pad is attached prior to draping the patient.

Fluoroscopy

First, obtain a true anterior-posterior (AP) view, which is obtained focusing by at the thoracolumbar junction for implantation of thoracolumbar percutaneous leads. The best view of the T12–L1 or L1–L2 interlaminar space should be sought by tilting the C-arm cephalad or caudal. The endplates should be squared off and aligned, and space for two entry points should be visible. We recommend utilizing a spinal needle at the targeted interspace (T12–L1 or L1–L2) as a marker to assist in the frequent counting of vertebrae.[174]

Slightly contralateral oblique the C-arm to the introducer needle entry side to facilitate guidance of the stimulator lead, as its tendency is to travel contralaterally to the side of entry. The leads will be tracked in AP view up to desired location, midline. Last, an AP view is used to identify the border of the iliac crest for correct placement of the IPG.[174]

To monitor the depth of the Tuohy needle's advancement into the epidural space, we recommend the use of a lateral C-arm view, while alternating between a lateral and AP view. This is always good practice with lead advancement to ensure that the leads remain posterior in the epidural space. A contralateral oblique view may be beneficial to advancing the needle between the lamina at the ideal angle.[174–175]

Thoracolumbar Percutaneous Lead Placement

Once the level of entry has been identified (usually between T11–T12 and L2–L3) and imaging has been optimized, the next step is to identify the medial aspect of the ipsilateral pedicle at the level below the desired interlaminar entry point, because this will be the skin entry point and may be marked with a sterile marker. For a patient with higher BMI, the skin entry site may be distal to this site by as much as half the distance to the next pedicle.[174]

Local anesthetic (1% lidocaine with epinephrine) is injected into the skin and subcutaneous tissues at the entry point of the inserting probe. An initial stab incision with a 11 or 15 scalpel blade and dissection toward the thoracolumbar fascia layer can be done prior to needle placement, per surgeon's preference. Once the entry point is established, the next step is to use a styleted 14-gauge Tuohy needle to enter the skin and subcutaneous layers toward the epidural space.[174]

The angle of entry should be 30° to 40°, with the goal of entering the epidural space at the targeted interlaminar level (T12–L1 or L2–L3). Insert the styleted Tuohy needle and advance the needle medially and cephalad with the bevel up or down until contact is made with the lamina, just lateral to the spinous process (Figure 19.1). Then, using a paramedian wall approach, walk the needle to the edge of the lamina, continuing to advance in medial and cephalad fashion. Remove the stylet and secure the LOR syringe to the needle. A combination of contrast dye and/or preservative-free saline may be utilized to prevent pneumocephalus with unintentional dural puncture. Engage the ligamentum flavum using ballottement or constant pressure on the LOR syringe, continuing to advance until LOR occurs, indicating entry into the epidural space, and then remove the LOR syringe (Figure 19.2). An alternative technique after LOR is to use the lead blank to feel for epidural space placement.[174]

After LOR, feed the percutaneous lead with the stylet through the needle into the epidural space. Begin advancing the percutaneous lead into the epidural space, obtaining a lateral view to confirm epidural space placement. Once a reliable dorsal epidural space entry is achieved, the lead is introduced and advanced with intermittent fluoroscopic views (lateral, contralateral oblique, and AP views). Under live fluoroscopy (pulse setting or low-dose, preferred), steer the lead into its targeted position. Steering is best accomplished using

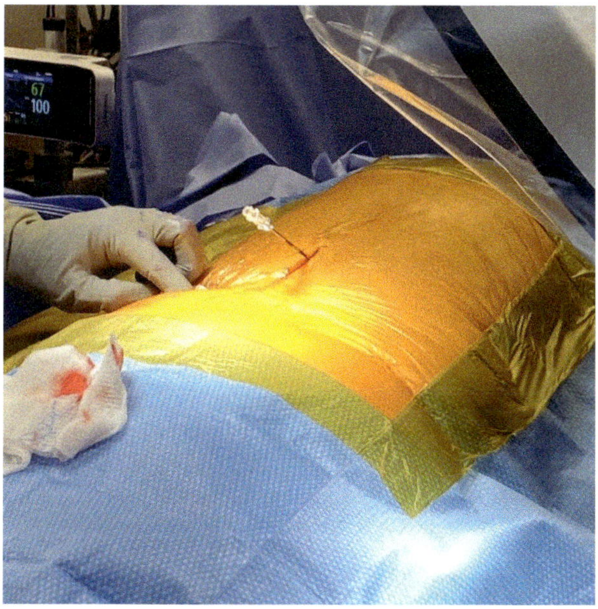

FIGURE 19.1. Initial placement of the Tuohy needle.
Image courtesy of Nevro.

the hand proximal to the needle for cranial/caudal movements, while the distal hand works to guide the lead medially or laterally by rolling the tail of the lead in the desired direction or pulling back as needed. A two-handed technique allows for more efficient and safe lead advancement (Figure 19.3).[174]

The optimal level of lead placement is determined by the results of the SCS trial and is correlated with the level of pain. In general, for low back pain, leads are placed between T6 and T8; for lower extremity pain, between T8 and L1; for foot pain, between T10 and L1, and for pelvic pain, between T5 and S3 (Figure 19.4). Table 19.6 lists lead placement levels for given pathologies and pain patterns when using paresthesia mapping.[176–177] In contrast, a paresthesia-free system, such as HF-10 stimulation, is anatomically guided, and the two leads are placed to intersect at the T9–T10 interspace. If a second lead is placed, it should be accomplished in a fashion similar to that for the first lead, with the ability to place on the contralateral or ipsilateral side and at the same entry level or a level above or below the initial entry based on the patient's anatomy and the device manufacturer's recommendation.

Cervical Percutaneous Lead Placement

For cervical percutaneous lead placement, many of the aforementioned steps are the same, with notable exceptions discussed here.

Position the patient with pillows under the chest to bring the thoracic spine into flexion. Again, the level of entry is variable, but more proximal entry points are acceptable depending on patient anatomy and surgeon preference, and a point as proximal as C7 to T1 has been described. The goal is to select an interlaminar space that can provide a wide

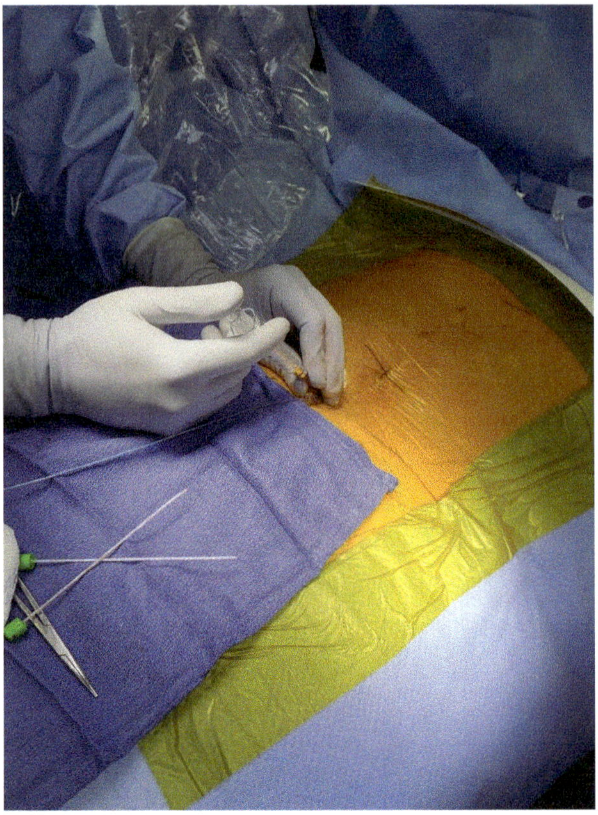

FIGURE 19.2. Loss-of-resistance (LOR) syringe attached to the Tuohy needle as the needle enters the epidural space.
Image courtesy of Nevro.

space for access while maintaining a shallow angle to reduce the risk of dural puncture. Fluoroscopy should be positioned to align the vertebral endplates of the optimal level of entry. Identify the medial aspect of the ipsilateral pedicle at the level below the desired interlaminar entry level and mark it with a sterile marker. Anesthetize the skin as previously described, and, if needed, perform a stab incision.

The styleted Tuohy needle is inserted at a 30° angle, while a RX Coude needle can be inserted at a 90° angle depending on the level of insertion and the distance between the skin entry point and the desired interlaminar entry space. Advance the needle medially with the bevel up or down until contact occurs with the lamina lateral to the spinous process while using AP, lateral, and contralateral oblique fluoroscopic view intermittently to confirm positioning (Figure 19.1). Using a cephalo-medial walk-off method, advance the needle slowly to the edge of the lamina, remove the stylet, and attach the LOR syringe. Very carefully advance the needle, walking off the lamina into the epidural space, engaging the ligamentum flavum using a ballottement pressure until LOR is noted, indicating entrance into the epidural space (Figure 19.2). Remove the LOR syringe and insert the percutaneous lead into the epidural space (Figure 19.3). Under live fluoroscopy guidance, steer the lead

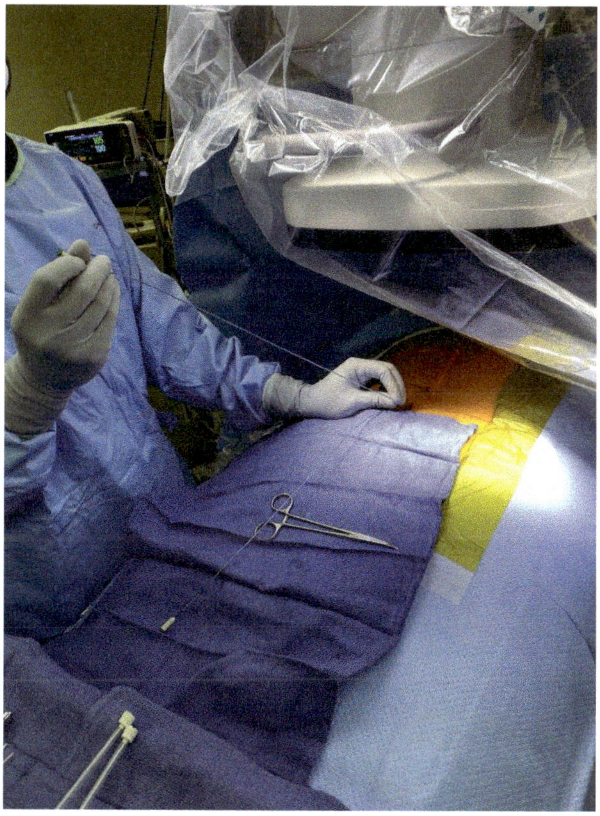

FIGURE 19.3. The surgeon threads the lead through the posterior epidural space as he tracks it, using live fluoroscopy, to the desired location.

Image courtesy of Nevro.

using a rolling motion as the lead is advanced or pulled back, as described above. If placing a second lead, repeat the procedure. Finally, optimal lead position is anywhere from the C3 to C7 level, based on specific anatomic pain coverage mapping (Figure 19.5, Table 19.6).[176–177]

Incision, Anchoring, and Implanting: Lumbar and Cervical SCS

As previously described, some surgeons will choose to make their incision and dissection prior to needle and lead placement. The argument in favor of this technique is efficiency with the implant, while others argue that needle and lead placement may need to be changed due to adhesions from the trial. Others still are more comfortable with lead placement being accomplished first, then incising and dissecting. There is no evidence suggesting one approach is superior to another.[174]

To start, mark the incision site with a sterile marker to outline the area. Anesthetize the skin and subcutaneous tissue with 1% lidocaine with epinephrine. Make the incision with a sharp No. 11 or No. 15 blade scalpel. Expose the fascial layer with sharp and blunt dissection and bipolar electrocautery as indicated for hemostasis. Cautery should be used

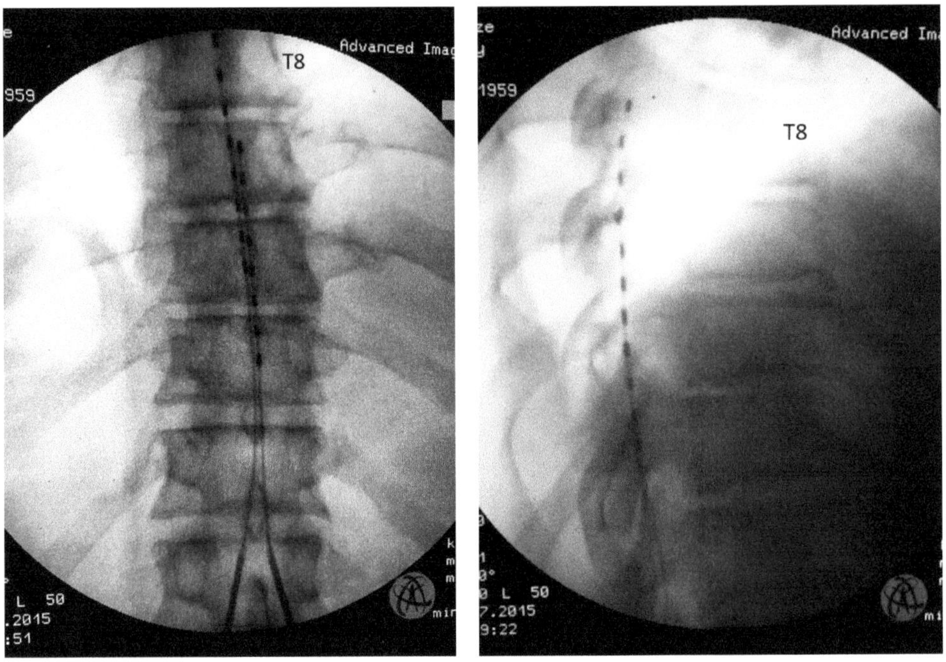

FIGURE 19.4. AP and lateral views of leads in proper position for thoracolumbar placement. Images courtesy of Nevro.

TABLE 19.6. Recommended Lead Placement Level, as Indicated by Location of Pain[a]

Lead Placement Level	Indication
C2–C3	Occipital neuralgia, cervical postlaminectomy syndrome, axial neck pain
C3–C4	Shoulder joint pain (leads usually placed more laterally)
C5–C6	Arm and hand pain, peripheral neuropathy involving upper extremities
C7	Hands, complex regional pain syndrome I/II
T1–T4	Intractable angina
T4–T5	Postmastectomy pain syndrome, postthoracotomy pain syndrome, postherpetic neuralgia
T5–T6	Chronic intractable abdominal pain, chronic pancreatitis
T6–T8	Low back pain, lumbar postlaminectomy syndrome, axial low back pain
T8–T11	Lower extremities
T10–L1	Foot
T12	Hip pain, groin pain
S2	Urogenital pain, rectum, inguinal neuralgia, post-hernia-repair pain
S3	Vulvodynia, endometriosis

[a] Adapted from Sabia et al and Carlson et al.[174,177]

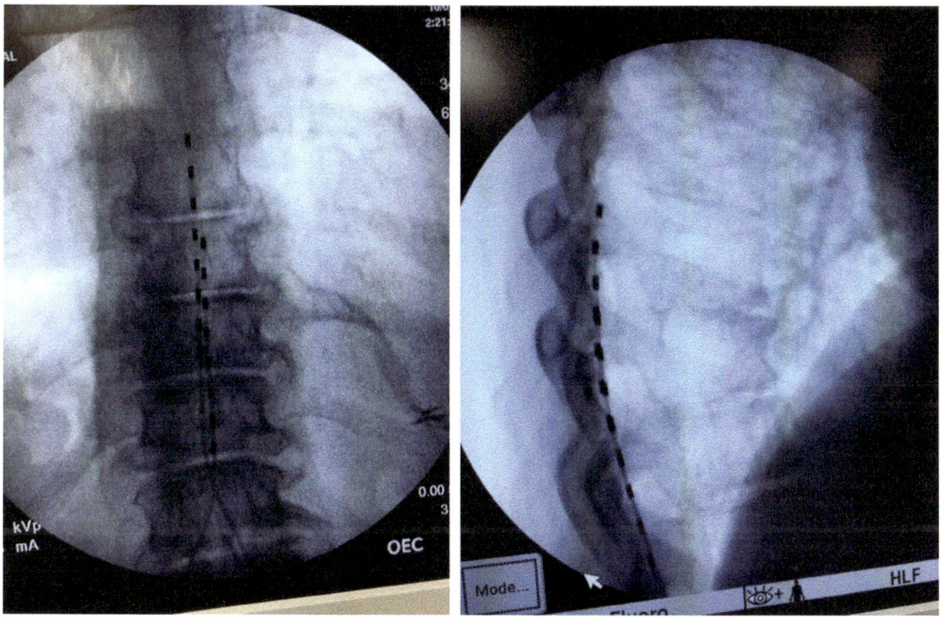

FIGURE 19.5. AP and lateral views of leads in proper position for cervical placement.
Images courtesy of Nevro.

with extreme caution because contacting the needles or leads could be extremely harmful to the patient. Weitlaner retractors or the Army-Navy retractors with surgical technician assistance may be helpful in direct visualization of the fascia for anchoring (Figure 19.6).[174]

Using a nonabsorbable braided nylon suture, such as Ethibond, anchor the leads to the fascial tissue. This may be accomplished either by tying to the fascia first or tying the lead to the fascia in one pass, depending on the surgeon's preference, with two or three loops. Once the suture is strongly secured by a gentle "pull test," the needles are removed. The connecting anchors are placed and secured to the leads using the manufacturer's locking system and suture loops. Bluntly dissect the adjacent tissue to create and place strain-relief loops, which minimize lead migration.[174]

Pocket Creation and Tunneling

The IPG pocket location is critical to long-term success of the procedure. Typically, the location is in the low back or superior gluteal region, but it can depend on manufacturer guidelines, patient's preference, and surgeon's preference. In planning the surgical pocket for the IPG, consider certain important anatomic landmarks, such as the cluneal nerves, if there is to be lower lateral lumbar placement, and the iliohypogastric nerve, if there is to be abdominal placement.[174]

Mark the skin using a sterile marker with a transverse line of the intended incision, which should be just slightly wider than the IPG to be implanted. Anesthetize the skin and pocket subcutaneous tissue with 1% lidocaine with epinephrine. Using a sharp No. 11 or No. 15 blade, make the incision along the marked line. Blunt dissection is recommended to

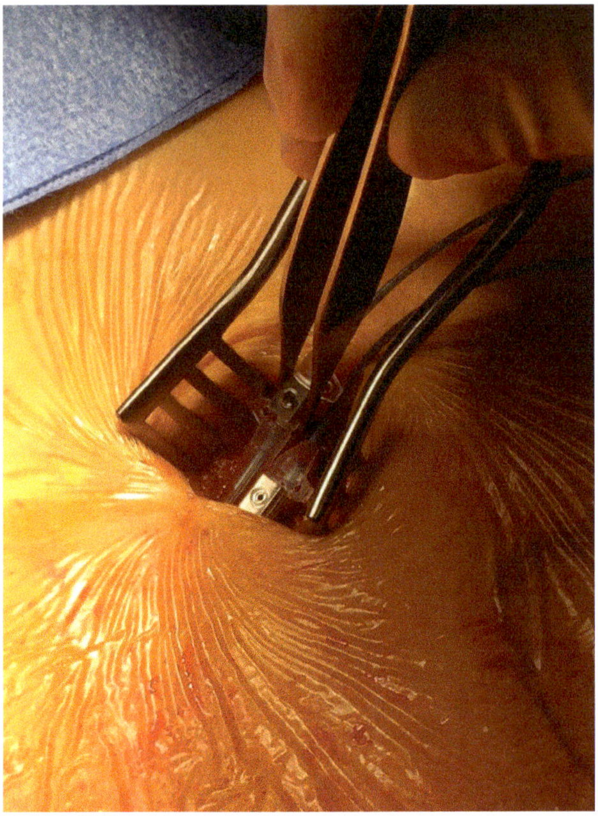

FIGURE 19.6. The surgeon secures the leads to the proprietary connectors. Weitlaner retractors help provide visualization of the fascia, to which the surgeon secures the connectors.
Image courtesy of Nevro.

extend the pocket within the fascial plane parallel to the skin surface. Bipolar cautery can be used to achieve hemostasis, again with precautions. The depth of the pocket should encompass the IPG without tension. A sizing device is used to ensure proper size of the pocket. It is important to note that pocket formation should be made in parallel to the surface of the skin, not extending beyond the maximal depth.[174]

Once the pocket has been made, attention is turned to tunneling the leads from the spine to the IPG pocket. Mark a dotted path with a sterile surgical marker from the midline spine to the pocket and infiltrate this trajectory with local anesthetic. The tunneling device enters at the fascial plane deep to subcutaneous soft tissue, but above the muscle tissue plane. The device is then advanced toward the IPG pocket, exercising caution that it does not violate the muscular layer. Holding the sheath in place, withdraw the tunneling device, leaving the sheath in place. Place the electrode through the sheath and advance it into the IPG pocket (Figure 19.7).[174]

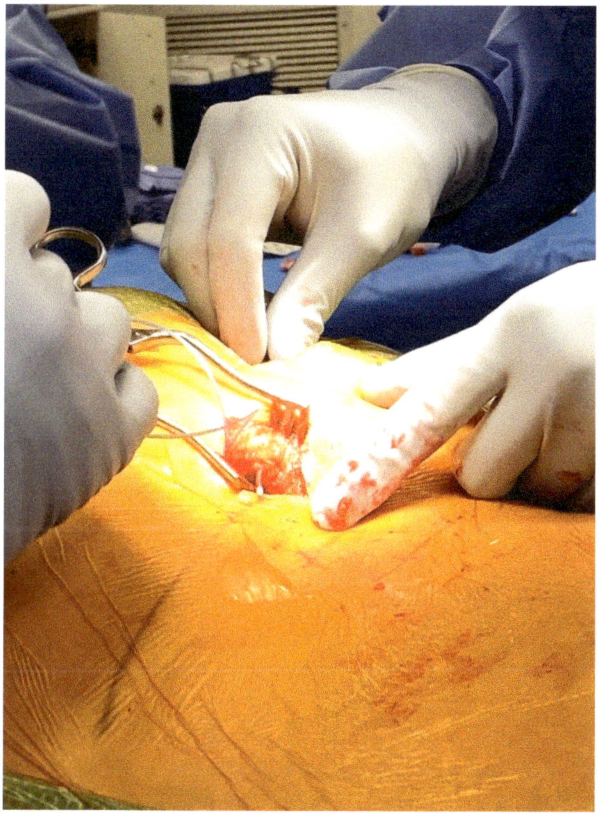

FIGURE 19.7. The pocket has been prepared while Weitlaner retractors hold open the incision. The tunneling device has brought the leads (assistant at left is holding them) to the pocket in preparation for attachment to the implantable pulse generator.

Image courtesy of Nevro.

IPG Placement

A rechargeable IPG is placed at 1 cm depth beneath the skin to prevent erosion, while still allowing for optimal charging. A primary cell (nonrechargeable) IPG can be placed deeper, at to 2 to 4 cm. Clean the leads and attach them to the IPG. Screw in the leads and do a pull test to confirm they are tightened within the device (Figure 19.8). An audible click will be heard. Next, copiously irrigate the pocket with saline and bacitracin and consider applying 1 g of vancomycin powder to surgical sites. Place the IPG in the pocket, with excess lead wire posterior to the IPG.[174]

Closure of the pocket and lead anchoring incision begins with deep fascial layers, using Vicryl. Next, close the subcuticular layer with suture (Figure 19.9). Finally, close the superficial layer with staples or running absorbable skin suture and finalize with skin glue. Sterile dressing is applied over the surgical wounds.

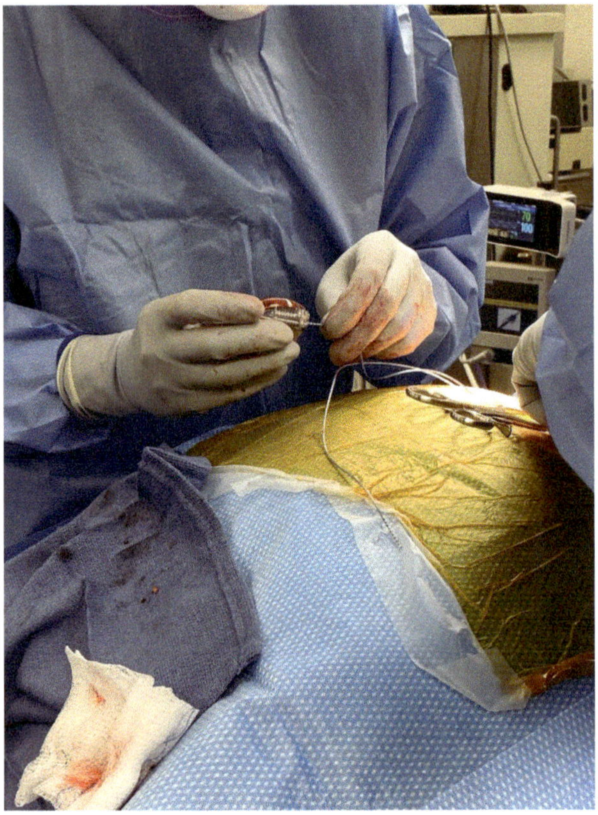

FIGURE 19.8. The leads are secured to the implantable pulse generator.
Image courtesy of Nevro.

Postoperative Management and Follow-up

Patients recover in a monitored postanesthesia care unit (PACU). Any changes in neurologic function require prompt evaluation. Typically, patients are discharged the same day. Upon discharge, they can resume most medications, except for anticoagulation and antiplatelet medication, as referenced in Table 19.5.[174,178] Discharge plans should be in accord with preoperative planning and ensure that the patient and caregiver understand the importance of adherence to postdischarge recommendations.

Patients should avoid strenuous activity for the first 48 hours, although ambulation is highly encouraged. Pain control may be managed with ice topically and acetaminophen as needed up to recommended maximum dosage in a scheduled fashion. A short course of opioid medication after the procedure may be indicated in selected patients. Activity limitations include sudden movements, bending, twisting, lifting, reaching, or pulling for 6 weeks. The wound is to be kept clean and dry for the first 48 hours, and the dressing can be changed as needed thereafter. The patient is instructed to report any fever, change in neurologic function, areas of increasing tenderness, swelling, or redness. A wound check at 3 or 4 days postoperatively is appropriate for the first

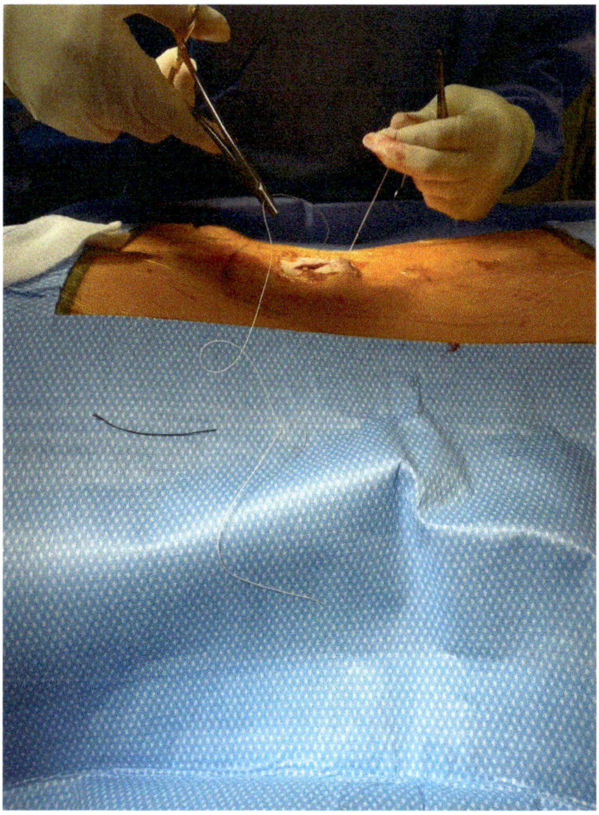

FIGURE 19.9. The incision for the pocket is closed in layers, first deep fascia with securing of the IPG to the fascia, then subcuticular layer, and finally the skin is closed with staples or glue. Here, a subcuticular running stitch has been employed.

Image courtesy of Nevro.

follow-up, with subsequent follow-up at 10 to 14 days for staple removal, if necessary. The patient can bathe or submerge after the wound has been checked at about 3 weeks postoperatively. In general, postoperative care is similar to that for other spine surgery interventions.

Complications and Management

Complications of SCS implantation have decreased with the improving technology and evolution of surgical and sterile techniques. Multiple studies have described the complications after SCS implantation.[174,179–183] The literature describes complication rates of between 14% and 43% of patients.[184] The complication rate requiring revision is between 23% and 33%, and explantation is required in 11%.[184–186] Some of the noted complications include: lead migration, lead fracture, seroma formation, infection, dural puncture, postdural headache, nerve injury, spinal cord injury, and epidural hematoma. Complications can be separated into intraoperative, technical, and biologic categories.

Intraoperative Complications

Intraoperative complications that are general to surgical procedures include local anesthetic toxicity, hemodynamic instability, and excessive sedation. Intraoperative complications specific to all interventional spinal procedures include inadvertent subarachnoid injection leading to total spinal block, dural puncture (~ 0.1%), spinal cord injury, and nerve damage.[187] SCS implantation carries additional potential for perforated viscus (especially with passing of the tunneling trocar) and dehiscence (deep and superficial), in addition to increased risk of the potential complications of all interventional spine procedures due to the invasiveness of the procedure.[174]

Technical Complications

The most common complication of SCS implantation is lead migration, which occurs in an estimated 11% to 13% of cases.[174,186] Lead fracture occurs in 5% to 9% of procedures.[188] Hardware malfunction and unexpected battery failure occur at a rate of 6.5% and 1.6%, respectively.[186] Other technical complications include misplacement of the lead(s) and undesirable paresthesia. Technical complications can be avoided by optimization and careful surgical technique during the procedure.

Biologic Complications

The most common biologic complication is infection, with superficial infection occurring about 5% of the time and deep infection 0.1% of the time.[180] As already discussed, there are specific recommendations for minimizing infections, such as sterile technique, preoperative skin scrubbing/showers, preoperative antibiotics, and intraoperative antibiotics. Also note that patients who receive an occlusive dressing with antibiotic powder or postoperative antibiotics for 7 days may have a lower infection rate. Pain over the IPG implantation site occurs in 0.9% to 5.8% of patients.[188] Epidural abscess is a possible, rare complication and is considered a medical emergency.[189] Other potential biologic complications include seroma (0.2%), skin erosion and exposure of hardware, neuraxial hematoma, incisional hematoma (0.1%), headache, cerebrospinal fluid hygroma, immunogenic reaction to hardware and/or leads, and epidural fibrosis.[174,187] There is also potential for temporary urologic complications, including renal failure or urinary retention, and gastrointestinal complications, including nausea, diarrhea, gastroesophageal reflux, or flatulence.[174] Incidence of SCS removal or reimplantation was 0.3% at 90 days and 3.4% at 1 year, according to a retrospective study by Labaran and colleagues in 12,297 patients. The study also examined emergency room utilization for SCS-related complications, finding 4.2% of patients and 17.2% of patients had visited the emergency department at 90 days and 1 year, respectively. Ultimately, the study found the percentage of subsequent surgery increased relatively linearly with time, reporting that subsequent surgery was performed in 0.9% at 90 days, 7.1% at 1 year, 11.7% at 2 years, and 15.5% at 3 years.[187]

Despite the possible complications, surgical techniques for SCS implantation are considered by numerous guidelines and society recommendations to be safe interventions. Serious adverse events, such as neurologic damage, are quite rare; hardware-related and biologic complications are manageable and at times reversible; and when proper sterile technique and surgical care are utilized, complications can be reduced to a minimum. Specifically, vigilance with surgical technique, sterile methods, and preoperative antibiotic precautions are most important, along with copious irrigation and adequate hemostasis in the pocket and incision site, and they have the highest level of evidence in preventing postoperative infections and complications. In addition, adequate use of strain-relief loops during lead anchoring has the highest likelihood of preventing lead migration.

Conclusion

SCS implantation has been a clinically effective treatment for a wide variety of chronic pain conditions for numerous years; however, it has been considered controversial according to many guidelines and specialty societies. For the past decades, particularly after the introduction of high-frequency and other new waveforms, SCS research has substantially grown, with level I evidence, and the status of SCS has been elevated from investigational to a safe and effective treatment. Device technology and surgical technique have evolved, understanding of the mechanisms of action has expanded, and interventional pain physicians have become more comfortable incorporating SCS use into their clinical practice, leading to a boom of data and furthering clinical research.

Now there is high-level, well-established evidence consistently reporting that SCS is a safe, minimally invasive, cost-effective treatment option with high patient satisfaction in numerous chronic pain conditions, including FBSS, chronic neuropathic pain, CRPS, chronic intractable axial spinal pain with or without radiculopathy, and others. Spinal cord stimulation has been shown to improve pain at short- and long-term follow-up, reduce disability, improve functional scores, decrease opioid utilization, and improve QoL in complex chronic pain patients. Therefore, it is feasible to consider SCS intervention earlier in the chronic pain treatment algorithm, on a case by case basis, as it is known that healthcare resource utilization increases with longer pain-to-SCS-implant time. The future of spinal cord stimulation is bright, with the technological advancements of multiple waveforms and programming stimulation algorithms targeting different anatomic sites and an expanding understanding of its mechanisms of action. Spinal cord stimulation offers the opportunity to modulate pain with precision and efficacy, as the field of neuromodulation continues to adapt and to deliver chronic pain patients an effective treatment in the modern healthcare era.

References

1. Gildenberg PL. History of electrical neuromodulation for chronic pain. *Pain Med.* 2006;7(suppl 1):S7–S13.
2. Shealy CN, Mortimer J, Reswick JB. Electrical inhibition of pain by stimulation of the dorsal columns: preliminary clinical report. *Anesth Analg.* 1967;46:489–491.
3. Melzack R, Wall PD. Pain mechanisms: a new theory. *Science.* 1965;150:971–979.

4. Isagulyan E, Slavin K, Konovalov N, et al. Spinal cord stimulation in chronic pain: technical advances. *Korean J Pain*. 2020;33(2):99–107.
5. Cohen SP. Epidemiology, diagnosis, and treatment of neck pain. *Mayo Clin Proc.* 2015;90:284–299.
6. Ferguson SA, Merryweather A, Thiese MS, et al. Prevalence of low back pain, seeking medical care, and lost time due to low back pain among manual material handling workers in the United States. *BMC Musculoskelet Disord.* 2019;20:243.
7. Dahlhamer J, Lucas J, Zelaya C, et al. Prevalence of chronic pain among adults—United States, 2016. *MMWR Morb Mortal Wkly Rep*. 2018;67:1001.
8. Karri J, Joshi M, Polson G, et al. Spinal cord stimulation for chronic pain syndromes: a review of considerations in practice management. *Pain Physician*. 2020;23:599–616.
9. Foreman RD, Linderoth B. Neural mechanisms of spinal cord stimulation. *Int Rev Neurobiol.* 2012;107:87–119.
10. Durbhakula S, Malik K. Spinal cord stimulation. In: *Essentials of Pain Medicine*. Elsevier; 2018:663–676.
11. Caylor J, Reddy R, Yin S, et al. Spinal cord stimulation in chronic pain: evidence and theory for mechanisms of action. *Bioelectronic Med.* 2019;5(12):1–41.
12. Fishman MA, Antony A, Esposito M, et al. The evolution of neuromodulation in the treatment of chronic pain: forward-looking perspectives. *Pain Med.* 2019;20(1):58–68.
13. Rosenow JM, Stanton-Hicks M, Rezai AR, et. al. Failure modes of spinal cord stimulation hardware. *J Neurosurg Spine*. 2006;5:183–190.
14. Deer TR, Pope JE. *Atlas of Implantable Therapies for Pain Management*. New York, NY: Springer; 2016:159–165.
15. Manola L, Holsheimer J, Veltink PH. Technical performance of percutaneous leads for spinal cord stimulation: a modeling study. *Neuromodulation*. 2005;8(2):88–99
16. Law JD. Targeting a spinal stimulator to treat the "failed back surgery syndrome." *Appl Neurophysiol.* 1987;50:437–438.
17. Bradley K. The technology: the anatomy of a spinal cord and nerve root stimulator: the lead and the power source. *Pain Med.* 2006;7(S1):S27–S34.
18. Oakley JC. Spinal cord stimulation: patient selection, technique, and outcomes. *Neurosurg Clin North Am*. 2003;14:365–380.
19. Barolat G. Reply to a letter to the editor (2001;4:35–36). *Neuromodulation*. 2001;4(2):75.
20. Holsheimer J, Wesselink WA. Effect of anode-cathode configuration on paresthesia coverage in spinal cord stimulation. *Neurosurgery*. 1997;41:654–660.
21. *Up To Date, Clinical Guidelines 2021*. www.uptodate.com.
22. Foreman RD, Linderoth B. Mechanisms of spinal neuromodulation. In: Hayek S, Deer T, Levy R, eds. *Neurostimulation for the Treatment of Chronic Pain*. Vol 1. Elsevier; 2011.
23. Miller JP, Eldabe S, Buchser E, et al. Parameters of spinal cord stimulation and their role in electrical charge delivery: a review. *Neuromodulation*. 2016;19(4):373–384.
24. Heijmans L, Joosten EA. Mechanisms and mode of action of spinal cord stimulation in chronic neuropathic pain. *Postgrad Med.* 2020;132(3):17–21.
25. Alò K, Varga C, Krames E, et al. Factors affecting impedance of percutaneous leads in spinal cord stimulation. *Neuromodulation*. 2006;9(2):128–135.
26. Washburn S, Catlin R, Bethel K, et al. Patient-perceived difference between constant current and constant voltage spinal cord stimulation systems. *Neuromodulation*. 2014;17(1):28–35.
27. Abejon D, Feler CA. Is impedance a parameter to be taken into account in spinal cord stimulation? *Pain Physician*. 2007;10(4):533.
28. Benyamin R, Grider JS, Vallejo R, et al. Spinal cord stimulation: principles and applications. In: Kaye AD, David SF, eds. *Principles of Neurophysiological Assessment, Mapping and Monitoring.* New York, NY: Springer; 2014.
29. Chakravarthy K, Richter H, Christo PJ, et al. Spinal cord stimulation for treating chronic pain: reviewing preclinical and clinical data on paresthesia-free high frequency therapy. *Neuromodulation.* 2018;21:10–18.

30. Linderoth B, Stiller CO, Gunasekera L, et al. Gamma-aminobutyric acid is released in the dorsal horn by electrical spinal cord stimulation: an in vivo microdialysis study in the rat. *Neurosurgery.* 1994;34(3):484–489.
31. D'Mello RD, Dickenson AH. Spinal cord mechanisms of pain. *Br J Anesth.* 2008;101(1):8–16.
32. Linderoth B, Foreman RD. Conventional and novel spinal stimulation algorithms: hypothetical mechanisms of action and comments on outcomes. *Neuromodulation.* 2017;20(6):525–533.
33. Zhang TC, Janik JJ, Grill WM. Modeling effects of spinal cord stimulation on wide-dynamic range dorsal horn neurons: influence of stimulation frequency and GABAergic inhibition. *J Neurophysiol.* 2014;112:552–567.
34. Vallejo R, Kelly CA, Gupta A, et al. Modulation of neuroglial interactions using differential target multiplexed spinal cord stimulation in an animal model of neuropathic pain. *Mol Pain.* 2020;16:1–13.
35. Sato KL, Johanek LM, Sanada LS, Sluka KA. Spinal cord stimulation reduces mechanical hyperalgesia and glial cell activation in animals with neuropathic pain. *Anesth Analg.* 2014;118(2):464.
36. Watkins LR, Milligan ED, Maier SF. Glial activation: a driving force for pathological pain. *Trends Neurosci.* 2001;24(8):450–455.
37. Falowski S. An observational case series of spinal cord stimulation waveforms visualized on intraoperative neuromonitoring. *Neuromodulation.* 2018;22:219–228.
38. De Ridder D, Vancamp T, Falowski S, et al. All bursts are equal, but some are more equal (to burst firing): burstDR stimulation versus Boston burst stimulation. *Expert Rev Med Devices.* 2020;04, epub.
39. De Ridder D, Vanneste S, Plazier M, Van Der Loo E, Menovsky T. Burst spinal cord stimulation: toward paresthesia-free pain suppression. *Neurosurgery.* 2010;665:986–990.
40. De Ridder D, Vanneste S. Confusion about burst stimulation. *Neuromodulation.* 2020;23(1): 140–141.
41. Crosby ND, Weisshaar L, Smith JR, et al. Burst and tonic spinal cord stimulation differentially activate GABAergic mechanisms to attenuate pain in a rat model of cervical radiculopathy. *IEEE Trans Biomed Eng.* 2015;62:1604–1613.
42. De Ridder D, Vanneste S. Burst and tonic spinal cord stimulation: different and common brain mechanisms. *Neuromodulation.* 2016;19:47–59.
43. De Ridder D, Plazier M, Kamerling N, et al. Burst spinal stimulation for limb and back pain. *World Neurosurg.* 2013;80:642–649.
44. Yearwood T, Falowski S, Venkatesan L. Comparison of neural activity during tonic and burst spinal cord stimulation: a SUNBURST substudy. Poster presented at: NANS-NIC, 2016.
45. Arle JE, Mei L, Carlson KW, et al. High-frequency stimulation of dorsal column axons: potential underlying mechanisms of paresthesia-free neuropathic pain relief. *Neuromodulation.* 2016;19:385–397.
46. Hagedorn JM, Layno-Moses A, Sanders DT, et al. Overview of HF10 spinal cord stimulation for the treatment of chronic pain and an introduction to the Senza Omnia system. *Pain Manage.* 2020;.
47. Cuellar JM, Alataris K, Walker A, et al. Effect of high-frequency alternating current on spinal afferent nociceptive transmission. *Neuromodulation.* 2013;16:318–327.
48. Kapural L, Yu C, Doust MW, et al. Novel 10-kHz high-frequency therapy (HF10 therapy) is superior to traditional low-frequency spinal cord stimulation for the treatment of chronic back and leg pain: the SENZA-RCT randomized controlled trial. *Anesthesiology.* 2015;123(4):851–860.
49. Eisenberg E, Burstein Y, Suzan E, et al. Spinal cord stimulation attenuates temporal summation in patients with neuropathic pain. *Pain.* 2015;156(3):381–385.
50. Ahmed S, Yearwood T, De Ridder D, et al. Burst and high frequency stimulation: underlying mechanisms of action. *Expert Rev Med Devices.* 2018;15(1):61–70.
51. Vallejo R, Bradley K, Kapural L. Spinal cord stimulation in chronic pain. *Spine.* 2017;42(suppl 14):S53–S60.
52. Shiyeng L, Feng Y, Farber J, et al. Dependence of c-Fos expression on amplitude of high frequency SCS in an animal model. Las Vegas: North American Neuromodulation Society Meeting; 2018.
53. Zannou AL, Khadka N, Truong DQ, et al. Temperature increases by kilohertz frequency spinal cord stimulation. *Brain Stimul.* 2019;12(1):62–72.
54. Song Z, Villsanen H, Meyerson BA, et al. Efficacy of kilohertz-frequency and conventional spinal cord stimulation in rat models of different pain conditions. *Neuromodulation.* 2014;17:226–234.

55. Chakravarthy K, Malayil R, Kirketeig T, et al. Burst spinal cord stimulation: a systematic review and pooled analysis of real-world evidence and outcomes data. *Pain Med.* 2019;20(1):47–57.
56. Cedeño DL, Smith WJ, Kelley CA, et al. Spinal cord stimulation using differential target multiplexed programming modulates neural cell-specific transcriptomes in an animal model of neuropathic pain. *Mol Pain.* 2020;(0): 1–18
57. www.medtronic.com.
58. Parker K, Karantonis D, Single P. Hypothesis for the mechanism of action of ECAP-controlled closed-loop systems for spinal cord stimulation. *Healthcare Technol Lett.* 2020;7(3):76–80.
59. Mekhail N, Levy R, Deer T, et al. Long term safety and efficacy of closed-loop spinal cord stimulation to treat chronic back and leg pain (Evoke): a double-blind, randomised controlled trial. *Lancet Neurol.* 2020;19(2):123–134.
60. Russo M, Brooker C, Cousins MJ, et al. Sustained long-term outcomes with closed-loop spinal cord stimulation: 12-month results of the prospective, multicenter, open-label Avalon study. *Neurosurgery.* 2020;15;87(4): 485–495.
61. Levy R, Deer T, Poree L, et al. Multicenter, randomized, double-blind study protocol using human spinal cord recording comparing safety, efficacy and neurophysiological responses between patients being treated with compound action potential-controlled closed-loop spinal cord stimulation (the Evoke study). *Neuromodulation.* 2019;23:317–326.
62. Gmel GE, Escapa RS, Parker J, et al. The effect of spinal cord stimulation frequency on the neural response and perceived sensation in patients with chronic pain. *Front Neurosci.* 2021;15:625–635.
63. Levy R, Chakravarthy K, Poree L, et al. SCS pulsed stimulation patterns (PSP): multiple mechanisms of action in a single, novel waveform. Abstract In: North American Neuromodulation Society (NANS) 2020.
64. Centers for Medicare & Medicaid Services (CMS). 2021. www.cms.go..
65. *Official Disability Guidelines (ODG) 2021.* www.odgbymcg.com.
66. *American College of Occupational and Environmental Medicine (ACOEM) practice guidelines 2021.* www.mdguidelines.com
67. Aetna. *Clinical Policy Bulletin 2021.* www.aetna.com.
68. Blue Cross Blue Shield (BCBS). *Clinical Policy Bulletin 2021.* www.bcbs.com.
69. Atkinson L, Sundaraj SR, Brooker C, et al. Recommendations for patient selection in spinal cord stimulation. *J Clin Neurosci.* 2011;18:1295–1302.
70. Lamer TJ, Moeschler SM, Gazela HM, et al. Spinal cord stimulation for the treatment of intractable spine and limb pain: a systematic review of RCTs and meta-analysis. *Mayo Clin Proc.* 2019;94(8):1475–1487.
71. Sayed D, Rowe J. Percutaneous cervical spinal cord stimulation. In: *Deer's Treatment of Pain.* Springer; 2019.
72. Deer TR, Skaribas IM, Haider N, et al. Effectiveness of cervical spinal cord stimulation for the management of chronic pain. *Neuromodulation.* 2014;17:265–271.
73. Abdul Aziz S, Ghaleb H. Cervical spinal cord stimulator for the management of pain from brachial plexus avulsion [letter]. *Pain Med.* 2014;15(4)712–714.
74. Brill S, Aryeh I. Neuromodulation in the management of pain from brachial plexus injury. *Pain Physician.* 2008;11:81–85.
75. De Agostino R, Federspiel B, Cesnulis E, et al. High-cervical spinal cord stimulation for medically intractable chronic migraine. *Neuromodulation.* 2015;18:289–296.
76. Haider S, Owsu-Sarpong S, Peris Celda M, et al. A single center prospective observational study of outcomes with tonic cervical spinal cord stimulation. *Neuromodulation.* 2017;20(3):263–268.
77. Levine AB, Parrent AG, MacDougal KW. Cervical spinal cord and dorsal nerve root stimulation for neuropathic upper limb pain. *Can J Neurol Sci.* 2017;44(1):83–89.
78. Wolter T, Kiesselbach K. Cervical spinal cord stimulation: an analysis of 23 patients with long term follow-up plan. *Pain Physician.* 2012;1215(3):203–212.
79. Chivukula S, Tempel ZJ, Weiner GM, et al. Cervical and cervicomedullary spinal cord stimulation for chronic pain: efficacy and outcomes. *Clin Neurol Neurosurg.* 2014;127:33–41.

80. Vallejo R, Kramer J, Benyamin R. Neuromodulation of the cervical spinal cord in the treatment of chronic intractable neck and upper extremity pain: a case series and review of the literature. *Pain Physician*. 2007;10(2):305–311.
81. Amirdelfan K, Vallejo R, Benyamin R, et al. High-frequency spinal cord stimulation at 10 kHz for the treatment of combined neck and arm pain: results from a prospective multicenter study. *Neurosurgery*. 2020;87(2):176–185.
82. El Majdoub F, Neudorfer C, Richter R, et al. 10 kHz cervical SCS for chronic neck and upper limb pain: 12 months' results. *Ann Clin Transl Neurol*. 2019;.
83. Grider JS, Harned M. Cervical spinal cord stimulation using monophasic burst waveform for axial neck and upper extremity radicular pain: a preliminary observational study. *Neuromodulation*. 2019;.
84. North RB, Wetzel FT. Spinal cord stimulation for chronic pain of spinal origin: a valuable long-term solution. *Spine*. 2002;27(22):2584–2591.
85. North R, Shipley J. Practice parameters for the use of spinal cord stimulation in the treatment of chronic neuropathic pain. *Pain Med*. 2007;8:S200–S275.
86. Deer T, Slavin KV, Amirdelfan K, et al. Success Using Neuromodulation with BURST (SUNBURST) study: results from a prospective, randomized controlled trial using a novel burst waveform. *Neuromodulation*. 2018;21(1):56–66.
87. Song JJ, Popescu A, Bell RL. Present and potential use of spinal cord stimulation to control chronic pain. *Pain Physician*. 2014;17:235–246.
88. Kapural L, Yu C, Doust MW, et al. Novel 10kHz high-frequency therapy (HF10 therapy) is superior to traditional low-frequency spinal cord stimulation for the treatment of chronic back and leg pain: the SENZA-RCT randomized controlled trial. *Anesthesiology*. 2015;123:851–860.
89. North RB, Kidd DH, Farrokhi F, et al. Spinal cord stimulation versus repeated lumbosacral spine surgery for chronic pain: a randomized controlled trial. *Neurosurgery*. 2005;56:98–107.
90. Sharan AD, Riley J, Falowski S, et al. Association of opioid usage with spinal cord stimulation outcomes. *Pain Med*. 2017;19:699–707.
91. Sanders RA, Moeschler SM, Gazela HM, et al. Patient outcomes and spinal cord stimulation: a retrospective case series evaluating patient satisfaction, pain scores, opioid requirements. *Pain Pract*. 2016;16:899–904.
92. Rock AK, Truong H, Park YL, et al. Spinal cord stimulation. *Neurosurg Clin North Am*. 2018;12(3):.
93. Kumar K, Taylor RS, Jacques L, et al. Spinal cord stimulation versus conventional medical management for neuropathic pain: a multicenter randomised controlled trial in patients with failed back surgery syndrome. *Pain*. 2007;132:179–188.
94. Manca A, Kumar K, Taylor RS, et al. Quality of life, resource consumption and costs of spinal cord stimulation versus conventional medical management in neuropathic pain patients with failed back surgery syndrome (PROCESS trial). *Eur J Pain*. 2008;12(8):1047–1058.
95. Frey ME, Manchikanti L, Benyamin RM, et al. Spinal cord stimulation for patients with failed back surgery syndrome: a systematic review. *Pain Physician*. 2009;12:379–397.
96. British Pain Society. *Spinal Cord Stimulation for the Management of Pain: Recommendations or Best Clinical Practice*. British Pain Society; 2009. www.britishpainsociety.org.
97. Sweet J, Badjatiya A, Tan D, et al. Paresthesia-free high-density SCS for post-laminectomy syndrome in a pre-screened population: a prospective case series. *Neuromodulation*. 2016;19(3):260–267.
98. Schu S, Slotty PJ, Bara G, et al. A prospective, randomised, double-blind, placebo-controlled study to examine the effectiveness of burst stimulation patterns for the treatment of FBSS. *Neuromodulation*. 2014;17(5):443–450.
99. De Andres J, Monslave-Dolz V, Fabregat-Cid G, et al. Prospective randomized blind effect-on-outcome study of conventional vs high frequency spinal cord stimulation in patients with pain and disability due to failed back surgery syndrome. *Pain Med*. 2017;18:2401–2421.
100. Bolash R, Creamer M, Rauck R, et al. Wireless high-frequency spinal cord stimulation (10 kHz) compared with multi waveform low-frequency spinal cord stimulation in the management of chronic pain in failed back surgery syndrome subjects: preliminary results of a multicenter, prospective randomized controlled study. *Pain Med*. 2019;20:1971–1979.

101. Knife T, Pintea B, Link C, et al. High frequency (10 kHz) or burst spinal cord stimulation in FBSS patients with predominant back pain: preliminary data from a prospective observational study. *Neuromodulation.* 2016;19:268–275.
102. Muhammad S, Roeske S, Chaudhry SR, et al. Burst or high-frequency (10 kHz) SCS in failed back surgery syndrome patients with predominant back pain: one year comparative data. *Neuromodulation.* 2017;20:661–667.
103. De Voss CC, Bom MJ, Vanneste S, et al. Burst spinal cord stimulation evaluated in patients with failed back surgery syndrome and painful diabetic neuropathy. *Neuromodulation.* 2014;17:152–159.
104. Courtney P, Espinet A, Mitchell B, et al. Improved pain relief with burst spinal cord stimulation for two weeks in patients using tonic stimulation: results from a small clinical study. *Neuromodulation.* 2015;18:361–366.
105. De Ridder D, Lenders MW, De Vos CC, et al. A 2-center comparative study on tonic versus burst spinal cord stimulation: amount of responders and amount of pain suppression. *Clin J Pain.* 2015;31(5):433–437.
106. Kemler MA. Spinal cord stimulation in patients with chronic reflex sympathetic dystrophy. *N Engl J Med.* 2000;343(9):618–624.
107. Kemler MA, De Vet HC, Barendse GA, et al. The effect of SCS in patients with chronic reflex sympathetic dystrophy: two years follow up of the RCT. *Ann Neurol.* 2004;55(1):13.
108. Kemler MA, de Vet HC, Barendse GA, et al. Effect of spinal cord stimulation for chronic complex regional pain syndrome type I: five-year final follow-up of patients in a randomized controlled trial. *J Neurosurg.* 2008;108(2):292–298.
109. Kumar K, Rivzi S, Bishop S. Spinal cord stimulation is effective in management of complex regional pain syndrome I: fact or fiction. *Neurosurgery.* 2011;69:566–580.
110. Harke H, Gretenkort P, Ladleif HU, et al. Spinal cord stimulation in sympathetically maintained complex regional pain syndrome type I with severe disability. A prospective clinical study. *Eur J Pain.* 2005;9:363–363.
111. Van Ejis F, Geurts JW, Van Zundert J, et al. Spinal cord stimulation in complex regional pain syndrome type I of less than 12-month duration. *Neuromodulation.* 2012;15:144–150.
112. Sears NC, Machado AG, Nagel SJ, et al. Long-term outcomes of spinal cord stimulation with paddle leads in the treatment of complex regional pain syndrome and failed back surgery syndrome. *Neuromodulation.* 2011;14:312–318.
113. Geurts JW, Smits H, Kemler MA, et al. Spinal cord stimulation for complex regional pain syndrome type I: a prospective cohort study with long-term follow up. *Neuromodulation.* 2013;16:523–529.
114. Gopal H, Fitzgerald J, McCrory CJ. SCS for FBSS and CRPS: a review of 80 cases with on-table trial of stimulation. *Back Musculoskelet Rehab.* 106;29(1):7–13.
115. Visnjevac O, Costandi S, Patel BA, et al. A comprehensive outcome-specific review of the use of spinal cord stimulation for complex regional pain syndrome. *Pain Pract.* 2017;17:533–545.
116. Kriek N, Groeneweg JG, Stronks DL, et al. Preferred frequencies and waveforms for SCS in patients with CRPS: a multicentre, double-blind, randomized and placebo-controlled crossover trial. *Eur J Pain.* 2017;21(3):507–519.
117. Hoydonckx Y, Costanzi M, Bhatia A. A scoping review of novel spinal cord stimulation models for complex regional pain syndrome. *Can J Pain.* 2019;3(1):100–110.
118. Graybill J, Conermann T, Kabazie AJ, et al. Spinal cord stimulation for treatment of pain in a patient with post thoracotomy pain syndrome. *Pain Physician.* 2011;14:441–445.
119. Kurklinsky S, Palmer SC, Arroliga MJ, et al. Neuromodulation in postherpetic neuralgia: case reports and review of the literature. *Pain Med.* 2018;19:1237–1244.
120. Aiyer R, Barkin RL, Bhatia A, et al. A systematic review on the treatment of phantom limb pain with spinal cord stimulation. *Pain Manage.* 2017;7:59–69.
121. Sayed D, Kallewaard JW, Rotte A, et al. Pain relief and improvement in quality of life with 10 kHz SCS therapy: summary of clinical evidence. *CNS Neurosci Ther.* 2020;26(4):403–415.

122. Van Buyten JP, Al-Kaisy A, Smet I, et al. High-frequency spinal cord stimulation for the treatment of chronic back pain patients: results of a prospective multicenter European clinical study. *Neuromodulation*. 2013;16(1):59–65.
123. Al-Kaisy A, Palmisani S, Smith TE, et al. 10 kHz high-frequency spinal cord stimulation for chronic axial low back pain in patients with no history of spinal surgery: a preliminary, prospective, open label and proof-of-concept study. *Neuromodulation*. 2017;20(1):63–70.
124. Al-Kaisy A, Palmisani S, Smith TE, et al. Long-term improvements in chronic axial low back pain patients without previous spinal surgery: a cohort analysis of 10-kHz high-frequency spinal cord stimulation over 36 months. *Pain Med*. 2018;19(6):1219–1226.
125. Al-Kaisy A, Van Buyten JP, Caragnillo R, et al. 10 kHz SCS therapy for chronic pain, effects on opioid usage: post hoc analysis of data from two prospective studies. *Sci Rep*. 2019;9:11441.
Sayed D, Foster J, Nairizi A, et al. 10 kHz high-frequency spinal cord stimulator for chronic thoracic pain: a multicenter case series and guide for optimal lead placement. *Pain Physician*. 2020;23(4):369–376.
126. Stauss T, El Majdoub F, Sayed D, et al. A multicenter real world review of 10 kHz SCS outcomes for the treatment of chronic trunk and/or limb pain. *Ann Clin Transl Neurol*. 2019;6:496–507.
Sayed D, Salmon J, Khan TW, et al. Retrospective analysis of real-world outcomes of 10 kHz SCS in patients with upper limb and neck pain. *J Pain Res*. 2020;15(13):1441–1448.
127. Luecke T, Edgar D, Huse D. 10 kHz spinal cord stimulation for the treatment of chronic back and/or leg pain: summary of clinical studies. *SAGE Open Med*. 2020;8:1–10.
128. Al-Kaisy A, Van Buyten JP, Kapural L, et al. 10 kHz spinal cord stimulation for the treatment of non-surgical refractory back pain: subanalysis of pooled data from two prospective studies. *Anesthesia*. 2020;75:775–784.
129. De Voss CC, Meier K, Zaalberg PB, et al. Spinal cord stimulation in patients with painful diabetic neuropathy: a multicentre randomised clinical trial. *Pain*. 2014;155(11):2426.
130. Slangen R, Schapper NC, Faber CC, et al. Spinal cord stimulation and pain relief in painful diabetic peripheral neuropathy: A prospective two-center randomized controlled trial. *Diabetes Care*. 2014;37:3016–3024.
131. Petersen EA, Stauss T, Scowcroft J, et al. 10 kHz spinal cord stimulation for treatment of painful diabetic neuropathy: a multicenter randomized controlled trial. *Neurosurgery*. 2020;67(1):447–522.
132. Galan V, Scowcroft J, Chang P, et al. 10-kHz spinal cord stimulation treatment for painful diabetic neuropathy: results from post-hoc analysis of the SENZA-PPN study. *Pain Manage*. 2020;10(5):.
133. Mannheimer C, Eliasson T, Augustinsson LE, et al. Electrical stimulation versus coronary artery bypass surgery in severe angina pectoris: the ESBY study. *Circulation*. 1998;97(12):1157.
134. Norsell H, Pilhall M, Eliasson T, et al. Effects of spinal cord stimulation and coronary artery bypass grafting on myocardial ischemia and heart rate variability: further results from the ESBY study. *Cardiology*. 2000;94(1):12.
135. Ubbink DT, Vermeulen H. Spinal cord stimulation for non-reconstructable chronic critical leg ischemia. *Cochrane Database Syst Rev*. 2013;(2).
136. Saini HS, Shnoda M, Sainin I, et al. The effects of SCS on end organ perfusion: a literature review. *Cureus*. 2020;12(3):e7253.
137. Provenzano DA, Amirdelfan K, Kapural L, et al. Evidence gaps in the use of spinal cord stimulation treating spine conditions. *Spine*. 2017;42:580–592.
138. Hunter CW, Carlson K, Yang A, et al. Spinal cord stimulation for the treatment of failed neck surgery syndrome: outcomes of a prospective case series. *Neuromodulation*. 2018;21(5):496–503.
139. Simpson BA, Bassett G, Davies K, et al. Cervical spinal cord stimulation for pain: a report on 41 patients. *Neuromodulation*. 2003;6:20–26.
140. Burgher A, Kosek P, Surrett S, et al. Ten kilohertz SCS for the treatment of chronic upper extremity pain (UEP) results from prospective observational study. *J Pain Res*. 2020;13:2837–2851.
141. Simopoulos T, Aner M, Sharma S, et al. Explantation of percutaneous spinal cord stimulator devices: a retrospective descriptive analysis of a single-center 15-year experience. *Pain Med*. 2019;.
142. Reddy RD, Moheimani R, Yu GG, et al. A review of clinical data on salvage therapy in spinal cord stimulation. *Neuromodulation*. 2020;23(5):562–571.

143. Ghosh PE, Gill JS, Simopoulos T. The evolving role of high-frequency spinal cord stimulation as salvage therapy in neurostimulation. *Pain Pract.* 2020;20(7):706–713.
144. Kapural L, Sayed D, Kim B, et al. Retrospective assessment of salvage to 10 kHz spinal cord stimulation (SCS) in patients who failed traditional SCS therapy: RESCUE study. *J Pain Res.* 2020;13:2861–2867.
145. Pollard EM, Lamer TJ, Moeschler SM, et al. The effect of spinal cord stimulation on pain medication reduction in intractable spine and limb pain: a systematic review of RCTs and meta-analysis. *J Pain Res.* 2019;30(12):1311–1324.
146. Dougherty MC, Woodroffe RW, Wilson S, Gillies GT, Howard MA III, Carnahan RM. Predictors of reduced opioid use with spinal cord stimulation in patients with chronic opioid use. *Neuromodulation.* 2020;23(1):126–132.
147. Al-Kaisy A, Van Buyten JP, Amirdelfan K, et al. Opioid sparing effects of 10 kHz SCS: a review of clinical evidence. *Ann N Y Acad Sci.* 2020;1462(1):53–64.
148. Sharan AD, Riley J, Falowski S, et al. Association of opioid usage with spinal cord stimulation outcomes. *Pain Med.* 2018;19(4):699–707.
149. Simopoulos T, Sharma S, Wootton RJ, et al. Discontinuation of chronic opiate therapy after successful SCS is highly dependent upon the daily opioid dose. *Pain Pract.* 2019;19(8):794–799.
150. Lad SP, Petraglia FW, Kent AR, et al. Longer delay from chronic pain to spinal cord stimulation results in higher healthcare resource utilization. *Neuromodulation.* 2016;19(5):469–476.
151. Siegfried J, Lazorthes Y, Broggi G. Electrical spinal cord stimulation for spastic movement disorders. *Stereotact Funct Neurosurg.* 1981;44(1–3):77–92.
152. Barolat G, Myklebust JB, Wenninger W. Enhancement of voluntary motor function following spinal cord stimulation-case study. *Stereotact Funct Neurosurg.* 1986;49(6):307–314.
153. Dimitrijevic MM, Dimitrijevic MR, Illis LS, Nakajima K, Sharkey PC, Sherwood AM. Spinal cord stimulation for the control of spasticity in patients with chronic spinal cord injury: I. Clinical observations. *CNS Trauma.* 1986;3(2):129–143.
154. Gybels J, Van Roost D. Spinal cord stimulation for spasticity. *Adv Tech Stand Neurosurg.* 1987:63–96.
155. Midha M, Schmitt JK. Epidural spinal cord stimulation for the control of spasticity in spinal cord injury patients lacks long-term efficacy and is not cost-effective. *Spinal Cord.* 1998;36(3):190–192.
156. Nagel SJ, Wilson S, Johnson MD, et al. Spinal cord stimulation for spasticity: historical approaches, current status, and future directions. *Neuromodulation.* 2017;20(4):307–321.
157. Freeman D, Sturtevant D, Pino IP, Netoff T, Parr AM, Darrow DP. Spinal cord stimulation after chronic complete spinal cord injury enables volitional movement even in absence of stimulation. *Neurosurgery.* 2020;67(suppl 1):S447–S454.
158. Saito J, Koda M, Furuya T, et al. Combination of epidural spinal cord stimulation and treadmill training with body weight support attenuates spasticity in adult rats with spinal cord transection.
159. Parker J, Dietz BE. Spinal cord stimulation for the relief of spasticity from cerebral palsy. *Healthcare Technol Lett.* 2020;7(3):93–97.
160. McKenzie-Brown AM, Fishman S, Crowley M. Spinal cord stimulation: Placement and management. In: Post TW, ed. *UpToDate.* 2021.
161. Peters MJ, Morgan LC, Gluch L. Smoking cessation and elective surgery: the cleanest cut. *Med J Aust.* 2004;180:317–318.
162. Kreis PG. SCS screening trial: patient selection and preparation. In: Kreis PG, ed. *Spinal Cord Stimulation: Percutaneous Implantation Techniques.* New York, NY: Oxford University Press; 2009: 11–34.
163. Gatchel RJ. Comorbidity of chronic mental and physical health disorders: the biopsychosocial perspective. *Am Psychol.* 2001;59:792–805.
164. Gatchel RJ, Haggard R. Biopsychosocial prescreening for spinal cord and peripheral nerve stimulation devices. In: *Practical Management of Pain.* 5th ed. Elsevier; 2013: 933–938.

Schocket KG, Gatchel RJ, Stowell AW, et al. A demonstration of a presurgical behavioral medicine evaluation for categorizing patients for implantable therapies: a preliminary study. *Neuromodulation.* 2008;11(4):237–248.

165. Bruns D, Disorbio JM. Assessment of biopsychosocial risk factors for medical treatment: a collaborative approach. *J Clin Psychol Med Settings*. 2009;16(2):127–147.
166. Heckler DR, Gatchel RJ, Lou L, Whitworth T, Bernstein D, Stowell AW. Presurgical behavioral medicine evaluation (PBME) for implantable devices for pain management: a 1-year prospective study. *Pain Pract*. 2007;7(2):110–122.
167. Deer TR, Provenzano DA, Hanes M, et al. The Neurostimulation Appropriateness Consensus Committee (NACC) recommendations for infection prevention and management. *Neuromodulation*. 2017;20(1):31–50.
168. Narouze S, Benzon HT, Provenzano D, et al. Interventional spine and pain procedures in patients on antiplatelet and anticoagulant medications: guidelines from the American Society of Regional Anesthesia and Pain Medicine, the European Society of Regional Anaesthesia and Pain Therapy, the American Academy of Pain Medicine, the International Neuromodulation Society, the North American Neuromodulation Society, and the World Institute of Pain. *Reg Anesth Pain Med*. 2018;43(3):225–262.
169. Hogan QH. Lumbar epidural anatomy. A new look by cryomicrotome section. *Anesthesiology*. 1991;75:767–775.
170. Bernards CM. Sophistry in medicine: lessons from the epidural space. *Reg Anesth Pain Med*. 2005;30:56–66.
171. Meijenhorst GC. Computed tomography of the lumbar epidural veins. *Radiology*. 1982;145:687–691.
172. Shils JL, Arle JE. Neuromonitoring for SCS lead placement under general anesthesia. *J Clin Neurol*. 2018;14(4):444–453.
173. Falowski S, Dianna A. Neuromonitoring protocol for spinal cord stimulator cases with case descriptions. *Int J Acad Med*. 2016;2:132–144.
174. Carlson JD, Lee ET, Zakas G. Permanent percutaneous spinal cord stimulator implantation: cervical/lumbar. In: *Advanced Procedures for Pain Management*. Cham, Switzerland: Springer; 2018:203–225.
175. Kim RE, Baez-Cabrera LD, Furman MB. Thoracolumbar spinal cord stimulation. In: Furman MB, et al, eds. *Atlas of Image-Guided Spinal Procedures*. Elsevier; 2018:325–336.
176. Barolat G, Massaro F, He J, Zeme S, Ketcik B. Mapping of sensory responses to epidural stimulation of the intraspinal neural structures in man. *J Neurosurg*. 1993;78(2):233–239. doi:10.3171/jns.1993.78.2.0233. PMID:8421206.
177. Sabia M, Mathur R. *Interventional Pain Procedures: Handbook and Video Guide*. Springer; 2018.
178. Deer TR, Mekhail N, Provenzano D, et al. The appropriate use of neurostimulation of the spinal cord and peripheral nervous system for the treatment of chronic pain and ischemic diseases: the Neuromodulation Appropriateness Consensus Committee. *Neuromodulation*. 2014;17(6):515–550.
179. Eldrige JS, Weingarten TN, Rho RH. Management of cerebral spinal fluid leak complicating spinal cord stimulator implantation. *Pain Practice*. 2006;6(4):285–288.
180. Pope JE. Complications of spinal cord stimulation. In: *Reducing Risks and Complications of Interventional Pain Procedures*. 2012:3–10.
181. Hoelzer BC, Bendel MA, Deer TR, et al. Spinal cord stimulator implant infection rates and risk factors: a multicenter retrospective study. *Neuromodulation*. 2017;20(6):558–562.
182. Schmidt GL. The use of spinal cord stimulation/neuromodulation in the management of chronic pain. *JAAOS: J Am Acad Orthop Surg*. 2019;27(9):e401–e407.
183. Deer TR, Stewart CD. Complications of spinal cord stimulation: identification, treatment, and prevention. *Pain Med*. 2008;9(suppl 1):S93–S101.
184. Cameron T. Safety and efficacy of spinal cord stimulation for the treatment of chronic pain: a 20-year literature review. *J Neurosurg Spine*. 2004;100(3):254–267.
185. Kumar K, Wilson JR, Taylor RS, Gupta S. Complications of spinal cord stimulation, suggestions to improve outcome, and financial impact. *J Neurosurg Spine*. 2006;5(3):191–203.
186. Kumar K, Buchser E, Linderoth B, Meglio M, Van Buyten JP. Avoiding complications from spinal cord stimulation: practical recommendations from an international panel of experts. *Neuromodulation*. 2007;10(1):24–33.

187. Labaran L, Jain N, Puvanesarajah V, Jain A, Buchholz AL, Hassanzadeh H. A retrospective database review of the indications, complications, and incidence of subsequent spine surgery in 12,297 spinal cord stimulator patients. *Neuromodulation*. 2020;23(5):634–638.
188. Turner JA, Loeser JD, Deyo RA, Sanders SB. Spinal cord stimulation for patients with failed back surgery syndrome or complex regional pain syndrome: a systematic review of effectiveness and complications. *Pain*. 2004;108(1–2):137–147.
189. Sarubbi FA, Vasquez JE. Spinal epidural abscess associated with the use of temporary epidural catheters: report of two cases and review. *Clin Infect Dis*. 1997;25(5):1155–1158.

20

Peripheral Nerve Stimulator Implantation

Steven Zhou, Nasir Hussain, Timothy Deer, and Alaa Abd-Elsayed

Introduction

The evolution and rapid expansion of peripheral nerve stimulation (PNS) has made it one of the most exciting yet divisive therapies for pain available today. At its core, neuromodulation is electrical dosing of the nervous system to change its function. As knowledge has advanced, interventional therapies have steadily moved toward the periphery to directly target injured nerves of interest. PNS differs from spinal cord stimulation in that the nerve stimulator leads are often placed in close anatomic proximity to the individual nerves themselves. Although previously PNS was done using fluoroscopic guidance in most cases, the further growth of ultrasound-based techniques has improved the overall precision of lead placement and reduced complications. After conservative therapies have been exhausted, PNS offers an alternative therapy for chronic neuropathic or, in some settings, nociceptive pain.

In addition to PNS, which is the direct stimulation of nerves outside of the neuraxis, there also is peripheral nerve field stimulation (PNFS), which is targeted stimulation of smaller, mostly unnamed, nerves at the site of the pain.[1] While PNS often targets differing lengths of nerves of interest, PNFS (sometimes referred to as subcutaneous neurostimulation or targeted subcutaneous stimulation) uses electrodes positioned subcutaneously at the site of maximal pain. Unlike PNS, which targets a specific dermatome, PNFS involves subcutaneous modulation of smaller, distal, often ill-defined branches of nerves.[2] In light of recent exciting advances in PNS technology, this chapter explores the common nerves of interest being targeted by pain interventionalists, the research supporting PNS use, and a general overview of the implantation techniques utilized. While much research needs to be done, the field of neuromodulation is poised for an eruption in the near future as our knowledge continues to expand. While the potential of PNS and PNFS currently outpaces reality, it is our hope that it can one day be realized. At the present time, there is limited evidence about PNFS, and many additional studies are needed before any conclusions can be drawn about the utility of this therapeutic option.

Mechanism and Theories of Use

While the mechanism of action for PNS has not been fully elucidated, the field of neuromodulation is based on Melzack and Wall's landmark gate-control theory of pain,[3] which holds that pain perception is largely due to spinal cord signals generated by both large-diameter (non-nociceptive) and small-diameter (nociceptive) primary afferent fibers.[4] Activation of the larger non-nociceptive afferent fibers (via touch, vibration, pressure) is thought to "close" the gate through neurons in the dorsal horn. This then leads to the inhibition of excitatory neurons and pain. In contrast, when the small-diameter nociceptor fibers are activated, the gate "opens," which result in impedance of inhibitory interneurons. This dynamic balance between the non-nociceptive and nociceptive sensory fibers regulates the perception of pain. PNS, through direct stimulation of the peripheral nerves, has been found to reduce excitability, increase the nerves' electrical threshold, and lead to a transient slowing of the nerves' conduction velocity.[5,6] Several other theories also exist regarding the mechanism of action of PNS. Some literature suggests that PNS may also directly inhibit primary nociceptive afferent fibers and reduce long-term central pain sensitization.[1] It has also been hypothesized that PNS may alter local concentrations of biochemical mediators of pain and the inflammatory response (neuropeptides, endorphins), which may enhance the pain response and contribute to chronic pain.[4,7,8] Other theories suggest that PNS can further decrease ectopic discharges at the periphery, decreasing pain perception at the site of nerve injury.

The first peripheral nerve stimulators were devices originally designed for spinal cord stimulation in the epidural space. Therefore, complications, such as lead migration, lead fracture, connector failures, and others, invariably arose.[9] These first-generation stimulators were cuff-shaped, requiring open surgical access and leading to unwanted motor stimulation and perineural fibrosis.[5] Also, given that PNS leads are typically implanted in areas of the periphery that undergo large amounts of activity and movement, the practicality of stimulator use was limited. The devices were also especially problematic in areas like the arms or neck, with many having mechanical lead failure. With advances in technology, newer devices, including surgical paddle-type electrodes, can be implanted percutaneously, a development that significantly decreases the complication rate. Figure 20.1 shows an example of a modern lead design. While newer designs have improved from the originals, much work remains to design stimulators that are specifically tailored to the unique anatomy and pathophysiology of peripheral nerves.

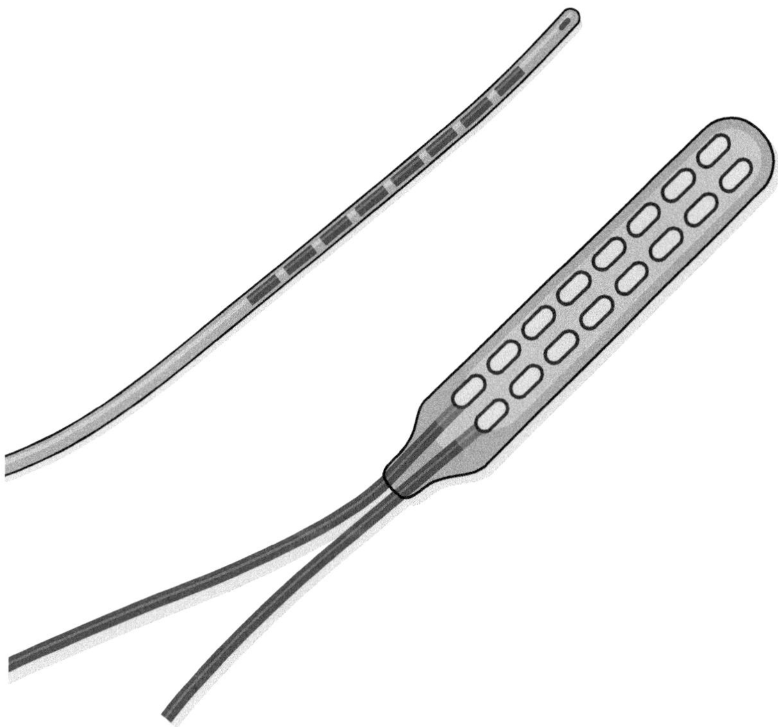

FIGURE 20.1. Modern lead design.

Patient Selection and Contraindications

Indications

While specific guidelines are sparse and mostly have been formulated from societal statements, PNS is generally indicated for chronic neuropathic pain originating from peripheral nerves. This category commonly includes complex regional pain syndrome (CRPS) type 2, neuropathic pain from mono- or plexopathies, and headaches.[1,10] The indications for PFNS are even more nebulous, since its exact mechanism of action is not clearly defined. Some uses for PNFS include chronic back pain (where it is often used in conjunction with a spinal cord stimulator) and phantom limb pain, although the evidence for both is lacking. Importantly, since current PNFS devices are generally not FDA approved and are used "off label," patient selection is even more crucial, because most interventions are not covered by insurance. This is largely due to the minimal evidence supporting PNFS.

As is true for any other pain treatment modality, the success of PNS and PNFS relies on patient selection.[11] The first step for any new chronic pain patient is taking a thorough history and physical exam, including a detailed pain history, pain distribution, and exacerbating/alleviating factors.[2] All previous medications and attempted interventions should be clearly defined and explored, along with clear documentation of the pain's effect on the patient's life. The typical patient for whom PNS may be an option is one who has already failed conventional medical treatment. Comorbid psychiatric illnesses should also be explored, since if they are poorly controlled, they can significantly reduce interventional success rates.[1,12] Often, it may be beneficial to perform a psychological evaluation or to explore concurrent psychiatric treatment as part of the presurgical optimization process before proceeding.[13] There is also support for more encompassing patient screening, including depression screening, McGill Pain Questionnaires, International Patient Satisfaction Index (IPSI), Visual Analog Scale (VAS), and the Pain Disability Index as adjuncts in the process.[4,12,13,14]

Follow-up

While PNS is generally safer than spinal cord stimulation or other neuraxial techniques, it must be noted that PNS still involves surgical procedures that require close follow-up. Those with a history of poor treatment adherence are at high risk of being lost to follow-up and may be poor candidates for PNS. Furthermore, PNS devices often require upkeep and manipulation even after implantation, further emphasizing the importance of follow-up.

Contraindications

Generally, there are only a few absolute contraindications to PNS. The most common contraindications include coagulopathies, immunocompromise, medication allergies, infections at the nerve of interest or injection site, comorbidities preventing fluoroscopic needle guidance, and patient refusal.[1,2] Since PNS is a peripheral procedure, risk of permanent damage is less likely than with other neuraxial procedures. Other considerations include prior radiation to the region, age, and likelihood of follow-up (as discussed in the previous paragraph). Clinicians should always utilize clinical judgment in both patient selection and location of lead placement. Specific contraindications may exist for different implantation sites (i.e., median nerve stimulation), and they should be explored in detail preoperatively.

Peripheral Nerve Stimulator Implantation

Procedure and Clinical Utility

While a detailed overview of all therapies is outside the scope of this chapter and new techniques are being developed daily, this section provides an overview of the current literature and current PNS practice. Specific topics covered include general indications for the specific procedure, a brief overview of the evidence, perioperative management, a brief explanation of the techniques utilized, postoperative management/follow-up, and the most common complications.

Percutaneous peripheral nerve stimulator implantation comes with a set of challenges. The anatomy involved is often complex and is greatly affected by patient positioning. Therefore, many techniques also require direct visualization, either by fluoroscopy/ultrasound or by anatomic relation to well-defined landmarks. This discussion touches on both percutaneous implantation techniques as well as the more established open surgical techniques.

Preoperative Planning

While the specific procedure for each nerve of interest is outside of the scope of this chapter, the general steps in PNS include obtaining a thorough history and physical examination, trial stimulator placement, and permanent stimulator implantation. In addition to the history and physical, preoperative planning often necessitates imaging of the area of interest. This may be a quick ultrasound scan of the relevant anatomy, but it may also include a CT scan or MRI for confirmation. If the physician believes that the patient will benefit from PNS, a trial stimulator placement is offered first, followed by permanent stimulator placement. A diagnostic block to confirm the diagnosis is recommended. Generally, regardless of whether trial or permanent PNS leads are being placed, the procedure can be performed under conscious sedation, which keeps the patient comfortable and relaxed yet still allows intraoperative testing of the positioned electrodes.[2] General anesthesia may be needed in specific cases and somatosensory-evoked potential monitoring should be considered.[15]

Perioperative antibiotics should be given less than 1 hour before incision and should cover common skin flora. Often, weight-based dosing of cefazolin is considered adequate for this purpose. Finally, special equipment, such as fluoroscopy and/or ultrasound, should be available to confirm electrode location.

Intraoperative Preparation and Procedure

Positioning of the patient is crucial and should take into account use of fluoroscopy and standard surgical preparation and draping. Hair in the involved area is typically removed or clipped, and the skin is carefully cleaned. For percutaneous trial lead placement, the skin is initially infiltrated with local anesthetic, and then a 3- to 5-mm entry incision is made.[2] A Tuohy needle is advanced into the subcutaneous space overlying the targeted nerve. The guidewire is advanced through the Tuohy needle, while fluoroscopic/ultrasound images are used to follow its trajectory. After the Tuohy needle is withdrawn, a plastic cannula is advanced over the guidewire using Seldinger technique; the guidewire is then withdrawn. The electrode lead is then advanced through the cannula and is connected to the generator. Electrode placement depth is critically important, because the electrode can provoke muscle contractions if it is placed too deep. Typically, one or two electrodes are implanted for PNS. With the device on, paresthesias are evaluated, and the amplitude, frequency, and pulse width of stimulation are adjusted as needed. After initial lead placement, patients typically undergo a trial period of 2 to 14 days.[2] During that time, care is taken to ensure the cables are kept clean and dry. Patients should also refrain from strenuous activities to prevent lead displacement.

A trial is deemed successful if the patient experiences a significant improvement in pain severity. If the trial is successful, a permanent stimulator is then placed, sometimes under general anesthesia to ensure proper cable tunneling. The leads are placed in a similar fashion to that described above. For staged trials, a 4- to 6-cm incision is made and dissection is carried down to expose the fascia.[16] For permanent placement, additional plastic anchors and nonabsorbable sutures are used at the site of entry to help stabilize the leads in the fascia.[1] A strain-relief loop is also created at the incision site to minimize lead migration and kinking.[1,2] Finally, a subcutaneous pocket is created for the implantable pulse generator. Before the layered closure is completed, antibiotic irrigation is typically performed (typically with vancomycin powder). Sterile dressings are then applied before the patient leaves the procedural suite, and subsequent device programming is completed in the recovery area.

The general steps for ultrasound-guided PNS implantation are similar to those for the fluoroscopy-guided technique. The ultrasound-guided technique has become increasingly popular, but it is limited to more superficial peripheral nerves. Before the procedure is scheduled, often an ultrasound is completed to evaluate the proposed trajectory, accessibility, and depth.[17] Body habitus is also a significant concern, because thinner patients may have a higher incidence of lead erosion, while more obese patients may present increased difficulty with initial lead placement. For ultrasound-guided approaches, it is beneficial to mark the nerve trajectory on the skin with a skin marker, along with any specific changes to depth. Placement should be completed under continuous short- and long-axis ultrasound views, and care should be taken to ensure that fascial planes are clearly visualized, the lead does not cross joints, and transection through large volumes of muscles is avoided.[17,16] In a purely percutaneous approach, the leads are then anchored at the skin. Figure 20.2 depicts ultrasound-guided lead placement.

It is important to note that there are slight differences between different systems; some are operated by a battery, some are wireless, some are temporarily placed, and others are permanently placed.

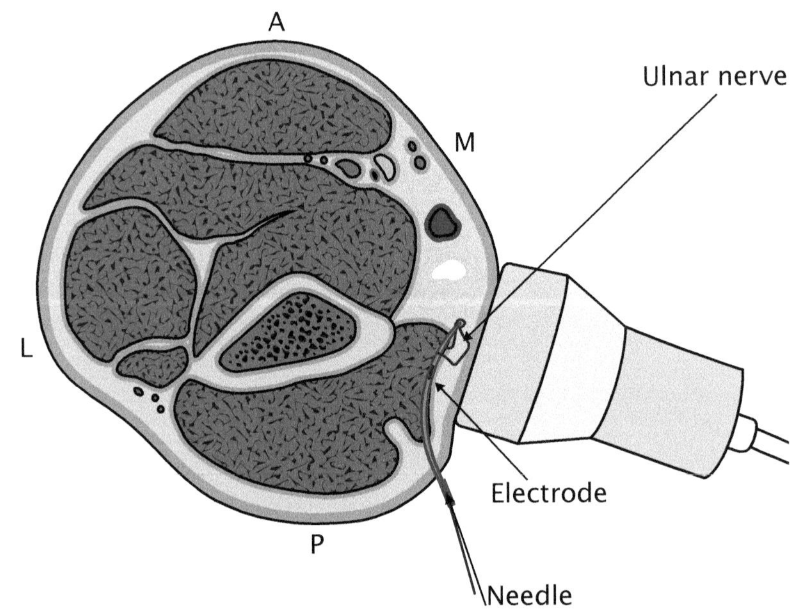

FIGURE 20.2. Lead placement via ultrasound guidance.
A = anterior, M = medial, L = lateral, P = posterior.

TABLE 20.1. Common Postoperative Complications of PNS and PNFS[24–29]

Complication	PNS	PNFS
Infection	3.6%–17.9%	4.4%
Erosion	4.5%–50%	2.2%
Migration	9%–25%	15.6%
Mechanical failure	3.6%	11%
Lack of efficacy	21%	4.7%–17%

Postoperative Care

Follow-up should generally be completed with the same physician who initially placed the device.[15] If significant improvement in pain is observed, attempts should be made in conjunction with the patients' primary care provider to gradually taper off other pain medications. Periodic adjustments to pain medication may need to be made by the physician as well. Importantly, postoperative complications of PNS should be monitored for and assessed at all follow-up visits. Although complications are generally rare, common complications include infection, lead erosion, migration, and mechanical failure.[2] Table 20.1 lists the most common complications of both PNS and PNFS.

Of note, most of the devices used in PNS are not MRI compatible. Careful evaluation of the device manufacturer's information should be completed for each device implanted.

Common Targets for PNS

There are many nerves that can be targeted using PNS, and there is evidence for the effectiveness of stimulation for each nerve. As expected, certain targeted nerves have higher-quality evidence supporting their use in comparison to others. Tables 20.2 to 20.7 furnish a high-yield summary of the common nerves targeted by PNS and broad evidence for PNS use. The tables have been organized by location of pain to allow quick reference by

TABLE 20.2. Facial Pain: Nerve Involvement, Indications for PNS, and Evidence

Nerve	Indications for PNS	Evidence
Trigeminal n. and supra/infraorbital n.'s	▪ Trigeminal neuropathy ▪ Postherpetic neuralgia ▪ Poststroke pain	▪ Multiple case reports/series of treatment by stimulation of trigeminal ganglion/nerve/branches for neuropathic craniofacial pain or trigeminal neuropathy, including both short- and long-term pain relief and reduction of opioid use[30–34] ▪ Broken down by cause, some evidence suggests PNS may work better for poststroke pain than for postherpetic neuralgia[35]
Occipital n.	▪ Occipital neuralgia ▪ Migraine	▪ Strong evidence for occipital neuralgia[5,36] ▪ Strong evidence with randomized sham-controlled trials for chronic migraines; significant reduction in headache scoring, increased headache-free days, decreased migraine-related disability[5,37,38,39]

TABLE 20.3. Upper Extremity Pain: Nerve Involvement, Indications for PNS, and Evidence

Nerve	Indications for PNS	Evidence
Suprascapular/ axillary n.	• Subacromial impingement syndrome • Complex regional pain syndrome (CRPS) • Post-stroke shoulder pain	• Case series with some evidence of improved pain control for upper limb neuropathic pain and CRPS[40] • Some evidence for improvement in chronic shoulder pain, disability scoring, shoulder ROM from subacromial impingement syndrome[41] • Randomized controlled trial of PNS versus usual care for chronic shoulder pain after stroke showed significant reduction in shoulder pain[42]
Ulnar n.	• Neuropathic/posttraumatic pain	• Case series and individual case reports suggesting improvement in pain control[17,16,43]
Median n.	• Neuropathic/ posttraumatic pain • Carpal tunnel syndrome	• Weak evidence from individual case reports[17,16,44] • Case series regarding pain improvement for carpal tunnel syndrome[45]
Radial n.	• Neuropathic/posttraumatic pain	• Weak evidence from individual case reports[16,44]
Brachial plexus	• Rotator cuff repair • Upper limb CRPS	• Weak evidence suggesting that brachial plexus nerve stimulation (roots or trunk) may improve pain after perioperative period and reduce opioid use post-operatively[46] • Case series suggesting improvement in pain for CRPS[47]

Note: Trials and case studies involving pain in the upper extremities are typically lumped together, and most often are not separated by individual nerves. Rather, case series often combine patients with chronic neuropathic upper extremity pain limited to specific nerves and separate patients during the report.

TABLE 20.4. Trunk Pain: Nerve Involvement, Indications for PNS, and Evidence

Nerve	Indications for PNS	Evidence
Intercostal n.'s	• Chronic abdominal pain • Postthoracotomy pain • Neuropathic pain	• Weak evidence from a case report for reduction in pain and decreased narcotic use in a patient with chronic abdominal pain of unknown cause[48] • Some evidence of utility of TENS for postthoracotomy pain, potential for PNS in future[49–51] • Weak evidence from a case series showing improvement in intercostal pain[52]
Cluneal n.'s	• Neuropathic pain	• Weak evidence from a case report for stimulation of superior cluneal n. and neuropathic pain[53]
Lumbar sympathetic chain	• Loin pain hematuria syndrome (LPHS)	• Weak evidence from a small case series with decreased pain scores and analgesic consumption for LPHS[54]

TABLE 20.5. Pelvic Pain: Nerve Involvement, Indications for PNS, and Evidence

Nerve	Indications for PNS	Evidence
Ilioinguinal/ iliohypogastric n.	▪ Inguinal neuralgia ▪ Chronic postherniorrhaphy inguinal pain (CPIP)	▪ Some evidence from case reports for treatment of inguinal pain and CPIP[35,55,56,57,58]
Genitofemoral n.	▪ Inguinal neuralgia	▪ Weak evidence from small case series of 3 patients suggesting improvement in pain, increased activity levels, and pain medication cessation[59]
Pudendal n.	▪ Peroneal neuralgia ▪ Bladder pain syndrome	▪ Weak evidence from case series for slight improvement in peroneal neuralgia[60,61] ▪ Some evidence for improvement in bladder pain syndrome for patients who previously failed sacral nerve stimulation, also showed significantly greater reduction in bladder pain and irritative urinary symptoms[62,63]

TABLE 20.6. Lower Extremity Pain: Nerve Involvement, Indications for PNS, and Evidence

Nerve	Indications for PNS	Evidence
Lateral femoral cutaneous n.	▪ Meralgia paresthetica	▪ Weak evidence from a case report[64]
Femoral n.	▪ Postamputation pain	▪ Some evidence from case series and a randomized crossover placebo-controlled trial suggesting improvement in postamputation pain, improved ADL, sometimes even after stimulator removal[65–67]
Sciatic n.	▪ Neuropathic pain ▪ Postamputation pain	▪ Some evidence from several case series and randomized crossover placebo-controlled trial suggesting improvement in postamputation pain, improved ADL, sometimes even after stimulator removal[65–67]
Genicular/IPS	▪ Anterior knee pain	▪ Weak evidence from an individual case report[68]
Peroneal n.	▪ Neuropathic pain	▪ Weak evidence from individual case reports[16,69]
Saphenous n.	▪ Neuropathic pain	▪ Weak evidence from an individual case report[9]
Posterior tibial n.	▪ Chronic pelvic pain ▪ Bladder pain syndrome	▪ Moderate evidence from randomized sham-controlled study showing significant improvement in pain scoring from stimulation versus sham treatment[70] ▪ Supported by smaller studies suggesting improved pain control[71–73] ▪ Conflicting evidence for use of posterior tibial nerve stimulation in bladder pain syndrome. One study found improvement in pain and irritative bladder symptoms, while two others did not[74–76]
Sural n.	▪ Neuropathic pain	▪ Weak evidence from a case report[77]
Lumbar plexus	▪ Neuropathic pain	▪ Weak evidence from a case series for improvement in lower limb neuropathic pain refractory to spinal cord stimulation[78]

Note: Deer et al did publish a randomized study showing a significant benefit in the lower extremities, but the specific nerves targeted were not included.[79] Therefore, conclusions regarding the efficacy of neuromodulation of specific nerves cannot be drawn from that study.

TABLE 20.7. Miscellaneous Indications for PNS: Nerve Involvement, Indications, and Evidence

Nerve	Indications for PNS	Evidence
Sphenopalatine ganglion (SPG)	▪ Cluster headaches ▪ Migraine	▪ Strong evidence for cluster headaches, including for acute response, disability, quality of life; possible benefit as prophylactic treatment[80–84] ▪ Weak evidence for migraines; small reduction in acute migraines, current prospective study ongoing[9,85]
Vagus n.	▪ Chronic pelvic pain from endometriosis ▪ Refractory epilepsy ▪ Treatment-resistant depression ▪ Obesity/satiety	▪ Weak evidence for vagal nerve stimulation (VNS) for chronic pelvic pain from a randomized crossover single-session vagal afferent nerve stimulation versus nonvagal auricular stimulation[86] ▪ Strong evidence for use of VNS for refractory epilepsy based on randomized clinical trials[9,87,88] ▪ Strong evidence from observational and open-label trials showing improvement in depression scoring and remission rate with VNS[9,89,90] ▪ Weight loss reported in multiple previous studies for epilepsy and depression[13] ▪ Weak evidence suggesting increased satiety and role for VNS in obesity[91,92]
Phrenic n.	▪ Congenital central hypoventilation syndrome ▪ Spinal cord injury ▪ Sleep apnea	▪ Strong evidence for long-term use of phrenic nerve stimulation for congenital central hypoventilation syndrome and spinal cord injuries—significant improvement in quality of life noted[93] ▪ Strong evidence for treatment of centrally mediated sleep apnea—FDA-approved[94]
Carotid sinus/n.	▪ Resistant hypertension ▪ Heart failure	▪ Strong evidence for baroreceptor activation therapy (BAT) in treatment of resistant hypertension via double-blind randomized placebo-controlled studies[9,95–97] ▪ Strong evidence for BAT in improving quality of life, exercise capacity, and NT-proBNP measurements in patients with heart failure[98]
Hypoglossal n.	▪ Obstructive sleep apnea (OSA)	▪ Strong evidence from randomized clinical trials for use in OSA—seems to work best in BMI < 40[99–102]
Sacral n.'s	▪ Refractory overactive bladder ▪ Refractory urinary incontinence ▪ Nonobstructive urinary retention ▪ Chronic fecal incontinence ▪ Chronic pelvic pain ▪ Bladder pain syndrome	▪ Strong evidence for sacral nerve stimulation for improvement in symptoms of overactive bladder, urinary incontinence, and nonobstructive urinary retention[103–104] ▪ Strong evidence for improvement in fecal incontinence[105,106] ▪ Some evidence from case series for improvement of chronic pelvic/urogenital pain[107–109] ▪ Strong evidence from longitudinal studies[110–112] for improvement in bladder pain syndrome
Splanchnic n.	▪ Pain from chronic pancreatitis	▪ Weak evidence from case reports for improvement in pain control and decreased narcotic use in chronic pancreatitis[113]

TABLE 20.8. Combination Targets for Hybrid Stimulation[114–117]

Pain Location	Spinal Lead Location	Peripheral Lead Location
Axial back/neck	Corresponding cord level	Cluneal or PNFS near cutaneous dorsal rami serving pain location
Thoracic radicular	Corresponding thoracic level	Intercostal or PNFS near pain location
Facial	Cervical (nucleus caudalis)	Corresponding nerve of the face
Shoulder	Cervical or high thoracic	Axillary nerve or suprascapular nerve
Abdominal	Mid to higher thoracic (T5, T6)	Ilioinguinal, hypogastric, or PNFS near pain location
Flank	Corresponding thoracic level	PNFS near pain location

practicing physicians. Furthermore, the evidence has been classified as either weak (primarily from case reports or series) or strong (primarily from randomized controlled trials).

PNFS

PNFS refers to the placement of electrodes near the area of pain without direct contact with the peripheral nerve.[4] The procedure is similar to PNS electrode implantation, except that multiple electrodes are used to provide adequate coverage.[2] The depth is also more shallow, as the leads do not need to be as close to the specific nerves, instead resting 10-15 mm below the skin surface.[18] The main benefits of using PNFS rather than traditional PNS include a reduction in potential nerve damage. However, due the superficial placement of the electrodes, adverse events can include electrode migration or failure. While there are currently poor prospective data on PNFS, most research so far has focused on low back pain, with a recent study of sacroiliac joint pain.

For chronic back pain specifically, Kloimstein et al evaluated the long-term efficacy of PNFS in patients with refractory chronic low back pain.[4,19] After implantation, patients reported stable decreases in pain at the 6-month follow-up, as well as improvements in secondary parameters, including the Oswestry Disability Questionnaire score and the Beck Depression Inventory. Of note, 9.6% of the patients experienced complications requiring surgical intervention. A further study by McRoberts et al confirmed these findings and found significant differences in VAS scores with nerve stimulation.[20] Long-term benefits have also been noted. A study by Gilmore et al found sustained pain control up to 12 months after the end of the 1 month of treatment and explantation.[21] Overall, there seems to be strong evidence for the utility of PNFS in the treatment of chronic low back pain.

PNFS has also been studied for sacroiliac joint pain, with Guentchev et al reporting a case series where patients reported improved pain control, satisfaction, and Oswestry Disability Index scores after implantation.[22] These effects also appeared to hold true for up to 12 months after implantation.

Hybrid Stimulation

Spinal cord stimulation (SCS) has been used in conjunction with PNS to maximize coverage over an area of pain. While specific discussion of SCS is outside the scope of this chapter, there are multiple published trials assessing the synergy of SCS with PNS. One such trial was completed by Mironer et al, who found that SCS combined with PNFS provided wider axial coverage than SCS or PNFS alone.[23] Table 20.8, which is adapted from the ASRA best practices for PNS, lists some common combination targets for hybrid stimulation.

Conclusions

From the evidence in this chapter, it is clear that PNS offers exciting possibilities for safe and efficacious pain control in multiple parts of the body, but much work remains to bring PNS into the mainstream of neuromodulation and interventional pain management.

References

1. Timothy R. Deer, Michael S. Leong, Asokumar Buvanendran, Vitaly Gordin, Philip S. Kim, Sunil J. Panchal, Albert L. Ray. Comprehensive treatment of chronic pain by medical, interventional, and integrative approaches. *The American Academy of Pain Medicine Textbook on Patient Management*. Springer; 2013: 583–600.
2. Petersen EA, Slavin KV. Peripheral nerve/field stimulation for chronic pain. *Neurosurg Clin North Am*. 2014;25(4):789–797.
3. Gildenberg PL. History of electrical neuromodulation for chronic pain. *Pain Med*. 2006;7(suppl 1):S7–S13. https://doi.org/10.1111/j.1526-4637.2006.00118.x.
4. Chakravarthy K, Nava A, Christo PJ, Williams K. Review of recent advances in peripheral nerve stimulation (PNS). *Curr Pain Headache Rep*. 2016;20(11):60. doi:10.1007/s11916-016-0590-8. PMID:27671799.
5. Goroszeniuk T, Pang D. Peripheral neuromodulation: a review. *Curr Pain Headache Rep*. 2014;18:412. https://doi.org/10.1007/s11916-014-0412-9.
6. Ignelzi RJ, Nyquist JK. Direct effect of electrical stimulation on peripheral nerve evoked activity: implications in pain relief. *J Neurosurg*. 1976;45:159–165.
7. Papuc E. The role of neurostimulation in the treatment of neuropathic pain. *Ann Agric Environ Med*. 2013;1:14–17.
8. Slavin KV. Peripheral nerve stimulation for neuropathic pain. *Neurotherapeutics*. 2008;5(1):100–106.
9. Slavin KV. Stimulation of the peripheral nervous system: the neuromodulation frontier. *Progress in Neurological Surgery*. Vol. 29. Karger; 2016.
10. Bittar RG, Teddy PJ. Peripheral neuromodulation for pain. *J Clin Neurosci*. 2009;16:1259–1261.
11. Gildenberg PL. General principles and selection of techniques in the management of pain of benign origin. In: Gildenberg PL, Tasker RR, eds. *Textbook of Stereotactic and Functional Neurosurgery*. New York, NY: McGraw-Hill; 1998:1321–1336.
12. Fishbain D, Goldberg M, Meagher BR, et al. Male and female chronic pain patients characterized by DSM-III psychiatric diagnostic criteria. *Pain*. 1986;26:181–197.
13. Campbell CM, Jamison RN, Edwards RR. Psychological screening/phenotyping as predictors for spinal cord stimulation. *Curr Pain Headache Rep*. 2013;17:307.
14. Tait RC, Pollard CA, Margolis RB, et al. The Pain Disability Index: psychometric and validity data. *Arch Phys Med Rehabil*. 1987;68:438–441.
15. Deer TR, Lamer TJ, Pope JE, et al. The Neurostimulation Appropriateness Consensus Committee (NACC) safety guidelines for the reduction of severe neurological injury. *Neuromodulation*. 2017;20:13–30. doi:10.1111/ner.12564.

16. Huntoon MA, Burgher AH. Ultrasound-guided permanent implantation of peripheral nerve stimulation (PNS) system for neuropathic pain of the extremities: original cases and outcomes. *Pain Med.* 2009;10(8):1369–1377. https://doi.org/10.1111/j.1526-4637.2009.00745.x.
17. Singh V, Sandhu D, Xiang N. Techniques for peripheral nerve stimulator implantation of the upper extremity. *Pain Med.* 2020;21(suppl 1):S27–S31. https://doi.org/10.1093/pm/pnaa185.
18. Mørch CD, Nguyen GP, Wacnik PW, Andersen OK. Mathematical model of nerve fiber activation during low back peripheral nerve field stimulation: analysis of electrode implant depth. *Neuromodulation.* 2014;17(3):218–225.
19. Kloimstein H, Likar R, Kern M, et al. Peripheral nerve field stimulation (PNFS) in chronic low back pain: a prospective multicenter study. *Neuromodulation.* 2014;17(2):180–187.
20. McRoberts WP, Wolkowitz R, Meyer DJ, et al. Peripheral nerve field stimulation for the management of localized chronic intractable back pain: results from a randomized controlled study. *Neuromodulation.* 2013;16(6):565–575.
21. Gilmore, C. A., Kapural, L., McGee, M. J., & Boggs, J. W. Percutaneous Peripheral Nerve Stimulation for Chronic Low Back Pain: Prospective Case Series With 1 Year of Sustained Relief Following Short-Term Implant. *Pain practice : the official journal of World Institute of Pain.* 2020; 20(3): 310–320.
22. Guentchev M, Preuss C, Rink R, Peter L, Wocker EL, Tuettenberg J. Technical note: treatment of sacroiliac joint pain with peripheral nerve stimulation. *Neuromodulation.* 2015;18(5):392–396.
23. Mironer YE, Hutcheson JK, Satterthwaite JR, LaTourette PC. Prospective, two-part study of the interaction between spinal cord stimulation and peripheral nerve field stimulation in patients with low back pain: development of a new spinal-peripheral neurostimulation method. *Neuromodulation.* 2011;14(2):151–155.
24. Slavin KV. Technical aspects of peripheral nerve stimulation: hardware and complications. *Prog Neurol Surg.* 2011;24:189–202.
25. Mobbs RJ, Nair S, Blum P. Peripheral nerve stimulation for the treatment of chronic pain. *J Clin Neurosci.* 2007;14:216–223.
26. Verrills P, Rose R, Mitchell B, et al. Peripheral nerve field stimulation for chronic headache: 60 cases and long-term follow-up. *Neuromodulation.* 2014;17:54–59.
27. Melvin EA Jr, Jordan FR, Weiner RL, et al. Using peripheral stimulation to reduce the pain of C2-mediated occipital headaches: a preliminary report. *Pain Physician.* 2007;10:453–460.
28. Falowski S, Wang D, Sabesan A, et al. Occipital nerve stimulator systems: review of complications and surgical techniques. *Neuromodulation.* 2010;13:121–125.
29. McRoberts WP, Wolkowitz R, Meyer DJ, et al. Peripheral nerve field stimulation for the management of localized chronic intractable back pain: results from a randomized controlled study. *Neuromodulation.* 2013;16:565–575.
30. Van Buyten JP, Hens C. Chronic stimulation of the gasserian ganglion in patients with trigeminal neuropathy: a case series. *J Neurosurg Rev.* 2011;1:73–77.
31. Young RF. Electrical stimulation of the trigeminal nerve root for the treatment of chronic facial pain. *J Neurosurg.* 1995;83(1):72–78.
32. Holsheimer J. Electrical stimulation of the trigeminal tract in chronic, intractable facial neuralgia. *Arch Physiol Biochem.* 2001;109(4):304–308.
33. Taub E, Munz M, Tasker RR. Chronic electrical stimulation of the gasserian ganglion for the relief of pain in a series of 34 patients. *J Neurosurg.* 1997;86(2):197–202.
34. Slavin KV, Colpan ME, Munawar N, et al. Trigeminal and occipital peripheral nerve stimulation for craniofacial pain: a single-institution experience and review of the literature. *Neurosurg Focus.* 2006;21(6):E5.
35. Carayannopoulos A, Beasley R, Sites B. Facilitation of percutaneous trial lead placement with ultrasound guidance for peripheral nerve stimulation trial of ilioinguinal neuralgia: a technical note. *Neuromodulation.* 2009;12(4):296–301.
36. Weiner RL, Reed KL. Peripheral neurostimulation for control of intractable occipital neuralgia. *Neuromodulation Technol Neural Interface.* 1999;2:217–221.
37. Saper JR, Dodick DW, Silberstein SD, McCarville S, Sun M, Goadsby PJ; ONSTIM Investigators. Occipital nerve stimulation for the treatment of intractable chronic migraine headache: ONSTIM feasibility study. *Cephalalgia.* 2011;31(3):271–285.

38. Silberstein SD, Dodick DW, Saper J, et al. Safety and efficacy of peripheral nerve stimulation of the occipital nerves for the management of chronic migraine: results from a randomised, multi-center, double blinded, control study. *Cephalalgia.* 2012;32(16):1165–1179.
39. Dodick DW, Silberstein SD, Reed KL, et al. Safety and efficacy of peripheral nerve stimulation of the occipital nerves for the management of chronic migraine: long-term results from a randomized, multicenter, double-blinded, controlled study. *Cephalalgia.* 2015;35(4):344–358.
40. Bouche B, Manfiotto M, Rigoard P, et al. Peripheral Nerve Stimulation of Brachial Plexus Nerve Roots and Supra-Scapular Nerve for Chronic Refractory Neuropathic Pain of the Upper Limb. *Neuromodulation.* 2017;20(7):684–689. doi:10.1111/ner.12573.
41. Wilson RD, Harris MA, Gunzler DD, Bennett ME, Chae J. Percutaneous peripheral nerve stimulation for chronic pain in subacromial impingement syndrome: a case series. *Neuromodulation.* 2014;17(8):771–776. doi:10.1111/ner.12152
42. Wilson RD, Gunzler DD, Bennett ME, Chae J. Peripheral nerve stimulation compared with usual care for pain relief of hemiplegic shoulder pain: a randomized controlled trial. *Am J Phys Med Rehabil.* 2014;93(1):17–28.
43. Kothari S, Goroszeniuk T. Percutaneous permanent electrode implantation to ulnar nerves for upper extremity chronic pain: 6-year follow up. *Reg Anesth Pain Med.* 2006;31(5 suppl):16.
44. Stevanato G, Devigili G, Eleopra R, et al. Chronic post-traumatic neuropathic pain of brachial plexus and upper limb: a new technique of peripheral nerve stimulation. *Neurosurg Rev.* 2014;37(3):473–480. doi:10.1007/s10143-014-0523-0
45. Deer TR, Levy RM, Rosenfeld EL. Prospective clinical study of a new implantable peripheral nerve stimulation device to treat chronic pain. *Clin J Pain.* 2010;26(5):359–372.
46. Ilfeld BM, Finneran JJ 4th, Gabriel RA, et al. Ultrasound-guided percutaneous peripheral nerve stimulation: neuromodulation of the suprascapular nerve and brachial plexus for postoperative analgesia following ambulatory rotator cuff repair. A proof-of-concept study. *Reg Anesth Pain Med.* 2019;44(3):310–318. doi:10.1136/rapm-2018-100121
47. Frederico TN, da Silva Freitas T. Peripheral nerve stimulation of the brachial plexus for chronic refractory CRPS pain of the upper limb: description of a new technique and case series. *Pain Med.* 2020;21(suppl 1):S18–S26. doi:10.1093/pm/pnaa201.
48. Johnson RD, Green AL, Aziz TZ. Implantation of an intercostal nerve stimulator for chronic abdominal pain. *Ann R Coll Surg Engl.* 2010;92(3):W1–W3. doi:10.1308/147870810X12659688851474
49. Miller-Jones CM, Phillips D, Pitchford EA, Smallpeice CJ. Transcutaneous nerve stimulation in post-thoracotomy pain relief. *Anaesthesia.* 1980;35(10):1018.
50. Solak O, Turna A, Pekcolaklar A, et al. Transcutaneous electric nerve stimulation for the treatment of postthoracotomy pain: a randomized prospective study. *Thorac Cardiovasc Surg.* 2007;55(3):182–185.
51. Erdogan M, Erdogan A, Erbil N, Karakaya HK, Demircan A. Prospective, randomized, placebo-controlled study of the effect of TENS on postthoracotomy pain and pulmonary function. *World J Surg.* 2005;29(12):1563–1570.
52. Oswald J, et al. Prospective case series on the use of peripheral nerve stimulation for focal mononeuropathy treatment. *Pain Manage.* 2019;9(6):551–558. doi:10.2217/pmt-2019-0028.
53. Abd-Elsayed A. Wireless peripheral nerve stimulation for treatment of peripheral neuralgias. *Neuromodulation.* 2020;23(6):827–830. doi:10.1111/ner.13131.
54. Goroszeniuk T, Khan R, Kothari S. Lumbar sympathetic chain neuromodulation with implanted electrodes for long-term pain relief in loin pain haematuria syndrome. *Neuromodulation.* 2009;12(4):284–291. doi:10.1111/j.1525-1403.2009.00237.x
55. Bouche B, Eisenberg E, Meignier M, et al. Facilitation of diagnostic and percutaneous trial lead placement with ultrasound guidance for peripheral nerve stimulation ilioinguinal neuralgia. Abstracts from the 10th World Congress of the International Neuromodulation Society. *Neuromodulation.* 2011;14:563.
56. Banh DP, Moujan PM, Haque Q, Han TH. Permanent implantation of peripheral nerve stimulator for combat injury-related ilioinguinal neuralgia. *Pain Physician.* 2013;16(6):E789–E791.
57. Shaw A, Sharma M, Zibly Z, Ikeda D, Deogaonkar M. Sandwich technique, peripheral nerve stimulation, peripheral field stimulation and hybrid stimulation for inguinal region and genital pain. *Br J Neurosurg.* 2016;30(6):631–636. doi:10.1080/02688697.2016.1199777

58. Elahi F, Reddy C, Ho D. Ultrasound guided peripheral nerve stimulation implant for management of intractable pain after inguinal herniorrhaphy. *Pain Physician.* 2015;18(1):E31–E38.
59. Stinson LW Jr, Roderer GT, Cross NE, Davis BE. Peripheral Subcutaneous Electrostimulation for Control of Intractable Post-operative Inguinal Pain: A Case Report Series. *Neuromodulation.* 2001;4(3):99–104. doi:10.1046/j.1525-1403.2001.00099.x
60. Peters KM, Killinger KA, Jaeger C, Chen C. Pilot study exploring chronic pudendal neuromodulation as a treatment option for pain associated with pudendal neuralgia. *Low Urin Tract Sympt.* 2015;7:138–142. doi:10.1111/luts.12066.
61. Carmel M., Lebel M., Tu LM. Pudendal nerve neuromodulation with neurophysiology guidance: a potential treatment option for refractory chronic pelvi-perineal pain. *Int Urogynecol J.* 2010;21:613–616. doi:10.1007/s00192-009-1054-z.
62. Peters KM, Killinger KA, Boguslawski BM, Boura JA. Chronic pudendal neuromodulation: expanding available treatment options for refractory urologic symptoms. *Neurourol Urodyn.* 2010;29:1267–1271. doi:10.1002/nau.20823.
63. Peters KM, Feber KM, Bennett RC. A prospective, single-blind, randomized crossover trial of sacral vs pudendal nerve stimulation for interstitial cystitis. *BJU Int.* 2007;100(4):835-839. doi:10.1111/j.1464-410X.2007.07082.x.
64. Langford B, Mauck WD. Peripheral nerve stimulation: a new treatment for meralgia paresthetica. *Pain Med.* 2020;326(8). doi:10.1093/pm/pnaa326.
65. Rauck RL, Cohen SP, Gilmore CA, et al. Treatment of post-amputation pain with peripheral nerve stimulation. *Neuromodulation.* 2014;17(2):188–197. doi:10.1111/ner.12102
66. Gilmore C, Ilfeld B, Rosenow J, et al. Percutaneous peripheral nerve stimulation for the treatment of chronic neuropathic postamputation pain: a multicenter, randomized, placebo-controlled trial. *Reg Anesth Pain Med.* 2019;44(6):637–645. doi:10.1136/rapm-2018-100109
67. Phan T, Murphy D, Lester D. Effects of percutaneous peripheral nerve stimulation on ambulation in an amputee with refractory pain. Presented at AAPM&R Conference; October 25–28, 2018; Orlando, FL.
68. McLean B. Identification of the infrapatellar branch of the saphenous nerve for treatment using a peripheral nerve stimulator: a technical report. *Cureus.* 2019;11(5):e4668. doi:10.7759/cureus.4668.
69. Ferreira-Dos-Santos G, Hurdle MFB, Gupta S, Clendenen SR. Ultrasound-Guided Percutaneous Peripheral Nerve Stimulation for the Treatment of Lower Extremity Pain: A Rare Case Report. *Pain Pract.* 2019;19(8):861-865. doi:10.1111/papr.12810
70. Kabay S, Kabay SC, Yucel M, Ozden H. Efficiency of posterior tibial nerve stimulation in category IIIB chronic prostatitis/chronic pelvic pain: a Sham-Controlled Comparative Study. *Urol Int.* 2009;83(1):33–38. doi:10.1159/000224865
71. Kim SW, Paick JS, Ku JH. Percutaneous posterior tibial nerve stimulation in patients with chronic pelvic pain: a preliminary study. *Urol Int.* 2007;78:58–62. doi:10.1159/000096936.
72. Istek A, Gungor Ugurlucan F, Yasa C, Gokyildiz S, Yalcin O. Randomized trial of long-term effects of percutaneous tibial nerve stimulation on chronic pelvic pain. *Arch Gynecol Obstet.* 2014;290:291–298. doi:10.1007/s00404-014-3190-z.
73. Gokyildiz S, Kizilkaya Beji N, Yalcin O, Istek A. Effects of percutaneous tibial nerve stimulation therapy on chronic pelvic pain. *Gynecol Obstet Invest.* 2012;73:99–105. doi:10.1159/000328447.
74. Klingler HC, Pycha A, Schmidbauer J, Marberger M. Use of peripheral neuromodulation of the S3 region for treatment of detrusor overactivity: a urodynamic-based study. *Urology.* 2000;56:766–771. doi:10.1016/S0090-4295(00)00727-5.
75. Zhao J, Bai J, Zhou Y, Qi G, Du L. Posterior tibial nerve stimulation twice a week in patients with interstitial cystitis. *Urology.* 2008;71:1080–1084. doi:10.1016/j.urology.2008.01.018.
76. Ragab MM, Tawfik AM, Abo El-enen M, et al. Evaluation of percutaneous tibial nerve stimulation for treatment of refractory painful bladder syndrome. *Urology.* 2015;86:707–711. doi:10.1016/j.urology.2015.06.041.
77. Langford B, Mauck WD. Advancement in neuromodulation technology with the innovation of design-specific peripheral nerve stimulators: sural nerve stimulation for radiculopathy. *Pain Med.* 2020;21(6):1297–1300. doi:10.1093/pm/pnaa077.

78. Petrovic Z, Goroszeniuk T, Kothari S. Percutaneous lumbar plexus stimulation in the treatment of intractable pain. *Reg Anesth Pain Med.* 2007;32(5 suppl 1):11.
79. Deer T, Pope J, Benyamin R, et al. Prospective, Multicenter, Randomized, Double-Blinded, Partial Crossover Study to Assess the Safety and Efficacy of the Novel Neuromodulation System in the Treatment of Patients With Chronic Pain of Peripheral Nerve Origin. *Neuromodulation.* 2016;19(1): 91–100. doi:10.1111/ner.12381
80. Fontaine D, Santucci S, Lanteri-Minet M. Managing cluster headache with sphenopalatine ganglion stimulation: a review. *J Pain Res.* 2018;11:375–381. Published 2018 Feb 16.
81. Ansarinia M, Rezai A, Tepper SJ, et al. Electrical stimulation of sphenopalatine ganglion for acute treatment of cluster headaches. *Headache.* 2010;50(7):1164–1174. doi:10.1111/j.1526-4610.2010.01661.x
82. Schoenen J, Jensen RH, Lantéri-Minet M, et al. Stimulation of the sphenopalatine ganglion (SPG) for cluster headache treatment. Pathway CH-1: a randomized, sham-controlled study. *Cephalalgia.* 2013;33(10):816–830. doi:10.1177/0333102412473667
83. Jürgens TP, Barloese M, May A, et al. Long-term effectiveness of sphenopalatine ganglion stimulation for cluster headache [published correction appears in Cephalalgia. 2016 Sep 1;:]. *Cephalalgia.* 2017;37(5):423–434. doi:10.1177/0333102416649092
84. Goadsby PJ, Sahai-Srivastava S, Kezirian EJ, et al. Safety and efficacy of sphenopalatine ganglion stimulation for chronic cluster headache: a double-blind, randomised controlled trial. *Lancet Neurol.* 2019;18(12):1081–1090. doi:10.1016/S1474-4422(19)30322-9
85. Tepper SJ, Rezai A, Narouze S, Steiner C, Mohajer P, Ansarinia M. Acute treatment of intractable migraine with sphenopalatine ganglion electrical stimulation. *Headache.* 2009;49:983–989.
86. Napadow V, Edwards RR, Cahalan CM, et al. Evoked pain analgesia in chronic pelvic pain patients using respiratory-gated auricular vagal afferent nerve stimulation. *Pain Med.* 2012;13(6): 777–789. doi:10.1111/j.1526-4637.2012.01385.x
87. Müller K, Fabó D, Entz L, et al. Outcome of vagus nerve stimulation for epilepsy in Budapest. *Epilepsia.* 2010;51(suppl S3):98–101.
88. Englot DJ, Chang EF, Auguste KI. Vagus nerve stimulation for epilepsy: a meta-analysis of efficacy, and predictors of response. *J Neurosurg.* 2011;115:1248–1255.
89. Rush AJ, George MS, Sackeim HA, et al. Vagus nerve stimulation (VNS) for treatment-resistant depressions: a multicenter study. *Biol Psychiatry.* 2000;47(4):276–286. doi:10.1016/s0006-3223(99)00304-2
90. Bajbouj M, Merkl A, Schlaepfer TE, et al. Two-year outcome of vagus nerve stimulation in treatment-resistant depression. *J Clin Psychopharmacol.* 2010;30(3):273-281. doi:10.1097/JCP.0b013e3181db8831
91. Ogbonnaya S, Kaliaperumal C. Vagal nerve stimulator: evolving trends. *J Nat Sci Biol Med.* 2013;4(1):8–13. doi:10.4103/0976-9668.107254.
92. Bodenlos JS, Kose S, Borckardt JJ, et al. Vagus nerve stimulation acutely alters food craving in adults with depression. *Appetite.* 2007;48(2):145–153. doi:10.1016/j.appet.2006.07.080
93. Glenn WW, Brouillette RT, Dentz B, et al. Fundamental considerations in pacing of the diaphragm for chronic ventilatory insufficiency: a multi-center study. *Pacing Clin Electrophysiol.* 1988;11(11 Pt 2): 2121–2127. doi:10.1111/j.1540-8159.1988.tb06360.x
94. Costanzo MR, Javaheri S, Ponikowski P, et al. Transvenous Phrenic Nerve Stimulation for Treatment of Central Sleep Apnea: Five-Year Safety and Efficacy Outcomes. *Nat Sci Sleep.* 2021;13:515–526. Published 2021 Apr 29. doi:10.2147/NSS.S300713
95. Ng MM, Sica DA, Frishman WH. Rheos: an implantable carotid sinus stimulation device for the nonpharmacologic treatment of resistant hypertension. *Cardiol Rev.* 2011;19(2):52–57. doi:10.1097/CRD.0b013e3181f87921
96. Scheffers IJ, Kroon AA, Schmidli J, et al. Novel baroreflex activation therapy in resistant hypertension: results of a European multi-center feasibility study. *J Am Coll Cardiol.* 2010;56(15):1254–1258. doi:10.1016/j.jacc.2010.03.089
97. Bisognano JD, Bakris G, Nadim MK, et al. Baroreflex activation therapy lowers blood pressure in patients with resistant hypertension: results from the double-blind, randomized, placebo-controlled rheos pivotal trial. *J Am Coll Cardiol.* 2011;58(7):765–773. doi:10.1016/j.jacc.2011.06.008
98. Zile MR, Lindenfeld J, Weaver FA, et al. Baroreflex Activation Therapy in Patients With Heart Failure With Reduced Ejection Fraction. *J Am Coll Cardiol.* 2020;76(1):1–13. doi:10.1016/j.jacc.2020.05.015

99. Van de Heyning PH, Badr MS, Baskin JZ, et al. Implanted upper airway stimulation device for obstructive sleep apnea. *Laryngoscope*. 2012;122:1626–1633.
100. Strollo PJ Jr, Soose RJ, Maurer JT, et al; STAR Trial Group. Upper-airway stimulation for obstructive sleep apnea. *N Engl J Med*. 2014;370:139–149.
101. Woodson BT, Gillespie MB, Soose RJ, et al; STAR Trial Investigators. Randomized controlled withdrawal study of upper airway stimulation on OSA: short- and long-term effect. *Otolaryngol Head Neck Surg*. 2014;151:880–887.
102. Rodenstein D, Rombaux P, Lengele B, Dury M, Mwenge GB. Residual effect of THN hypoglossal stimulation in obstructive sleep apnea: a disease-modifying therapy. *Am J Respir Crit Care Med*. 2013;187:1276–1278.
103. Noblett K, Siegel S, Mangel J, et al. Results of a prospective, multicenter study evaluating quality of life, safety, and efficacy of sacral neuromodulation at twelve months in subjects with symptoms of overactive bladder. *Neurourol Urodyn*. 2016; 35(2):246–251. doi:10.1002/nau.22707
104. Das AK, White MD, Longhurst PA. Sacral nerve stimulation for the management of voiding dysfunction. *Rev Urol*. 2000;2(1):43–60.
105. Hull T, Giese C, Wexner SD, et al. Long-term durability of sacral nerve stimulation therapy for chronic fecal incontinence. *Dis Colon Rectum*. 2013;56(2):234–245. doi:10.1097/DCR.0b013e318276b24c
106. Patton V, Wiklendt L, Arkwright JW, Lubowski DZ, Dinning PG. The effect of sacral nerve stimulation on distal colonic motility in patients with faecal incontinence. *Br J Surg*. 2013; 100(7):959–968. doi:10.1002/bjs.9114
107. Siegel S, Paszkiewicz E, Kirkpatrick C, Hinkel B, Oleson K. Sacral nerve stimulation in patients with chronic intractable pelvic pain. *J Urol*. 2001; 166(5):1742–1745.
108. Martellucci J, Naldini G, Carriero A. Sacral nerve modulation in the treatment of chronic pelvic pain. *Int J Colorectal Dis*. 2012;27(7):921–926. doi:10.1007/s00384-011-1394-2
109. Sokal P, Zielinski P, Harat M. Sacral roots stimulation in chronic pelvic pain. *Neurol Neurochir Pol*. 2015;49:307–312. doi:10.1016/j.pjnns.2015.07.003.
110. Al-Zahrani AA, Elzayat EA, Gajaweski JB. Long-term outcome and surgical interventions after sacral neuromodulation implant for lower urinary tract symptoms: 14-year experience at 1 centre. *J Urol*. 2011;185:981–986. doi:10.1016/j.juro.2010.10.054.
111. Gajewski JB, Al-Zahrani AA. The long-term efficacy of sacral neuromodulation in the management of intractable cases of bladder pain syndrome: 14 years of experience in one centre. *BJU Int*. 2011;107:1258–1264. doi:10.1111/j.1464-410X.2010.09697.x.
112. Ghazwani YQ, Elkelini MS, Hassouna MM. Efficacy of sacral neuromodulation in treatment of bladder pain syndrome: long-term follow-up. *Neurourol Urodyn*. 2011;30:1271–1275. doi:10.1002/nau.21037.
113. Goroszeniuk T, Khan R. Permanent percutaneous splanchnic nerve neuromodulation for management of pain due to chronic pancreatitis: a case report. *Neuromodulation*. 2011;14(3):253–257. doi:10.1111/j.1525-1403.2011.00347.x.
114. McRoberts P. Best Practices for Peripheral Nerve Stimulation. *ASRA Pain Medicine*. 2018. https://www.asra.com/news-publications/asra-updates/blog-landing/legacy-b-blog-posts/2018/12/02/best-practices-for-peripheral-nerve-stimulation
115. Cairns KD, McRoberts WP. Peripheral nerve stimulation for truncal pain. *Prog Neurol Surg*. 2011;24:58–69.
116. McRoberts WP, Cairns KD. Peripheral nerve and peripheral nerve field stimulation for the painful extremity. *Prog Neurol Surg*. 2011;24:156–170.
117. McRoberts WP, Deer TR, Abejon D, Barolat G. Stimulation of the extraspinal peripheral nervous system. In: Deer TR, Pope JE, eds. *Atlas of Implantable Therapies for Pain Management*. New York, NY: Springer Science; 2016:171–183.

21

Dorsal Root Ganglion Stimulation

Alyson M. Engle, Jonathan M. Hagedorn, and Timothy Ray Deer

Introduction

Neuromodulation is an established therapy for chronic, refractory neuropathic pain.[1] It was first made clinically available in 1967 as a salvage therapy for chronic pain states.[2,3] Analgesia is achieved by modulating pain pathways through the delivery of electrical current. Electrical current is supplied by electrodes located on thin wires, called electrode leads, which are positioned near the target. Early developments initially targeted stimulation of the dorsal column, later termed spinal cord stimulation (SCS). Therapeutic limitations of traditional SCS gave rise to advanced neurostimulation targeting focal pain generators in the dorsal root ganglion (DRG).

In 1949 the DRG was recognized as an important therapeutic target for selective neuromodulation,[4,5] and many chronic pain conditions are maintained in DRG where pathologic changes have occurred. This finding led to the development of pain interventions targeting pathologies in the DRG. Neurostimulation of the DRG was first explored in 1991 in animal models for the treatment of pain and inflammation.[6] However, it was only in 2016 that DRG neurostimulation devices received Food and Drug Administration (FDA) approval for treating intense focal pain of a defined area of the body.[7]

Similar to SCS, DRG neurostimulation uses an implantable pulse generator (IPG) and electrode leads that employ electrical field potentials to specific DRG targets.[4] The DRG device is implanted if the patient fails more conservative therapies due to ineffective pain relief or intolerable side effects. DRG neurostimulation allows physicians to provide personalized precision medicine by effectively delivering a drug-free therapy for extended periods of time at a specified target.

TABLE 21.1. DRG Stimulation: Indications and Levels of Evidence

CRPS* 1 and 2[9,13]	
▪ Lower extremity[†]	Level I, Grade A, Consensus Strong[†]
▪ Upper extremity[‡]	Level II, Grade A, Consensus Strong[‡]
Focal neuropathic pain secondary to peripheral nerve injuries or disease[9]	Level II, Grade A, Consensus Strong
Axial back pain[12,14]	No current consensus recommendations
Neuropathic groin pain[9,15]	Level II, Grade B, Consensus Strong
Pelvic pain[8]	Level III, Grade C, Consensus Moderate
Postherpetic neuralgia[16]	No current consensus recommendations
Chronic postoperative surgical pain[9,17] Postthoracotomy chest wall pain Postmastectomy chest wall pain	Level III, Grade C, Consensus Moderate
Postamputation pain[18]	Level III, Grade I, Consensus Moderate

*Complex regional pain syndrome (CRPS) types 1 and 2.

The opportunity to selectively neuromodulate DRG has several advantages over traditional SCS. DRG neurostimulation utilizes precise lead positioning near the affected DRG, has reduced contact size, and allows more flexibility in positioning, resulting in improved pain relief and fewer unwanted side effects.[8–11] In the ACCURATE study conducted by Deer and colleagues, there were higher treatment success rates in patients with CRPS or causalgia who were treated with DRG neurostimulation compared to SCS.[9] Huygen et al reported DRG stimulation at the L2–L3 levels relieved low back pain that could not be effectively treated with traditional SCS.[12] In addition, Hunter and colleagues demonstrated the efficacy of DRG stimulation in the treatment of chronic pelvic pain by targeting the L1/S2 DRGs.[8] Table 21.1 outlines the levels of evidence pertaining to each indication.

Patient Selection and Contraindications

To be considered for DRG stimulation, patients should be psychologically stable and without uncontrolled addiction. A history of sexual abuse is a relative contraindication to DRG stimulation for pelvic pain. There should also be a defined pathology related to the source of pain and identification of the mechanism of injury, such as surgical or trauma-related, and the specific nerve(s) affected. Medical comorbidities should be optimized before DRG stimulator placement, including, but not limited to, conditions that may poorly impact the procedural outcome. For example, patients with diabetes should have their hemoglobin A_{1c} checked and have acceptable blood sugar control before DRG stimulator placement to decrease their infection risk. Patients with immunosuppression also need to be optimized to decrease infection risk. Patients taking anticoagulants should be assessed to determine whether it is safe to hold the anticoagulant for placement of an epidural lead. Finally, there are limited data published on the safety of placing DRG leads above the C6 level.

Relative Contraindications

- Impaired wound-healing states (e.g., tobacco use, uncontrolled diabetes, immune incompetence)
- Uncontrolled comorbidities that may be exacerbated in the setting of DRG neurostimulation (e.g., cardiopulmonary disease)
- Inability of patient to understand and operate the device
- Spinal anatomic factors that limit safe lead placement

Absolute Contraindications

- Uncorrected coagulopathy
- Systemic infection or active infection at site of implantation
- Patient refusal or patient not able to provide informed consent (or medical power of attorney)
- Active psychosis
- Active substance abuse

Perioperative Management

Preoperative Planning

The target level(s) for implanting DRG stimulators are often the corresponding dermatomes where the pain is located. However, pain patterns may not always reflect the respective dermatomes if there is central sensitization or deafferentation, as is the case in many central pain states, such as phantom limb pain. The maximum number of leads that can be implanted per IPG is four. Table 21.2 provides a guide for target level selection in various pain states and the supportive evidence.

One of the primary concerns among implanters is the ability of the neuroforaminal space to accommodate the size of the electrodes without compromising the intraforaminal structures that house the DRG and nerve roots. Preoperative planning should include

TABLE 21.2. Selection of Dorsal Root Ganglion Level(s)

Pain location	Lead combinations	Recommended DRG	Clinically Relevant Evidence
Foot	L5/S1	S1	L5 ($N = 32$)[9] S1 ($N = 106$)[20]
Ankle	L4/L5/S1	L4	
Knee	L3/L4	L4	L4 ($N = 23$)[20] L3/L4 variations ($N = 12$)[21]
Groin	T12/L1/L2 T11/T12/L1 T11/T12	T11	L1, L2 ($N = 29$)[15] T12/L1 ($N = 8$ or 4 – confirm)[9] T11 ($N = 25$)[20]
Buttock	T12/L1/L2 > T12/S1	L2	L2 ($N = 12$)[20]
Back	T12/L1/2 > L5/S1	T12	T12 ($N = 28$)[20]
Pelvis	L1/S2	S2	S2 ($N = 6$)[20]

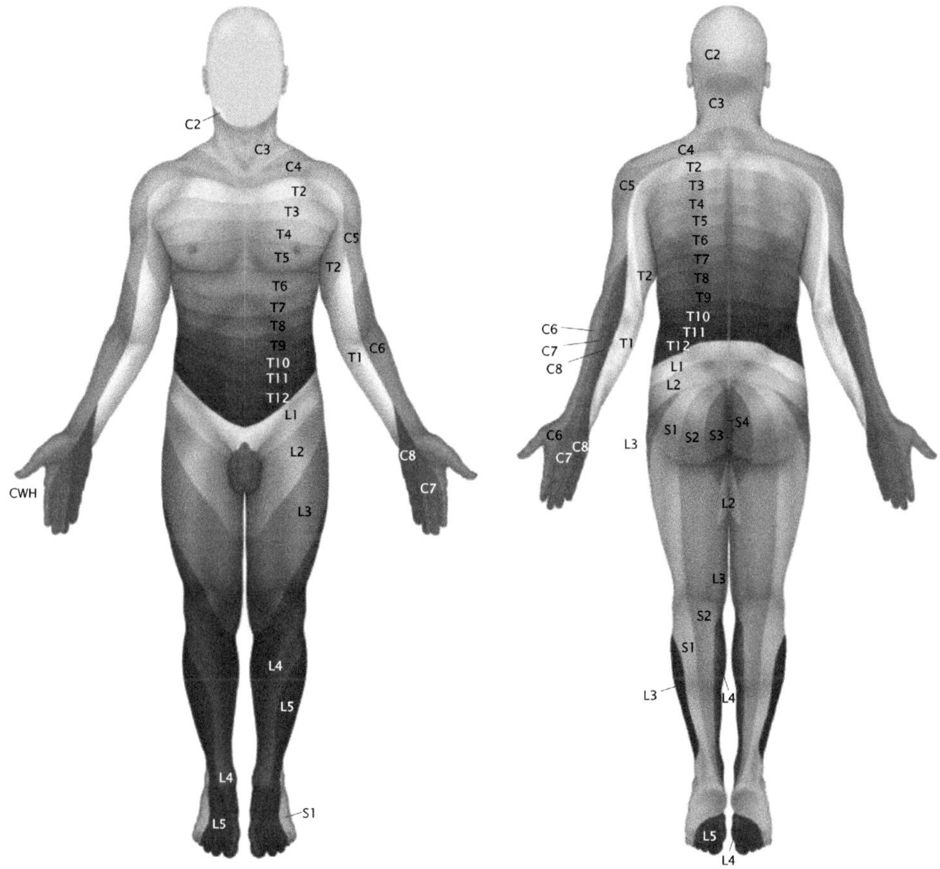

FIGURE 21.1. Dermatomal map. Source: Illustration by Corey Hunter, Figure 4 of NACC on Best Practices for DRG, 2018, *Neuromodulation*.[22]

imaging to screen for foraminal stenosis, lateral recess stenosis, and central canal stenosis to ensure DRG lead placement can be performed. Plain radiographs can aid in screening the neuroforamina. Parasagittal computed tomography (CT) scans can be used to detect foraminal stenosis due to bony encroachment. To assess for central and lateral spinal canal pathologies, magnetic resonance imaging (MRI) is needed. Parasagittal MRI allows visualization of the epidural fat, scar tissue, intervertebral disks, and vertebral abnormalities. The degree of foraminal narrowing may be assessed by a lack of perineural fat on T1-weighted sagittal images.[19] For patients with contraindications to MRI, CT myelography with 3D reconstruction is an alternative imaging modality.

Antibiotics

Infection of an implanted device is a serious complication, and prevention is the first step in management. Prevention begins with the evaluation of comorbidities and risk factors in the preoperative setting. Risk factors for infection include active smoking, insulin-dependent diabetes, obesity, chronic steroid use, autoimmune dysfunction, preexisting infection, poor hygiene, decubitus ulcers, incontinence, debilitated status, malnutrition, and extremely thin body habitus. Prior to DRG trial or implantation, the Neuromodulation Appropriateness Consensus Committee (NACC) guidelines recommend optimizing a patient's blood sugar, smoking cessation, and decolonization of any MSSA (methicillin-sensitive *Staphylococcus aureus*) or MRSA (methicillin-resistant *S. aureus*) carriers with mupirocin nasal ointment and chlorohexidine baths. Best practices also recommend preoperative utilization of weight-based antibiotics for both neurostimulation trials and implants. Nearly two-thirds of infections related to implanted devices are caused by *S. aureus* or coagulase-negative staphylococci.[23] The implanting physician should be familiar with the updated guidelines and best practice recommendations for reducing surgical site infections published in 2017 by the Centers for Disease Control and Prevention (CDC) and NACC.[24,25]

Anticoagulation

The provider should evaluate the patient's risk for a bleeding complication during the preoperative visit. Identification of coagulopathy begins with assessing the patient's comorbidities (e.g., liver dysfunction) and medications, such as anticoagulant and antiplatelet agents. For patients taking anticoagulants, the interventionist should be familiar with the most recent guidelines published by the American Society of Regional Anesthesia and Pain Medicine (ASRA) for interventional spine and pain procedures.[26,27]

Anesthesia

The patient is positioned prone on the operating room table with a pillow under the abdomen to flex the thoracolumbar spine and minimize lumbar lordosis. The procedure can be performed under various anesthetic techniques, including local anesthetic only, monitored anesthesia care (mild, moderate, or deep sedation), or general anesthesia. When general anesthesia is employed, neuromonitoring with somatosensory evoked potentials (SSEPs) and motor evoked potentials is recommended to detect nerve irritation early and to prevent permanent neurologic sequelae.

Intraoperative Neuromonitoring

Intraoperative neuromonitoring (IONM) can aid in detecting nerve irritation. SSEPs and motor evoked potentials are employed during neuromonitoring. The NACC recommendations on neurologic risk reduction state that it is critical to be able to detect neural injury during stimulator placement to reduce the risk of neurologic injury.[28] IONM is also helpful to confirm proper DRG lead positioning.[29]

Technique

Electrode leads can be placed surgically or percutaneously.[30] Both techniques require proper anatomic positioning of the lead(s) to achieve therapeutic efficacy and to avoid complications. The anatomic locations of the cathode can determine the dispersion of current in the depth and dispersion of electricity in the DRG nerve targets. Therefore, careful planning of placement of the contact leads in proximity to the DRG is essential, given the more lateral positioning in the lumbar spine and the more medial positioning in the thoracic spine.

Standard sterile technique is used in the surgical field. Chloraprep is the preferred sterile skin preparation with adequate dry time. The thoracolumbar spine is then draped with a full-body sterile drape. Fluoroscopic guidance with AP view is used to identify the appropriate landmarks for skin and epidural insertion. The target DRG and needle entry site are marked on the skin. Needle entry of the epidural space is desired at the midline of the interlaminar space. The length of lead required to extend from the target foraminal level to the implant site for the IPG is then determined. Next, subcutaneous injection of local anesthetic (7 to 10 mL of lidocaine 1% with 1:100,000 epinephrine) is performed. There is also an option to anesthetize the deeper needle entry tract with a 22-gauge spinal needle.

The inferior endplate of the vertebral level should be squared off using caudad or cephalad tilt. Tuohy needle enters the skin with the bevel facing toward the target level positioned either at the vertebral target level or one level below that target level. Insertion of a 14-gauge Tuohy needle is performed, with the needle advanced at an angle less than 45° under intermittent fluoroscopy. The Tuohy is advanced until it feels to be engaged in the ligamentum flavum, and confirmation of the location of needle is accomplished with fluoroscopy by visualizing the needle tip depth as it approaches the ventral interlaminar line in the contralateral oblique (CLO) view and/or the spinolaminar line in the lateral view. Most practitioners will try to touch the lamina and walk off the lamina to engage the ligamentum flavum. Loss-of-resistance technique is then employed to locate the epidural space.

Once loss of resistance is achieved and imaging confirms epidural needle location, the guidewire is inserted through the needle. If resistance is met, either confirm the needle is completely in the epidural space or remove the needle and re-enter with a more acute angle. It is important to note that extreme caution should be exercised when manipulating the guidewire or leads in the epidural space, to avoid dural tear or permanent nerve damage.

After confirmation of correct epidural placement. Inserting the sheath without the lead may increase the risk of dural puncture. Prevention includes confirming that the lead tip is slightly protruding from the end of the delivery sheath and the stylet is fully inserted in the lead. The lead is then inserted through the Tuohy needle and the lead stabilizer is tightened (clockwise screwing motion) until the lead does not slide within the sheath. The delivery sheath, with the lead and stylet in place, is inserted through the Tuohy and is advanced into the epidural space toward the target neuroforamen. When the distal end of the sheath is in or at the target neuroforamen, the lead stabilizer is loosened (counterclockwise screwing motion) and the lead is gently advanced into the dorsal neuroforamen. Ideal lead positioning is typically location of the second and third contacts in the superior part of the vertical interpedicular zone, over the DRG, along the thoracolumbar spine. Dorsal lead positioning is confirmed with the lateral view on fluoroscopic imaging (Figure 21.2). If IONM is being used, it may also be used to guide correct DRG positioning.[31]

Stimulation testing is employed after verifying that the electrodes extend beyond the sheath; otherwise, high impedance readings will prevent stimulation testing. To test the neurostimulator, connect the electrodes to the DRG stimulator's external pulse generator.

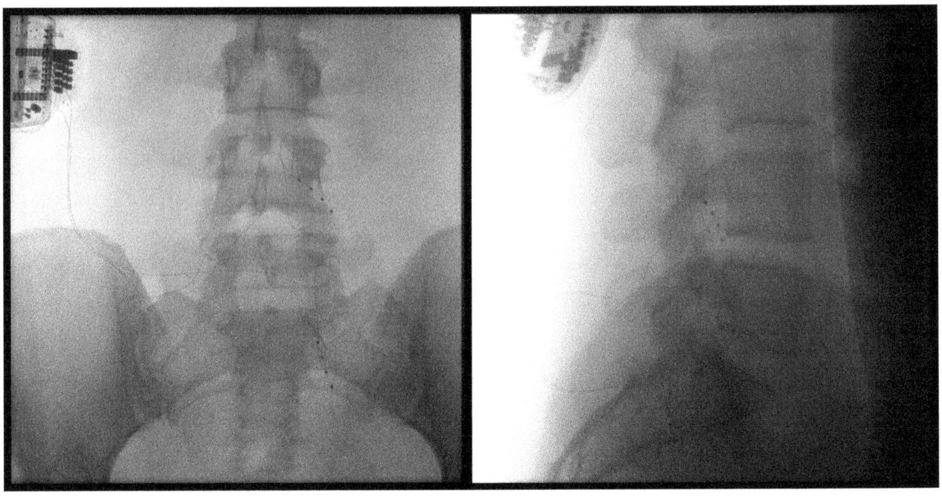

FIGURE 21.2. Right L4 and S1 dorsal root ganglion (DRG) lead placement on AP (left) and lateral (right) fluoroscopic views.

Next, strain-relief loops are formed by retracting the sheath to the needle bevel tip, followed by locking the lead in the sheath (Figure 21.3).[22] The lead is then advanced cephalad with the large curve of the sheath and the bevel of the needle both facing perpendicularly concave toward the surface of the skin until the lead makes an inflection in the cephalad direction. The lead is then unlocked from the sheath and advanced to create a cephalad loop. The formed loop should not be above the inferior endplate of the immediately adjacent cephalad vertebral body. The sheath is retracted back into the needle. The locked system is rotated to face the target DRG, while the needle bevel and curve are turned inferiorly and then are slightly advanced to create the apex of the inferior loop. The stylet is retracted about 12 to 15 cm, and the lead is advanced as the sheath is retracted into the needle, creating half of the inferior loop. The lead and sheath system is locked, rotated superiorly, and advanced toward the target DRG to compete the formation of the inferior strain-relief loop. The lead is then unlocked and retracted into the needle, maintaining the alignment.

After appropriate stimulation is ensured and the strain-relief loops are created, the needle and sheath are carefully removed. Under AP fluoroscopic view, the needle is moved into the sheath, and then the needle and sheath are removed together over the lead.

Next, the pocket skin incision is made, and blunt dissection is used to make an appropriately sized pocket for the IPG. The pocket can be made in the abdominal wall, the paravertebral region, or the gluteal cleft, per the patient's preference. The IPG should be placed below Scarpa's fascia.

A tunneling tool is used to the pass the leads from the spinal incision to the pocket. One should ensure that the tunneler is in the subcutaneous adipose tissue the entire time. The lead(s) are then threaded through the tunneler into the pocket. The tunneler is removed while maintaining a strain-relief loop in the lead to avoiding removing the lead(s) further from the epidural space. Next, the lead(s) are attached to the IPG, and the strain-relief loops are tucked behind the IPG. Both pockets must then be thoroughly irrigated with

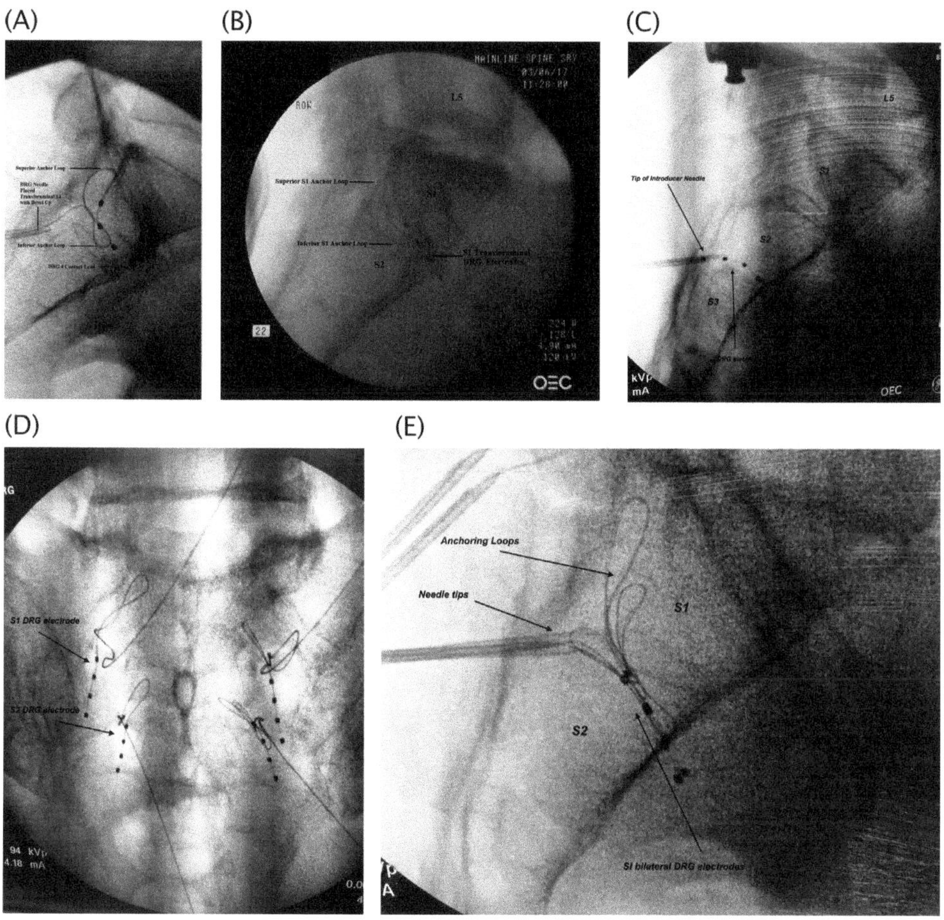

FIGURE 21.3. Dorsal root ganglion (DRG) lead placement in the sacral spine. A, S1 transforaminal placement of the needle during DRG lead placement. B, Lateral view of final DRG lead placement at S1 with superior and inferior anchoring loops. C, The lateral fluoroscopic image illustrates placement of a S2 DRG-stimulating electrode. The introducer needle has entered the S2 neuroforamen with the needle hub looking caudad. The electrode has been advanced into the neuroforamen, occupying its entire length, while the DRG introducer sheath is located at the very anterior aspect of the neuroforamen. D, This AP fluoroscopic image illustrates placement of bilateral S1 and S2 DRG electrodes. The neuroforamina are clearly visible, as well as multiple sacral anchoring loops for each DRG electrode. E, Lateral fluoroscopic image illustrating two anchored bilateral sacral (S1) DRG electrodes. The electrodes have been placed too far ventral and with both distal contacts outside the anterior S1 endplate. The sheaths have already been retracted and the needles are still in place. Sacral epidural anchoring loops can be identified for both sacral electrodes. This DRG stimulator electrode configuration represents a common suboptimal placement. The electrodes need to be further retracted dorsally, with all contacts in the neuroforamen or sacral canal.

Images obtained with permission from Deer et al, Figure 15 of NACC on Best Practices for DRG, 2018, *Neuromodulation*.[22]

warm normal saline with or without antibiotics. After hemostasis is confirmed, deep basal sutures are placed in both pockets using 3-0 Monocryl. Good hemostasis and fascial closure followed by subcuticular closure of each surgical incision and pocket are essential. Good skin approximation should be obtained for adequate healing. After skin closure, the wound should be covered with a sterile dressing. The patient should then be observed in the PACU.

Postoperative Management and Follow-up

Complications and Management

Overall, placement of neurostimulator devices is generally safe with proper technique and expertise, but it is not without risks of major and minor complications.[22,25,27,28,32] DRG neurostimulation complications can be categorized as procedural, equipment-related, and patient-specific complications. Prevention and management of complications should follow best practices and guidelines published by the CDC and the NACC.

Procedural Complications

General procedure-related complications include bleeding, infection, wound dehiscence, and neurologic injury. Complications specific to DRG neurostimulation implantation include cerebrospinal fluid (CSF) leakage, post-dural-puncture headache (PDPH), IPG malposition, implant pocket seroma, meningitis, epidural abscess, epidural hematoma, spinal cord injury, and death (see Box 21.1).

Bleeding

Bleeding into the epidural space is exceptionally rare with a DRG stimulator placement. More commonly, bleeding of the surrounding tissue can result from coagulopathy, ineffective intraoperative hemostasis, or trauma during epidural access. An epidural hematoma is a serious complication that requires prompt attention. Every interventional pain physician should be able to recognize the signs and symptoms of an acute epidural hematoma and appropriately manage the complication. An epidural hematoma can present with severe back pain, acute leg weakness or spasms, loss of distal extremity reflexes, or acute loss of bowel or bladder control. Any concern about an epidural hematoma is a neurosurgical emergency. The provider should immediately consult neurosurgery for evaluation and obtain imaging with MRI or non-contrast CT if MRI is unavailable or contraindicated.

Prevention of bleeding complications begins in the preoperative period. Identification of coagulopathy is based on comorbidities and use of anticoagulants, antiplatelet agents, nonsteroidal anti-inflammatory medications, and herbal supplements, such as garlic, ginseng, ginkgo, and turmeric. Patient-related factors that may increase the risk of bleeding include quantitative or qualitative platelet abnormalities, abnormalities in clotting factors, vitamin K deficiency, and hepatic synthesis dysfunction. Decisions about medications that affect clotting ability should follow the 2017 guidelines from NACC and ASRA for interventional spine and pain procedures in patients on antiplatelet and anticoagulant medications.[26,27]

Neurologic Injury

Neurologic injury is a rare but potentially devastating complication that can have serious permanent sequelae, including paralysis, hypesthesia, and incontinence. A large retrospective safety analysis ($N > 500$) reported that neurologic safety events accounted for 0.6%, lower than the reported 8% from the ACCURATE trial.[33,34] The adverse event rate of DRG neurostimulation is reported to be around 10.5%.[35] Neurologic injury can

BOX 21.1. Complications of DRG Neurostimulation Implantation

Procedural complications

- Bleeding
- CSF leakage
- Post-dural-puncture headache
- Seroma formation
- Neurologic injury
- Wound dehiscence
- Skin erosion
- Seroma
- Neuroma
- Infection
  - Superficial surgical site infection
  - Deep infection
  - Discitis
  - Epidural abscess
  - Meningitis

Equipment complications

- Catheter malfunction
  - Dislodgement
  - Malposition
  - Migration
  - Kinking
  - Fracture
- Device malfunction
  - Battery failure
  - IPG rotation

Patient-specific comorbidities

- Psychiatric comorbidities
- Cancer metastasis
- Smoking
- Uncontrolled diabetes
- Immunosuppression

result from direct needle trauma, infection, or bleeding that causes compression of nerve structures as well as decreased blood flow to the spinal cord, causing ischemia. Detection of neurologic injury during placement is critical for both patient safety and proper lead placement. Guidelines have suggested that placement of a lead in the spinal canal or at the DRG should be performed in the awake and conversant patient, or if performed in the anesthetized patient, IONM should be used during the surgical procedure.[28] IONM can reduce the risk of neurologic deficits by early detection of changes on electromyography (EMG) and in SSEPs.

CSF Leak

CSF leakage may result from intended dural puncture at the epidural entry site. The reported incidence of DRG neurostimulation procedure-related CSF leaks is around 2.7% for percutaneous lead placement.[33] During insertion, the electrode and guidewire are threaded through a large-bore Tuohy needle. Accidental dural puncture could occur during Tuohy needle insertion or electrode lead placement. If dural puncture occurs, CSF leak may cause symptoms, such as PDPH. PDPH is positional, with exacerbation of the headache in the upright position and alleviation in the supine position. Management of PDPH includes conservative therapy (e.g., hydration, abdominal binder, positioning, caffeine, sumatriptan, and theophylline). If conservative therapy fails to effectively manage the headache, then the next step is to perform an epidural blood patch with 15–20 cc of autologous blood at the puncture site. The epidural blood patch should be performed with aseptic technique under fluoroscopic guidance in order to avoid infection and damage to the neurostimulation device. Once the blood is injected and seals off the dural puncture, the symptoms should quickly resolve.

Prevention of CSF leaks includes consideration of preoperative risk factors and intraoperative meticulous technique. Steps to minimize the risk of dural puncture include choosing an appropriate path of entry, employing a shallow-angle technique, and utilizing the lateral view during loss of resistance.

Seroma Formation

Seroma develops when a pocket accumulates a collection of serosanguinous fluid, which could last a few days to a couple of months after stimulator implantation. Seroma formation is more common with poor surgical technique, including poor management of hemostasis and tissue trauma, but usually seroma is self-limiting, with no clinical consequence. Management includes observation and patient reassurance. Aspiration is avoided unless the fluid collection is excessive, persistent, and uncomfortable. Strict aseptic technique should be followed if aspiration is required. In some cases, postoperative abdominal binders may be used, but they should be used with caution so as not to cause local ischemia and wound breakdown.

Wound Dehiscence

Wound breakdown and dehiscence may result from poor suture technique, significant weight loss after implantation, improper IPG size-to-pocket ratio, improper IPG depth, and infection. Other factors are poor patient health (including uncontrolled diabetes), poor nutrition, chronic illness, obesity, high opioid intake, immunosuppression, smoking, direct compression (in a bed-bound or wheelchair-dependent patient), and untreated seroma or hematoma. Factors that may lead to wound breakdown should be considered in the preoperative evaluation in order to avoid dehiscence. For example, preexisting scars, ostomy sites, belt preference styles, and lifestyle concerns (e.g., wheelchair needs) should be considered when deciding on the surgical site, since such factors could lead to excessive pressure over the wound that causes dehiscence or device malposition.

Infection

Infection of an implanted device is a serious complication, with a reported incidence of 0.7% to 5.2%. Most infections present within the first 3 months after implantation.[36,37] The signs and symptoms of surgical site infection include pain at the surgical site, fever, chills, erythema, edema, fluctuant pocket, wound exudate, foul smell, induration at the incision or pump site, poor wound healing, and skin erosion. Most superficial infections do not require explantation of the device. In addition to assessing the superficial surgical site, the provider must rule out deeper infections, including epidural abscess and meningitis. Infection work-up includes a focused history and physical examination followed by the appropriate laboratory studies (e.g., white blood cell count, erythrocyte sedimentation rate, C-reactive protein) and aspiration of pocket fluid for cultures if relevant. If the provider is concerned about an epidural abscess, then an MRI or CT scan should also be ordered in addition to a neurosurgical evaluation. Deeper infections (e.g., epidural abscess and meningitis) require immediate explantation, hospital admission, and intravenous antibiotics based on culture sensitivities.[36] Postoperative discitis is a rare but serious complication that is often misdiagnosed. Early diagnosis and treatment are key to effective management, which begins with antibiotics, analgesics, bed rest, and, if needed, neurosurgical exploration with debridement of the disk space granulation tissue.[38]

Prevention of infection begins with evaluation and optimization in the preoperative setting, as discussed previously. Both trialing and implanting neurostimulation systems should adhere to the guidelines for reducing surgical site infections released by the CDC and NACC[24,25] (see Box 21.2).

Equipment-related Complications

Equipment-related complications include electrode lead or device malfunction. Complications requiring surgical revision have a reported annual incidence that ranges from 9.8% to 49.8%, with the majority being lead migration.[11,12,39] The implanter should be familiar with the NACC recommendations for mitigating complications and reducing these risks.

Electrode Lead-related Complications

Lead fracture or migration usually occurs in areas of high stress or due to lack of adequate strain-relief loops or lack of electrodes positioned through the ligaments.[36] Catheter migration, fracture, kink, occlusion, or dislodgement may present with increased pain, nerve irritation, CSF leak, or symptoms of spinal cord trauma. Imaging with plain radiography can aid in the detection of electrode migration or fractures. Based on clinical

BOX 21.2. Summary of Infection Management Practices from the NACC and CDC[24,25]

(CDC evidence rank, NACC consensus strength)

Perioperative measures

- Optimize glucose control before implantation of device (IB, strong)
- Discontinue tobacco use before implantation of device (IB, strong)
- Decolonize MSSA and MRSA carriers through the application of mupirocin nasal ointment and chlorohexidine baths (strong)
- Antibiotics
  - Prophylactic antibiotics for both trials and implants (IA, strong)
  - Weight-based antibiotic dosing is strongly recommended (IA, strong)
  - Use appropriate timing of prophylactic antimicrobial such that the bactericidal concentration is established in the serum and tissues at incision (IB, strong)
  - Vancomycin should not be used routinely (IB)
  - In clean and clean-contaminated procedures, do not administer additional prophylactic antimicrobial agent doses after the surgical incision is closed, even in the presence of a drain (IA, strong)
- If hair is removed, use electric clippers immediately before surgery (IA)
- Keep nails short and do not wear artificial nails for both trials and implants (IB, strong)
- Do not wear hand or arm jewelry for trials or implants (IB, strong)

Intraoperative measures

- Utilize chlorhexidine gluconate as preoperative skin antiseptic agent (IB, strong)
- Perform preoperative surgical scrub for a minimum of 2–5 min with an appropriate antiseptic prior to neuromodulation trials and implants (IB, strong)
- Limit operating room (OR) traffic (II, strong)
- Maintain positive pressure ventilation and HEPA filters in the OR for implants (IB, strong)
- Keep the OR doors closed during the procedure (IB, strong)
- Wear a surgical mask and fully cover hair for both trials and implants (IB, strong)
- Wear sterile gown and gloves for both trials and implants (IB, strong)
- Double glove (II, strong)
- If an incise drape is used, then iodophor-impregnated drape for implants is recommended (strong)
- Handle tissue gently, eradicate dead space, maintain hemostasis, and avoid electrocautery at tissue surface (IB)
- Irrigate with saline through bulb syringe prior to closure of surgical wound (strong)
- Employ implant strategies to limit operative time (strong)

Postoperative measures

- Apply an occlusive sterile dressing following trials and implants for 24 to 48 hours postoperatively (IB, strong)
- Do not routinely use topical antimicrobial agents for surgical wounds that are healing by primary intention (strong)
- If a dressing change is required, use hand washing (IB, strong) and sterile technique (II, moderate)
- Do not continue antimicrobial agents beyond 24 hours (strong)
- Understand maximum time criterion for defining a deep surgical site infection (SSI) of an implanted device: 1 year after implant (strong)
- Educate patient and family on proper incision care, signs of infection, and reporting symptoms (II, strong)
- When SSI is suspected, prescribe an antibiotic that covers the likely causative organisms, and consider local resistance patterns and culture results in choosing an antibiotic (strong)

Note: CDC Evidence rankings—IA, Strongly recommended for implementation and supported by well-designed experimental, clinical, or epidemiological studies. IB, Strongly recommended for implementation and supported by some experimental, clinical, or epidemiological studies and strong theoretical rationale. II, Suggested for implementation and supported by suggestive clinical or epidemiological studies or theoretical rationale.

presentation and imaging, the provider should be prepared to manage the complication or consult neurosurgery for management. Management may include a revision to replace leads that have been dislodged or fractured. Prevention includes placing the leads under direct fluoroscopic visualization, proper lead placement through the ligaments with contact points two and three under the medial and lateral pedicles, and creating sufficient strain-relief loops.

Equipment Malfunction

Mechanical device failure can occur in the setting of MRI, primarily with 90-cm leads, which are not MRI conditional yet. DRG neurostimulation systems with 50-cm leads are MRI conditional. If the IPG device fails, then replacement of the IPG is indicated. The only FDA-approved DRG neurostimulation system on the market as of 2020 was the Abbott Laboratories Proclaim IPG, which is a nonrechargeable primary-cell IPG (Proclaim DRG; Abbott Neurological, St. Jude Medical, Minneapolis, MN).[40] Battery failure occurs when the battery reaches the end of its life, necessitating battery replacement. Battery life depends on the number of leads placed and the programming needs of the patient.

Patient-specific Comorbidities

Underlying comorbidities that increase the risk for complications include psychosocial pathology (e.g., personality disorders, conversion disorder, poor coping mechanisms), uncorrected coagulopathy, anticoagulant medications, active infections, active smoking, diabetes, immunosuppression, and poor anatomy. Prevention is aimed at following the most recent guidelines and best practice recommendations released by the NACC (2018), CDC (2017), and ASRA (2018).[22,24,26]

Conclusion

DRG stimulation is a neuromodulation therapy for focal neuropathic pain syndromes. It is relatively safe when providers select the appropriate patient, plan preoperatively, and follow the guidelines and best practice recommendations released by the NACC (2018), CDC (2017), and the ASRA (2018).[22,24,26]

References

1. Taylor RS. Spinal cord stimulation in complex regional pain syndrome and refractory neuropathic back and leg pain/failed back surgery syndrome: results of a systematic review and meta-analysis. *J Pain Symptom Manage.* 2006;31(4 suppl):13–19. doi:10.1016/j.jpainsymman.2005.12.010.
2. Shealy CN, Mortimer JT RJ. Electrical inhibition of pain by stimulation of the dorsal columns: preliminary clinical report. *Anesth Analg.* 1967;46:489–491.
3. Slavin KV. Spinal stimulation for pain: future applications. *Neurotherapeutics.* 2014;11(3):535–542. doi:10.1007/s13311-014-0273-2.
4. Vuka I, Marciuš T, Došenović S, et al. Neuromodulation with electrical field stimulation of dorsal root ganglion in various pain syndromes: a systematic review with focus on participant selection. *J Pain Res.* 2019;12:803–830. doi:10.2147/JPR.S168814.
5. Soresi A. Control of "intractable pain" by spinal ganglia block. *Am J Surg.* 1949;77(1):72–78.
6. Bevan S, Yeats J. Protons activate a cation conductance in a sub-population of rat dorsal root ganglion neurones. *J Physiol.* 1991;433:145–161. https://dx.doi.org/10.1113%2Fjphysiol.1991.sp018419.
7. International Neuromodulation Society 12th World Congress Neuromodulation: Medicine Evolving Through Technology. Montreal, Canada. In: *Neuromodulation: Technology at the Neural Interface*; 2015:18:e107–e399. doi:10.1111/ner.12333.
8. Hunter CW, Yang A. Dorsal root ganglion stimulation for chronic pelvic pain: a case series and technical report on a novel lead configuration. *Neuromodulation.* 2019;22(1):87–95. doi:10.1111/ner.12801.
9. Deer TR, Levy RM, Kramer J, et al. Dorsal root ganglion stimulation yielded higher treatment success rate for complex regional pain syndrome and causalgia at 3 and 12 months: a randomized comparative trial. *Pain.* 2017;158(4):669–681. doi:10.1097/j.pain.0000000000000814.
10. Liem L, Russo M, Huygen FJPM, et al. A multicenter, prospective trial to assess the safety and performance of the spinal modulation dorsal root ganglion neurostimulator system in the treatment of chronic pain. *Neuromodulation.* 2013;16(5):471–482. doi:10.1111/ner.12072.
11. Liem L, Russo M, Huygen FJPM, et al. One-year outcomes of spinal cord stimulation of the dorsal root ganglion in the treatment of chronic neuropathic pain. *Neuromodulation.* 2015;18(1):41–49. doi:10.1111/ner.12228.
12. Huygen F, Liem L, Cusack W, Kramer J. Stimulation of the L2–L3 dorsal root ganglia induces effective pain relief in the low back. *Pain Pract.* 2018;18(2):205–213. doi:10.1111/papr.12591.
13. Van Buyten J, Smet I, Liem L, Russo M, Huygen F. Stimulation of dorsal root ganglia for the management of complex regional pain syndrome: a prospective case series. *Pain Pract.* 2015;15(3):208–216. https://doi.org/10.1111/papr.12170.
14. Huygen F, Kallewaard JW, Nijhuis H. Improved patient reported outcomes in chronic low back pain patients post-DRG stimulation. In: *North American Neuromodulation Society*. Las Vegas, NV; 2020.

15. Schu S, Gulve A, Eldabe S, et al. Spinal cord stimulation of the dorsal root ganglion for groin pain—a retrospective review. *Pain Pract.* 2015;15(4):293–299. doi:10.1111/papr.12194.
16. Yanamoto F, Murakawa K. The effects of temporary spinal cord stimulation (or spinal nerve root stimulation) on the management of early postherpetic neuralgia from one to six months of its onset. *Neuromodulation.* 2012;15(2):151–154. doi:doi:10.1111/j.1525-1403.2012.00438.x.
17. Bayman E, Brennan T. Incidence and severity of chronic pain at 3 and 6 months after thoracotomy: meta-analysis. *J Pain.* 2014;15:887–897.
18. Eldabe S, Burger K, Moser H, et al. Dorsal root ganglion (DRG) stimulation in the treatment of phantom limb pain (PLP). *Neuromodulation.* 2015;18(7):610–616. doi:10.1111/ner.12338.
19. Jenis LG, An HS. Lumbar foraminal stenosis. *Spine (Phila Pa 1976).* 2000;25(3):389–394. doi:10.1097/00007632-200002010-00022.
20. Morgalla MH, Fortunato M, Lepski G, Chander BS. Dorsal root ganglion stimulation (DRGS) for the treatment of chronic neuropathic pain: A single-center study with long-term prospective results in 62 cases. *Pain Physician.* 2018;21(4):E377–E387. doi:10.36076/ppj.2018.4.e377.
21. Hunter CW, Sayed D, Lubenow T, et al. DRG FOCUS: a multicenter study evaluating dorsal root ganglion stimulation and predictors for trial success. *Neuromodulation.* 2019;22(1):61–79. doi:10.1111/ner.12796.
22. Deer TR, Pope JE, Lamer TJ, et al. The Neuromodulation Appropriateness Consensus Committee on best practices for dorsal root ganglion stimulation. *Neuromodulation.* 2019;22(1):1–35. doi:10.1111/ner.12845.
23. Darouiche R. Treatment of infections associated with surgical implants. *N Engl J Med.* 2004;350:1422–1429.
24. Berriós-Torres SI, Umscheid CA, Bratzler DW, et al. Centers for Disease Control and Prevention guideline for the prevention of surgical site infection, 2017. *JAMA Surg.* 2017;152(8):784–791. doi:10.1001/jamasurg.2017.0904.
25. Deer TR, Provenzano DA, Hanes M, et al. The Neurostimulation Appropriateness Consensus Committee (NACC) recommendations for infection prevention and management. *Neuromodulation.* 2017;20(1):31–50. doi:10.1111/ner.12565.
26. Narouze S, Benzon HT, Provenzano D, et al. *Interventional Spine and Pain Procedures in Patients on Antiplatelet and Anticoagulant Medications.* 2nd ed. *Guidelines from the American Society of Regional Anesthesia and Pain Medicine, the European Society of Regional Anaesthesia and Pain Therapy,* Vol 43; 2018. doi:10.1097/AAP.0000000000000700.
27. Deer TR, Narouze S, Provenzano DA, et al. The Neurostimulation Appropriateness Consensus Committee (NACC) recommendations on bleeding and coagulation management in neurostimulation devices. *Neuromodulation.* 2017;20(1):51–62. doi:10.1111/ner.12542.
28. Deer TR, Lamer TJ, Pope JE, et al. The Neurostimulation Appropriateness Consensus Committee (NACC) safety guidelines for the reduction of severe neurological injury. *Neuromodulation.* 2017;20(1):15–30. doi:10.1111/ner.12564.
29. Falowski SM, Conti KR, Mogilner AY. Analysis of S1 DRG programming to determine location of the DRG and ideal anatomic positioning of the electrode. *Neuromodulation.* 2020;23(2):252–257. doi:10.1111/ner.13039.
30. Falowski S, Celii A, Sharan A. Spinal cord stimulation: an update. *Neurotherapeutics.* 2008;5(1):86–99. doi:10.1016/j.nurt.2007.10.066.
31. Falowski SM, Dianna A. A prospective analysis of neuromonitoring for confirmation of lead placement in dorsal root ganglion stimulation. *Oper Neurosurg.* 2018;14(6):654–659. doi:10.1093/ons/opx172.
32. Van Buyten JP. Neurostimulation for chronic neuropathic back pain in failed back surgery syndrome. *J Pain Symptom Manage.* 2006;31(4 suppl):25–29. doi:10.1016/j.jpainsymman.2005.12.012.
33. Deer T, Pope J, Hunter C, et al. Safety analysis of dorsal root ganglion stimulation in the treatment of chronic pain. *Neuromodulation.* 2019;. doi:10.1111/ner.12941.
34. Deer TR, Levy RM, Kramer J, et al. Dorsal root ganglion stimulation yielded higher treatment success rate for complex regional pain syndrome and causalgia at 3 and 12 months: a randomized comparative trial. 2017;0(0).

35. Deer TR, Levy RM, Kramer J, et al. Dorsal root ganglion stimulation yielded higher treatment success rate for complex regional pain syndrome and causalgia at 3 and 12 months: a randomized comparative trial. *Pain*. 2017;158(4):669–681. doi:10.1097/j.pain.0000000000000814.
36. Malinowski MN, Bremer N, Kim CH, Deer TR. *Intrathecal Drug Delivery: Indications, Risks, and Complications*. (Khelemsky Y., Malhotra A. GK, ed.). Springer; 2019. doi:10.1007/978-3-030-18005-8.
37. Flückiger B, Knecht H, Grossmann S, Felleiter P. Device-related complications of long-term intrathecal drug therapy via implanted pumps. *Spinal Cord*. 2008;46(9):639–643. doi:10.1038/sc.2008.24.
38. Luzzati R, Giacomazzi D, Danzi M, Tacconi L, Concia ESV. Diagnosis, management and outcome of clinically suspected spinal infection. *J Infect*. 2009;58(4):259–265.
39. Sivanesan E, Bicket MC, Cohen SP. Retrospective analysis of complications associated with dorsal root ganglion stimulation for pain relief in the FDA MAUDE database. *Reg Anesth Pain Med*. 2019;44(1): 100–106. doi:10.1136/rapm-2018-000007.
40. Abbott, St. Jude Medical. *Proclaim™ DRG Implantable Pulse Generator. Clinician's Manual*. Plano, TX: St. Jude Medical.

22

Intrathecal Drug Delivery

Jacqueline Weisbein and Priyanka Ghosh

Introduction

The first continuous spinal anesthetic was described in 1940 by Dr. William Leonard, who administered procaine with a control syringe attached to a malleable needle placed surgically in the lumbar spine. Since then, intrathecal drug delivery systems (IDDS) have become significantly streamlined and advanced, and they now consist of an intrathecal catheter placed percutaneously and tunneled to a small implanted pump, to deliver continuous medication to the intrathecal space. IDDS have been approved by the Food and Drug Administration (FDA) for chronic use in patients with moderate to severe pain from cancer or noncancer causes since the 1980s, with fixed continuous infusion rate pumps.[1]

Indications

Disease-specific indications for intrathecal pumps include both cancer and noncancer causes. Nine million people suffer from cancer-related pain each year, and 50% of cancer pain patients report inadequate pain relief, with 20% to 30% of cancer pain patients being refractory to opioid therapy and 25% of cancer pain patients dying with pain.[2] Since 2000, the Polyanalgesic Consensus Conference (PACC) has developed and updated guidelines for intrathecal drug therapy. The PACC guidelines strongly recommend, with a grade A recommendation, intrathecal therapy with ziconotide or opiates, in patients with cancer.[3] Cancer patients with either a single or multiple pain etiologies benefit from intrathecal therapy, especially patients with high tumor burden, chronic postsurgical pain, and diffuse metastatic disease. In a paradigm shift, intrathecal therapy is increasingly considered earlier in a patient's oncologic pain treatment due to studies signaling favorable analgesic and side-effect profiles.[4] Current literature increasingly includes multiple studies supporting IDDS in cancer-related pain due to the analgesic efficacy, therapy safety, healthcare savings, and opioid reduction that IDDS provide patients with cancer pain.

The FDA approval for IDDS includes moderate to severe trunk and limb pain, as well as intractable pain where more conservative therapies have failed. In the past, IDDS therapy for non-cancer-related pain was viewed as salvage therapy after failure of conservative therapies and even after the utilization of neuromodulation, but updated evidence now calls for consideration of IDDS therapy before administration of a course of high-dose systemic opiates, given the known dangers of high-dose opiates. There are many disease states for which there is strong evidence supporting the use of IDDS. The most commonly studied diseases include many spinal pathologies, such as multiple compression fractures, discogenic pain, diffuse multilevel spondylosis, failed back surgery syndrome (FBSS), and lumbar radicular pain.[11] Complex regional pain syndrome (CRPS), abdominal pain, trunk pain (including postherpetic neuralgia and postthoracotomy pain), severe osteoarthritis, rheumatoid arthritis, connective tissue disorders and other pain syndromes amenable to opiate therapy but complicated with intolerable side effects are also well-studied indications for utilization of IDDS.

Evidence

The work of Melzack and Wall showed that the spinal cord modulates and regulates painful stimuli.[5] By 1976, Yaksh et al had found that opioid analgesics administered into the spinal subarachnoid space of a rat were able to block spinal reflexes as well as the response to painful stimuli. When opioids bind to the receptors in the dorsal horn of the spinal cord, there is a reduction in substance P and glutamate, leading to a reduced amount of transmission of painful stimuli.[6]

In 1979, Josef Wang published data supporting the use of intrathecal morphine in 8 patients with intractable pain from infiltrating genitourinary cancers.[7] While much of the initial work with intrathecal pumps focused on pain management for malignant pain, eventually, in 1985, Auld et al published data supporting the use of intrathecal opiates for patients with nonmalignant pain, indicating that 65% of the 43 patients studied had relief over 2 years.[8]

Types of Intrathecal Pumps

Intrathecal pumps are approved by the FDA for chronic use in patients with moderate to severe pain from cancer or noncancer causes. Currently, two pumps are used: the Synchromed II from Medtronic and the Prometra II from Flowonix. (Internationally, there are still continuous-use pumps on the market.) While the Synchromed II is a peristaltic pump, the Prometra II is a voltage-gated pump. Both can be programmed to deliver specific doses based on the physician's or an assistant's direction. Both devices are MRI compatible;

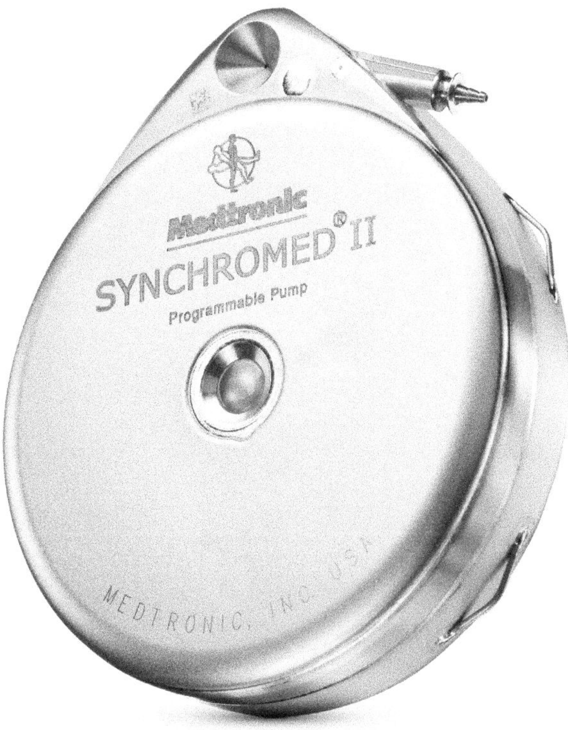

FIGURE 22.1. The Synchromed II pump by Medtronic uses peristaltic action to deliver drug from the reservoir through the catheter to the patient.
Image courtesy of Medtronic.

however, the Prometra II must be emptied of all medication prior to MRI evaluation and then refilled after the MRI. The process of accessing both pumps is done using a noncoring Huber needle to prevent infiltration of the pump with tissue or other skin cells. The intervals of refill can vary, depending on the practice, types of medications being used, and the concentration of the medication, but according to the FDA, refill should be done within 6 months.

Types of Medications

Currently, three medications are FDA-approved and labeled for intrathecal pump administration: morphine (Mitigo or Infumorph), ziconotide (Prialt), and baclofen (Lioresal or Gablofen). These medications are indicated for monotherapy administration through the pump. However, several medications are used off label, including, but not limited to, compounded dilaudid, fentanyl, bupivacaine, clonidine, and sufentanil. Thus, although only three medications have been FDA approved for monotherapy, many physicians opt to compound medications in order to administer combination therapy.

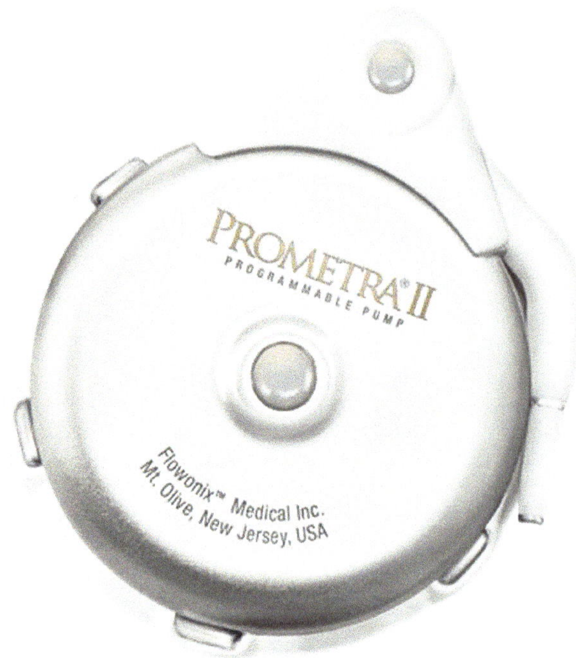

FIGURE 22.2. The Prometra II is a voltage-gated pump made by Flowonix. Image courtesy of Flowonix.

Patient Selection and Contraindications

Appropriate patient selection for intrathecal therapy is complex and requires the assessment of disease- and patient-specific factors to determine who will best benefit from the procedure. Selecting a patient for intrathecal therapy is a multistep process that includes initial evaluation of the patient's medical history and pain treatment history, the decision to treat an appropriate pain problem, psychological evaluation, and assessment of any absolute and relative contraindications.[9–11]

Cancer pain is one of the major indications for intrathecal therapy. In addition, there are many non-cancer-pain syndromes that can benefit from intrathecal therapy, including, but not limited to, FBSS, spinal or foraminal stenosis, diabetic peripheral neuropathy, CRPS, phantom limb pain, severe arthritis, and connective tissue disorders. Box 22.1 lists disease-specific indications for intrathecal drug delivery. The patient must also meet other, strict inclusion criteria, listed in Box 22.2, before intrathecal therapy is considered appropriate.[12]

Contraindications to implantation of IDDS include, but are not limited to, the presence of local or systemic infection, inability to implant the pump 2.5 cm (1 in) or less from the surface of the skin, insufficient body mass to accept pump bulk and weight, or spinal anomalies that complicate placement of the catheter.

Once it is determined that a patient may be a candidate for an intrathecal pump, a trial should be performed. There are various ways of performing a trial, but the two most common are a single-shot trial and the catheter trial. Both should be done using normal sterile technique. The advantage of a single-shot trial is that a small Quincke needle (25

BOX 22.1. Indications for Intrathecal Pumps

Primary or metastatic tumors causing pain from tissue invasion
Neuropathy or nerve irritation from chemotherapy or radiation therapy
Failed back surgery syndrome (FBSS)
Spinal canal or foraminal stenosis causing neuropathy
Complex regional pain syndrome (CRPS)
Severe arthritis including osteoarthritis and rheumatoid arthritis
Peripheral neuropathy refractory to conservative treatments

or 22 gauge) can be used to access the intrathecal space and a bolus of medication can be administered after barbotage with cerebrospinal fluid (CSF). The small gauge of the needle used decreases the risk of a post-dural-puncture headache (PDPH). However, many insurance carriers still require a catheter trial.

A catheter trial involves placement of a modified Tuohy needle to get intrathecal access. Then a catheter is advanced through the needle into the intrathecal space, after which a bolus or continuous flow of medication can be administered. While a continuous infusion trial may be similar to a continuous intrathecal flow of medication, an outpatient system to adequately support this type of trial can be difficult to find, depending on the location of practice.

It is typically recommended to trial with the medication intended to be utilized in administration of the pump. Thus, if any side effects of the medication are noted, changes can be made. Regardless of the type of trial, it is imperative to advise patients on the risks of respiratory depression, nausea, vomiting, itching, urinary retention, and altered mentation. If the patient is opiate naïve, it is recommended to use the lowest dose, as indicated in the PACC guidelines.

BOX 22.2. Patient Selection Criteria

More conservative treatment options have failed, or other options are unacceptable or not indicated.

Oral or transdermal medications produce unacceptable side effects or an unacceptable level of relief.

The patient's spinal anatomy will allow for the placement of a spinal catheter.

The patient is medically stable, with no untreated bleeding disorders, infectious processes or disorders that would preclude implantation of intrathecal catheter and a surgical foreign body.

The patient is mentally stable, with no untreated severe depression or anxiety disorders. No diagnosed significant personality disorders.

The region of pain can be covered by the anatomic congruent placement of an intrathecal catheter.

Perioperative Management

As for any surgical procedure, assessment of the patient's health prior to the procedure is imperative. Typical labs ordered include a complete blood count, comprehensive metabolic panel, prothrombin time, and INR, as well as urinalysis with reflex culture if indicated. Depending on the health of the patient, an electrocardiogram may also be required.

Perioperative antibiotics should be administered per the facility's guidelines. Currently, the standard of care for those undergoing surgical implants is administration of 2 g of cefazolin (Ancef) perioperatively unless there is a known allergy to penicillin. A test dose of antibiotic can be given if there is concern, or 1 g of vancomycin can be administered instead. Unless there is concern about a patient who might be immunocompromised from an underlying condition or cancer, postoperative antibiotics are not indicated.

Anticoagulant therapy is common in many patients who may be good candidates for intrathecal pump implantation. The elevated risk of bleeding with patients on anticoagulants can be especially dangerous in an intrathecal procedure because it can lead to spinal or epidural hematoma. Guidelines have been carefully crafted from the literature and each anticoagulant has specific recommendations, which are similar in both the PACC guidelines and the American Society of Regional Anesthesia and Pain Medicine (ASRA) guidelines.

Anesthetic technique for intrathecal pump placement is usually determined by conversation between the surgeon and anesthesiologist. Generally, monitored sedation (MAC) is the chosen technique because it allows patient comfort while also allowing easy, direct patient communication. If MAC is not suitable for the patient, then general anesthesia is acceptable, with consideration of an intermittent wake-up test to assess neurological irritation, particularly if needle insertion is at the conus or above. Many surgeons place the catheter with the patient under MAC and responsive, to determine if any paresthesias have developed. Neuromonitoring is another option for patients who are heavily sedated or under general anesthesia, to reduce the risk of nerve injury or irritation.

Technique

Currently, both the Prometra II and Synchromed II pumps are indicated for placement of the reservoir in the abdomen. The procedure is described here.

1. Mark the intended pump implantation site, usually an abdominal site, while the patient is awake and standing or sitting. Ensure that the pump site is away from bony prominences, especially the iliac crest and ribs, and ensure that there is sufficient, but not excess, subcutaneous fat for comfortable pump implantation, so that it still allows pump access. Marking while the patient is standing or sitting up ensures that the pump will not lie below the belt line or in a layer of pannus that might fold when a patient moves. Then proceed with positioning the patient in the lateral decubitus position, with the site of the pump placement up (i.e., if the pump is to be implanted in the right lower quadrant, the patient should be placed in the left lateral decubitus position; Figures 22.3 and 22.4).

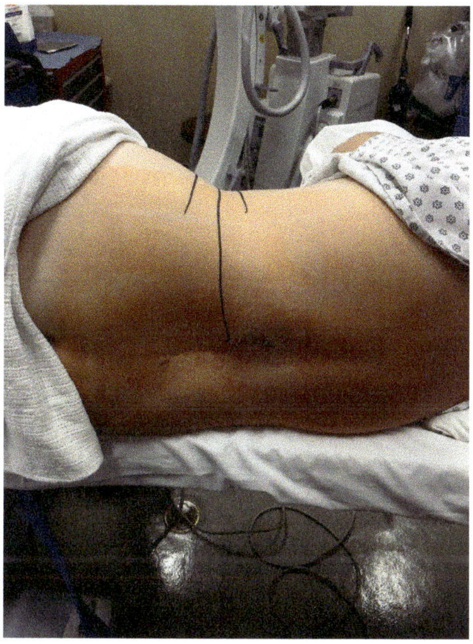

FIGURE 22.3. Patient lying in the right lateral decubitus position for placement of the pump. Image courtesy of J. Weisbein, DO.

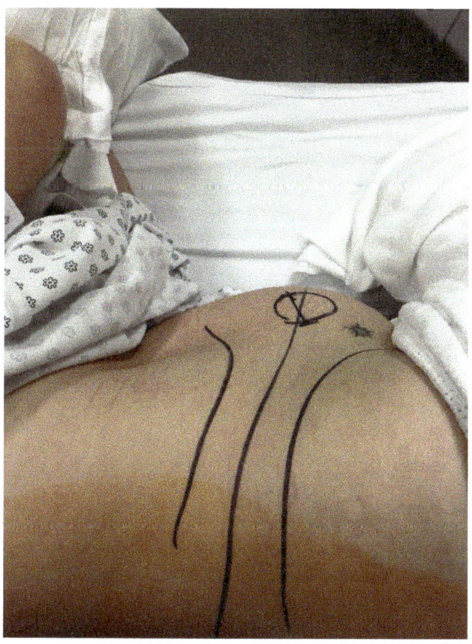

FIGURE 22.4. The patient's abdomen with markings for the costal margin and the ilium. Image courtesy of J. Weisbein, DO.

   a. Note: If an abdominal site is not possible, a smaller 20-mL pump may be placed in the superior gluteal region; however, this is not the FDA-approved location for either device.
2. Once the patient is positioned in the lateral decubitus position, obtain views of the lumbar spine in a lateral cross-table trajectory for an AP image. It is important to include radiographic views of the intended skin and interlaminar insertion site, as well as the site for the final intrathecal catheter tip, in these initial images.
3. After determining the starting position, administer local anesthesia in the skin and subcutaneous tissue to anesthetize the site. At this point, you can make an incision and dissect it down to the lumbodorsal fascia prior to placement of the modified Tuohy spinal needle or just insert the spinal introducer needle with stylet. For the purposes of this text, the space is accessed first and then the incision is made.
4. After adequate local anesthesia, insert the introducer needle using a shallow angle (approximately 30° to 45°) and use a paramedian approach to contact the lamina of the vertebral body caudal to the target interlaminar space. The needle is then drawn back and "walked-off" cephalad, using the loss-of-resistance technique, into the epidural space. Once in the epidural space, utilize the lateral fluoroscopic view to monitor needle depth as it is advanced into the intrathecal space.
   a. Note: Generally, the L2 to L4 interlaminar spaces are utilized as entry points.
5. Once you are at the intended interlaminar level and have proceeded with dural puncture, confirm the free flow of CSF. If there is not free flow, rotate the needle to assess for flow; if there is still no CSF flow, then slightly advance the needle. Once you get CSF flow, immediately replace the stylet to stop excess CSF flow, which could cause PDPH.
   a. Caution: It is important that the patient be able to verbally communicate with you during this part of the procedure, to avoid any inadvertent nerve damage.
6. Turn the bevel of the needle cephalad and carefully withdraw the inner stylet and insert the catheter. Ensure that the catheter guidewire is fully in the catheter, which is important for insertion and positioning of the catheter. Advance the catheter, under live fluoroscopic guidance, until the radiopaque tip is seen at the target level. Note: The catheter tip should generally terminate at the spinal cord level matching the dermatomal level of pain (i.e., for low back pain, between T8 and T10).
7. Once the catheter tip is at its desired level, withdraw the spinal needle slightly, but continue to protect the full intrathecal catheter. Make an incision parallel to the axis of the spine, over the spinous processes, extending from the needle's entry point approximately 5 to 8 cm.
8. After the incision has been made, dissect down to the lumbodorsal fascia. Be sure to debride all the fatty tissue from the area surrounding the needle, making sure of clean exposure of the fascia and ligament. Then fully remove the spinal needle and catheter stylet. Reconfirm CSF flow.
9. Attach the anchoring device with sutures. Again, reconfirm CSF flow to make sure the catheter remains intrathecal. Once the catheter is anchored, leave a strain-relief loop in the catheter before it is tunneled to the pocket (Figure 22.5).

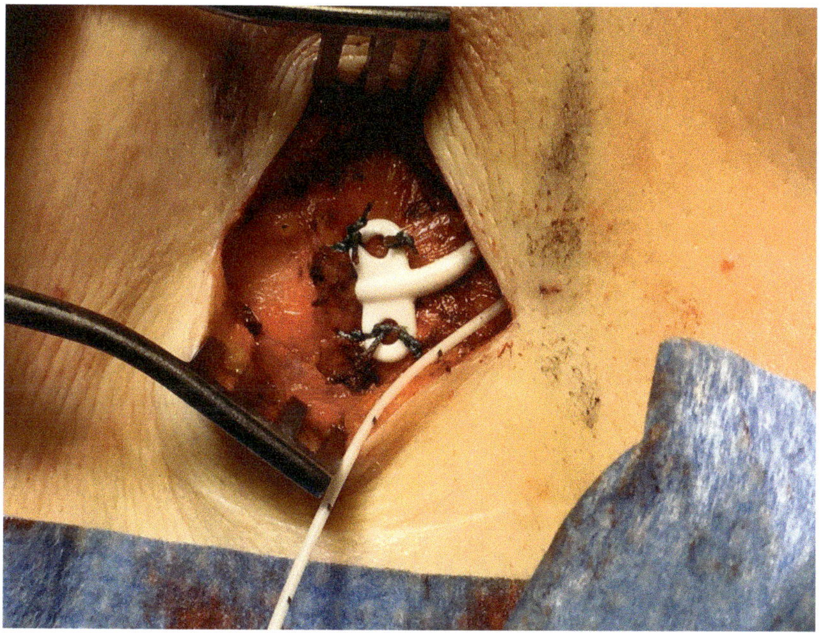

FIGURE 22.5. This is the Medtronic V-winged anchor sutured to the lumbodorsal fascia. Note that the entry of the anchor is diving into the fascial layer and the sutures are situated to allow the anchor to lie flat in the tissue.

Image courtesy of J. Weisbein, DO.

10. After confirming the catheter is intrathecal and is securely anchored, ensure that the patient has no adverse effects from the procedure thus far. At this point, optional sedation can be given for the pocket creation.
11. As stated above, proceed to the site marked on the abdomen in Step 1 for pocket creation. Utilize a generous amount of local anesthesia to anesthetize the skin over this area.
12. After the skin is anesthetized, use a No. 11 or No. 15 blade to make an incision 1 to 3 cm deep. Using this depth for pocket creation, continue to dissect with blunt dissection or sharp surgical instruments to create a pocket slightly larger than the total volume of the pump (typically the width of the fingers on the hand from the palmar insertion). Once the pocket has been created, test the pocket to ensure that the pump fits properly.
13. After confirming pocket fit and that the catheter has appropriate CSF flow and is appropriately secured, utilize the supplied tunneling device and tunnel the catheter from the spinal incision to the pocket created. During tunneling rod advancement, you should be able to palpate the tunneling rod through its entire passage; this avoids tunneling at depths that damage tissue or organs.
14. Once the catheter is tunneled to the pump site and CSF flow is reconfirmed, attach the catheter to the pump and place the pump in the pocket, then suture the pump in place. Take another film to assess the catheter's course once it is attached to the pump system.
15. After ensuring adequate hemostasis, irrigate all wounds with antibiotic solution and perform a 3-level closure at all incision sites.

Postoperative Management

Postoperatively, after the patient has woken up from anesthesia, a neurologic exam should be performed if any new symptoms or complaints occur. Patients should also be counseled about the immediate postoperative complications, so they are able to monitor for any signs and symptoms. Immediate postprocedure complications include, but are not limited to, bleeding, infection, CSF leakage, seroma formation, broken or damaged catheters, and issues with the subcutaneous pockets.

An abdominal binder may be placed perioperatively to assist patients with comfort and placement of ice. While varying thoughts on when to start therapy exist, many would agree that an opiate holiday prior to placement of the device is imperative to assist in keeping the patient at lower levels of systemic medication. The addition of some oral medication in the immediate postoperative period may be indicated to assist in pain management.

Complications and Management

Patients and physicians should vigilantly monitor the pump site for any postoperative complications, including, but not limited to, infection, wound dehiscence, seroma, or pump flipping. Also, there can be catheter threading that disrupts the spinal cord or the conus medullaris and causes new painful radiculopathy, a CSF leak can cause PDPH, and other, more serious complications, such as epidural abscess or meningeal infection, are possible postoperatively.

In the case of wound dehiscence, if there is visible hardware, explant of the system, because it is potentially infected and this is the safest course of action. Additionally, if there is significant indication of infection, the pump and catheter should both be removed to prevent further systemic infection. If the dehiscence appears superficial, wound care can be done with conservative techniques like Steri-Strips, Manuka honey, or specialized wound-healing bandages.

If there is concern about inadequate analgesia, a catheter evaluation and dye study can be performed to determine if there are any leaks or filling defects. If any defects are noted, a catheter revision is indicated.

If a patient develops neurologic findings after the use of IDDS, there should be work-up for development of a granuloma. A granuloma typically occurs at the tip of the catheter, creating a mass that can press on the spinal cord and present with neurologic changes. Work-up for granuloma includes catheter evaluation/dye study as well as focal MRI of the tip of the catheter. Should a granuloma be found, the catheter should be revised to prevent further neurologic compromise.[13]

Last, the long-term use of opiates is known to suppress hormone production in both sexes. With the administration of intrathecal opiates, it has been noted that both sexes will develop hypogonadotropic hypogonadism. Approximately 15% or patients develop central hypocorticism and about 15% of patients develop growth hormone deficiency. Therefore, endocrine consultation may be required for these patients in the long term.[14]

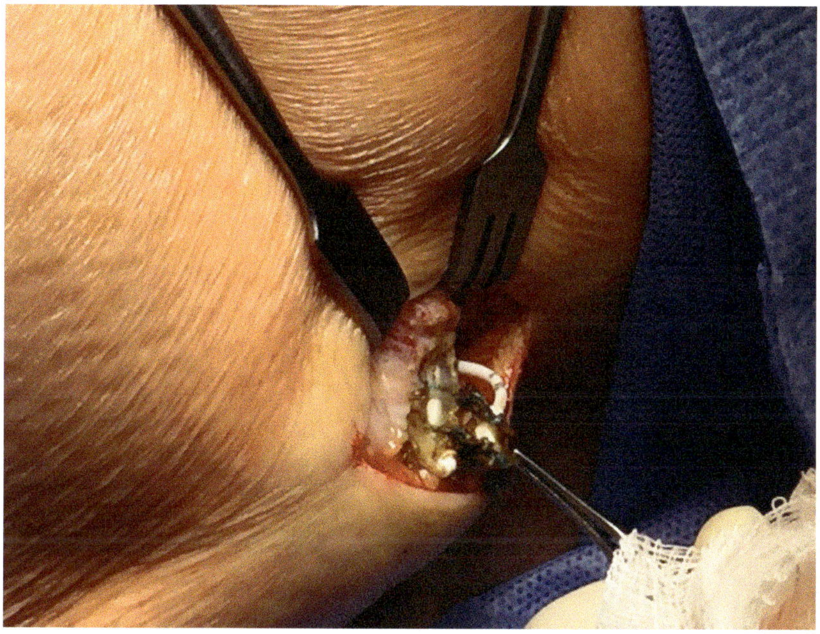

FIGURE 22.6. Older catheter that has become tangled in the spinal incision.

Image courtesy of J. Weisbein, DO.

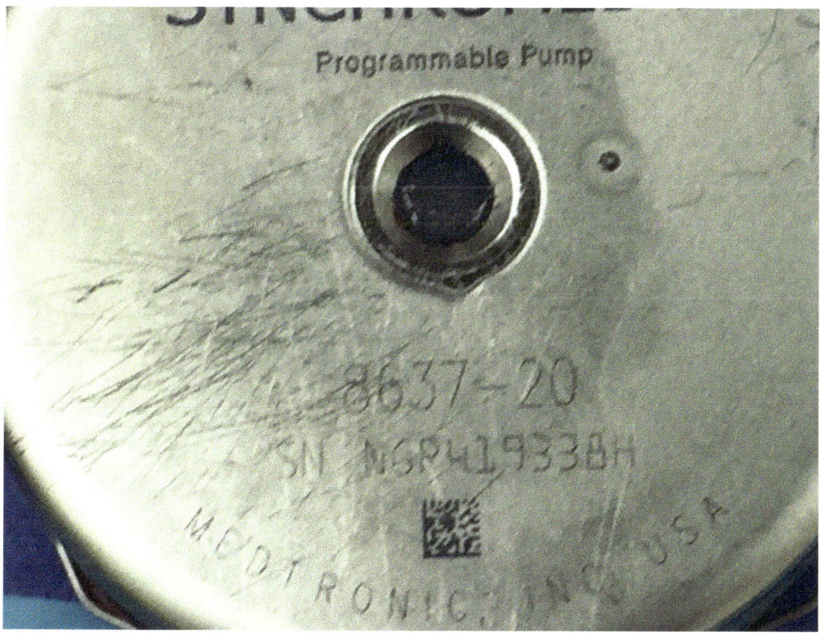

FIGURE 22.7. Pump explanted from a patient whose attempts to self-access the pump caused an infection of the pocket.

Image courtesy of J. Weisbein, DO.

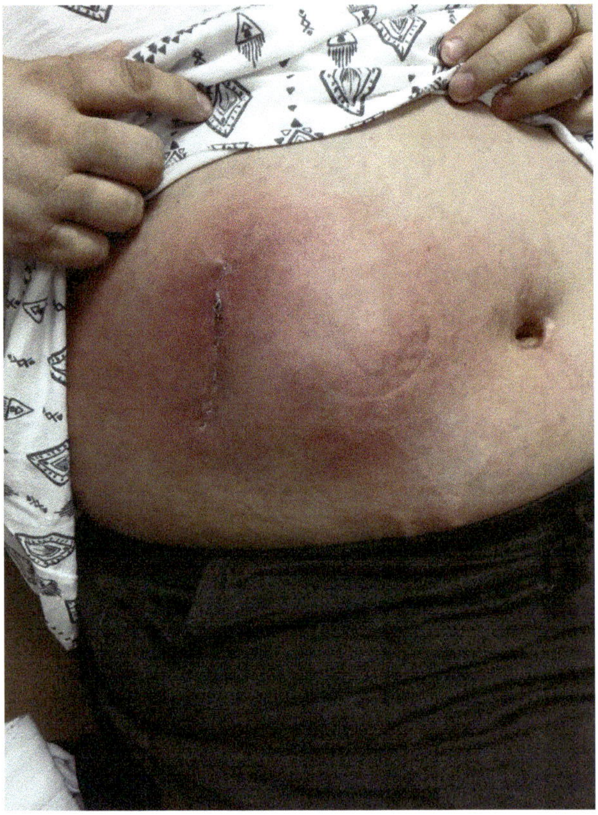

FIGURE 22.8. Infected pump pocket prior to removal.
Image courtesy of J. Weisbein, DO.

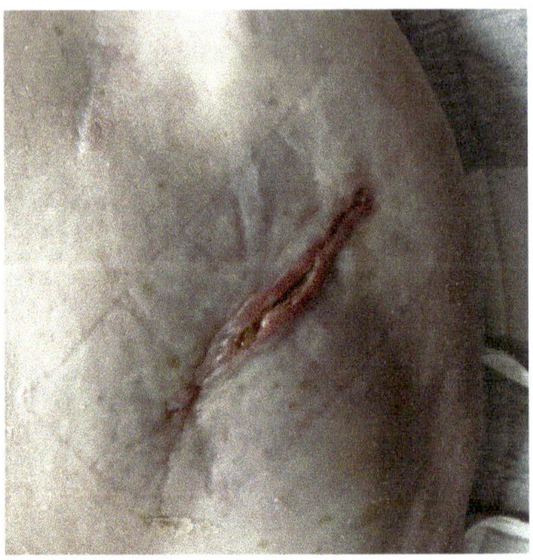

FIGURE 22.9. Superficial wound dehiscence.
Image courtesy of J. Weisbein, DO.

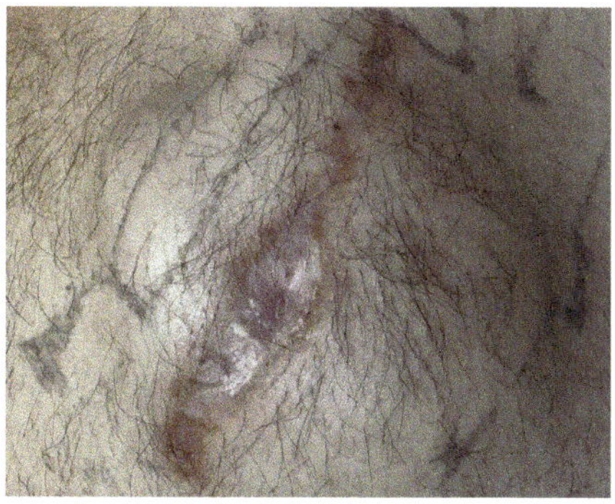

FIGURE 22.10. Superficial wound dehiscence with granulation.
Image courtesy of J. Weisbein, DO.

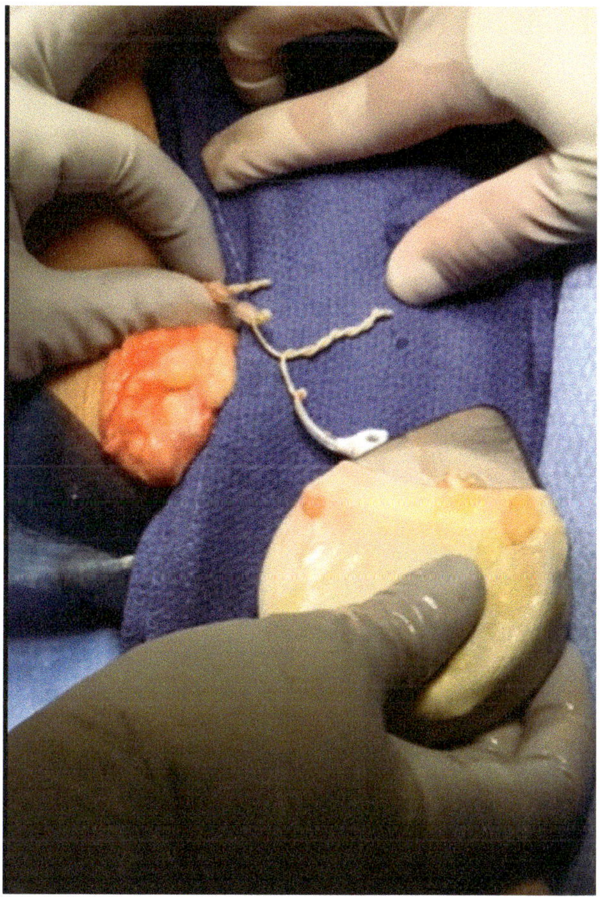

FIGURE 22.11. Intrathecal pump with twisted catheter from pump flipping in the abdominal pocket.
Image courtesy of J. Weisbein, DO.

Conclusion

IDDS allow systemic administration of opiates and other medications with greater accuracy, because 100% of the medication is delivered to the opiate receptors in the dorsal horn of the spinal cord. Unlike oral and IV medication, medications delivered by IDDS bypass the liver, thus allowing for greater absorption as well. The delivery of medication by a preprogrammed device removes issues regarding administration of doses at appropriate intervals and allows patients requiring stronger medication to receive it with fewer side effects. Although IDDS therapy was initially studied for malignant pain, the utilization of IDDS for those with nonmalignant pain has allowed much more consistent and appropriate use of opiates.

References

1. Onofrio BM, Yaksh TL, Arnold PG. Continuous low-dose intrathecal morphine administration in the treatment of chronic pain of malignant origin. *Mayo Clin Proc.* 1981;56(8):516–520. PMID:6894954.
2. Harsh V, Viswanathan A. Surgical/radiological interventions for cancer pain. *Curr Pain Headache Rep.* 2013;17:331. https://doi.org/10.1007/s11916-013-0331-1.
3. Deer TR, Pope JE, Hayek SM, et al. The Polyanalgesic Consensus Conference (PACC): recommendations on intrathecal drug infusion systems best practices and guidelines. *Neuromodulation.* 2017;20(2):96–132. doi:10.1111/ner.12538.
4. Stearns LM, Abd-Elsayed A, Perruchoud C, et al. Intrathecal drug delivery systems for cancer pain: an analysis of a prospective, multicenter product surveillance registry. *Anesth Analg.* 2020;130(2):289–297. doi:10.1213/ANE.0000000000004425.
5. Melzack R, Wall PD. Pain mechanisms: a new theory. *Science.* 1965;150(3699):971–979. doi:10.1126/science.150.3699.971. PMID:5320816.
6. Yaksh TL, Rudy TA. Analgesia mediated by a direct spinal action of narcotics. *Science.* 1976;192(4246):1357–1358. doi:10.1126/science.1273597. PMID:1273597.
7. Wang JK, Nauss LA, Thomas JE. Pain relief by intrathecally applied morphine in man. *Anesthesiology.* 1979;50(2):149–151. doi:10.1097/00000542-197902000-00013. PMID: 373503.
8. Auld AW, Maki-Jokela A, Murdoch DM. Intraspinal narcotic analgesia in the treatment of chronic pain. *Spine (Phila Pa 1976).* 1985;10(8):777–781. doi:10.1097/00007632-198510000-00014. PMID:3841231.
9. Grider JS, Harned ME, Etscheidt MA. Patient selection and outcomes using a lowdose intrathecal opioid trialing method for chronic nonmalignant pain. *Pain Physician.* 2011;14:343–351.
10. Hamza M, Doleys D, Wells M, et al. Prospective study of 3-year follow-up of low-dose intrathecal opioids in the management of chronic nonmalignant pain. *Pain Med.* 2012;13(10):1304–1613. doi:10.1111/j.1526-4637.2012.01451.x. PMID:22845187.
11. Deer TR, Smith HS, Cousins M, et al. Consensus guidelines for the selection and implantation of patients with noncancer pain for intrathecal drug delivery. *Pain Physician.* 2010;13(3):E175–E213.
12. Prager JP. Neuraxial medication delivery: the development and maturity of a concept for treating chronic pain of spinal origin. *Spine (Phila Pa 1976).* 2002;27(22):2593–2606. doi:10.1097/01.BRS.0000032243.78028.84. PMID:12435999.
13. Ver Donck A, Vranken JH, Puylaert M, Hayek S, Mikhail N, Van Zundert J. Intrathecal drug administration in chronic pain syndromes. *Pain Pract.* 2014; 14(5): 461–476
14. Abs R, Verhelst J, Maeyaert J, et al. Endocrine consequences of long-term intrathecal administration of opioids. *J Clin Endocrinol Metab.* 2000 Jun;85(6):2215–2222. doi:10.1210/jcem.85.6.6615. PMID: 10852454.

Index

For the benefit of digital users, indexed terms that span two pages (e.g., 52–53) may, on occasion, appear on only one of those pages.

Tables, figures, and boxes are indicated by *t*, *f*, and *b* following the page number